T0058428

The Complete Medicinal Herbal

A Practical Guide to the Healing Properties of Herbs

Penelope Ody

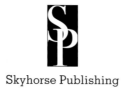

Skyhorse Publishing

Skyhorse Publishing books may be purchased in bulk at special discounts for sales promotion, corporate gifts, fund-raising, or educational purposes. Special editions can also be created to specifications. For details, contact the Special Sales Department, Skyhorse Publishing, 307 West 36th Street, 11th Floor, New York, NY 10018 or info@skyhorsepublishing.com.

Skyhorse® and Skyhorse Publishing® are registered trademarks of Skyhorse Publishing, Inc.®, a Delaware corporation.

Visit our website at www.skyhorsepublishing.com.

10 9 8 7

Library of Congress Cataloging-in-Publication Data is available on file.

Cover design by Rain Saukas
Cover photographs: iStockphoto.com
Interior images: iStockphoto.com except as follows:
p. 60, *Harpagophytum procumbens*: H. Zell
p. 63, *Hypericum perforatum*: courtesy of Penelope Ody
p. 81, *Nardostachys grandiflora*: Joseph Dalton Hooker
p. 126, *Withania Somnifera*: Wowbobwow12

Print ISBN: 978-1-63450-843-8
Ebook ISBN: 978-1-5107-1157-0

Printed in China

IMPORTANT NOTICE

CONTENTS

INTRODUCTION   vii

HERBS PAST & PRESENT   1

Origins of Western Herbalism   2

A Science of Life   3

Chinese Herbal Medicine   5

Out of the Dark Ages   9

North American Traditions   10

From Plants to Pills   12

Medicinal Meals   13

A–Z OF MEDICINAL HERBS
Arranged by Latin name, a visual directory of more than 100 herbs   17

Ayurvedic Herbs   128

Bush Herbs   130

Fungi   132

South American Herbs   134

HERBAL REMEDIES   139

Harvesting & Drying Herbs   140

Making Herbal Remedies   142

Other Herbal Remedies   148

Herbal First Aid   150

HOME REMEDIES   152

Aches & Pains   154

Headaches & Migraines   159

Infections   162

Respiratory Problems   165

Ears, Eyes, Mouth & Throat   170

Skin & Hair — 174

Heart, Blood & Circulation — 180

Digestive Problems — 185

Allergic Conditions — 194

Urinary Disorders — 197

Nervous Disorders — 200

Gynecological Problems — 208

Pregnancy & Childbirth — 213

Male Reproductive Problems — 219

Problems of the Elderly — 222

Endocrine & Glandular Problems — 225

Children's Complaints — 229

Ayurvedic Tonics — 238

Chinese Tonics — 242

    Qi Tonics — 242

    Blood Tonics — 243

    Yang Tonics — 245

    Yin Tonics — 246

Western Tonics — 247

    Energy Tonics — 248

    Nerve Tonics — 249

    Mind Tonics — 250

OTHER MEDICINAL HERBS — 253

CONSULTING AN HERBALIST — 257

GLOSSARY — 259

INDEX — 262

INTRODUCTION

One of the earliest Chinese herbals – Shen Nong's *Materia Medica,* dating from the first or second century AD – lists 365 healing remedies, most of them plants but including a few mineral and animal extracts. The Greek physician Dioscorides, writing in the first century AD, mentioned about 400 herbs. Today, the list of plants with known medicinal properties is much longer: around 5,800 in the Chinese *Materia Medica,* 2,500 known in India, at least 800 regularly collected from the tropical forests of Africa, almost 300 currently detailed for the medical profession in Germany (one of the few Western countries with official herbal monographs), and many thousands more known only to traditional healers in the more remote corners of our world. To produce a truly complete medicinal herbal would fill many volumes and be the work of several lifetimes. Yet, despite this bewildering array of healing plants, the average Western herbalist generally finds that a working knowledge of 150 to 200 plants is more than enough to cope with most human ailments.

Herbs may be defined as any plant that can be put to culinary or medicinal use and include those we associate with conventional drugs, such as foxglove and opium poppy, as well as everyday plants, such as garlic or sage. The herbs in this book are a representative cross section of these potent plants, ranging from exotic Eastern herbs, such as *ma huang* and ginseng, to more mundane apples and cabbages.

Interest in herbal remedies has grown steadily in the past decades. In the years since 1993, when the first edition of this book appeared, there has been a significant increase in sales of ready-made herbal remedies and more interest from the conventional medical profession in using herbal extracts as an alternative to powerful and potentially hazardous drugs. That interest has been fueled by concerns over the growing number of antibiotic-resistant micro-organisms that conventional treatments find increasingly difficult to tackle. In the West, people often cite the risk of side effects from powerful conventional drugs as a reason for turning to gentler, plant medicines. In the developing world, a lack of hard currency to pay for pharmaceutical imports is encouraging a reappraisal of traditional folk remedies.

This trend towards more natural medicines has gained added impetus from our growing concern with environmental issues, such as the destruction of rain forests and the loss of rare species. Although the therapeutic effects of many herbs have not been scientifically proven, research continues to identify the active ingredients that may one day form the basis of drugs to fight cancer or AIDS.

And yet, in extracting these chemicals and seeking to turn herbal remedies designed to help the body heal itself into powerful drugs to obliterate symptoms, we forget one of the basic tenets of traditional healing: a belief that the cause of disharmonies and "dis-ease" should be treated rather than the effects. We forget, too, that traditional health care has as much to do with preventing disease as with curing it.

The use of simple herbal remedies can encourage us once again to take responsibility for our own health. Instead of trying to obliterate symptoms when they become severe, we need to be sufficiently in tune with our bodies to recognize those symptoms as they develop and treat likely causes, whether physical, emotional, or spiritual, to restore balance.

In this book I do not simply aim to give a wealth of detail about a limited number of plants or provide cure-all lists of remedies that can be taken to alleviate symptoms. I have tried instead to look at how some herbs have been used by the traditional healers of many cultures and I have suggested a therapeutic approach for ailments that focuses on healing the whole person. For some, these suggestions may represent an effective solution. For others, they will only be the starting point for a wider exploration of the healing power of herbs.

Penelope Ody

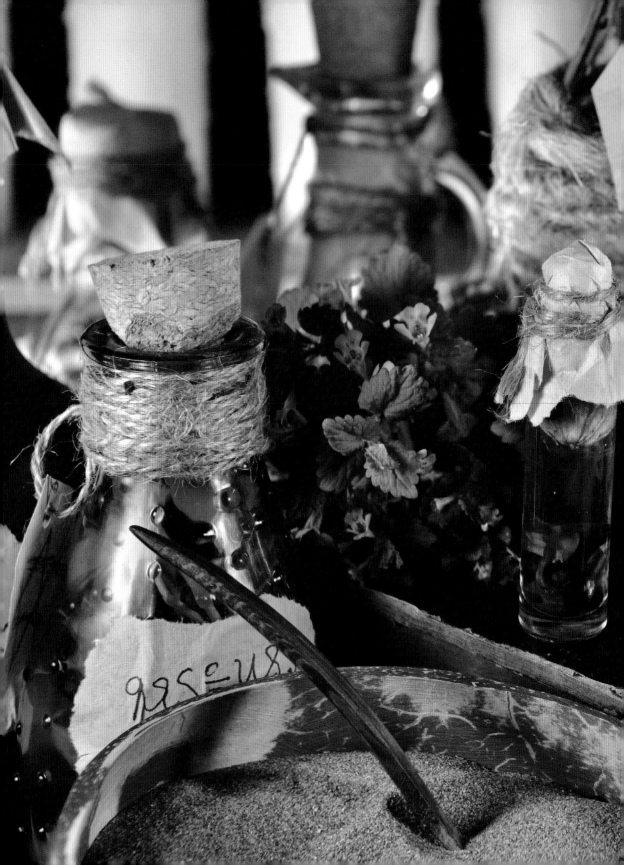

HERBS PAST & PRESENT

From ancient times, herbs have played a vital role in the healing traditions of many cultures. This section looks at the major herbal systems in different parts of the world throughout the ages. Some of these systems may seem incomprehensible to us in modern Western society, but the alternative way of looking at health care, which they represent, can be just as valid today as it was 5,000 years ago.

ORIGINS OF WESTERN HERBALISM

Hippocrates may be known today as the father of medicine, but for centuries medieval Europe followed the teachings of Galen, a second-century physician, who wrote extensively about the body's four humors – blood, phlegm, black bile, and yellow bile – and classified herbs by their essential qualities of hot, cold, dry, or damp. These theories were later expanded by the seventh-century Arab physicians, such as Avicenna, and today Galenic theories continue to dominate *Unani* medicine, practiced in the Muslim world and India. Galen's descriptions of herbs as, for example, "hot in the third degree" or "cold in the second" were still being used well into the eighteenth century.

HERBS IN ANCIENT CIVILIZATIONS

Surviving Egyptian papyri dating back to 1700 BC record that many common herbs, such as garlic and juniper, have been used medicinally for around 4,000 years. In the days of Ramesses III, Indian hemp (marijuana) was used for eye problems just as it may be prescribed for glaucoma today, while poppy extracts were used to quiet crying children.

By the time of Hippocrates (468–377 BC), European herbal tradition had already absorbed ideas from Assyria and India with Eastern herbs, such as basil and ginger, among the most highly prized, while the complex theory of humors and essential body fluids had begun to be formulated. Hippocrates categorized all foods and herbs by fundamental qualities – hot, cold, dry or damp. Good health was maintained by keeping these qualities in balance, as well as taking plenty of exercise and fresh air.

Pedanius Dioscorides wrote his classic text the *De Materia Medica* (*Peri hulas iatrikes* or *About medicinal trees*) around 60 AD, and it remained the standard textbook for 1,500 years. Dioscorides was reputed to have been either the physician to Antony and Cleopatra or an army surgeon during the reign of Emperor Nero. His herbal covers around 600 medicinal trees. These were grouped by character, such as aromatics or "herbs with a sharp quality," and appearance or part used, such as roots, herbs, or "ground trees." Many of the actions Dioscorides described are familiar today: parsley as a diuretic, fennel to promote milk flow, and white horehound mixed with honey as an expectorant.

ROMAN REMEDIES

The Greek theories of medicine reached Rome around 100 BC. As time passed, they became more mechanistic, presenting the body as a machine to be actively repaired rather than following the Hippocratic dictum of allowing most diseases to cure themselves. Medicine became a lucrative business with complex and highly-priced herbal remedies.

Opposing this practice was Claudius Galenus (131–199 AD), who was born in Pergamom in Asia Minor and was court physician to Emperor Marcus Aurelius. Galen reworked many of the old Hippocratic ideas and formalized the theories of humors. His books soon became the standard medical texts not only of the Romans, but also of later Arab and medieval physicians, and his theories still survive in *Unani* medicine today.

ISLAMIC INFLUENCES

With the fall of Rome in the fifth century, the center of classical learning shifted East and the study of Galenical medicine was focused in Constantinople and Persia. In the Arab world, Galenism was adopted with enthusiasm by the Arabs and merged with both folk beliefs and surviving Egyptian learning. It was this mixture of herbal ideas, practice, and traditions that was reimported back into Europe with the invading Arab armies.

Probably the most important work of the time was the *Kitab al-Qanun* or *Canon of Medicine* by Avicenna (Abdallah Ibn Sina, born at Bokhara in 910). This was based firmly on Galenical principles, and by the twelfth century had been translated into Latin and brought back into the West to become one of the leading textbooks in Western medical schools.

The Arabs were great traders and introduced many herbs and spices from the East, such as nutmeg, cloves, saffron, and senna, to the *materia medica* of Dioscorides and Galen.

THE GREEK FOUR-ELEMENT MODEL

Early Greeks saw the world as being composed of four elements: earth, air, fire, and water. These elements were also related to the seasons, to the four fundamental qualities (hot, cold, dry, and damp), the four body fluids or humors, and the four temperaments. In almost all individuals, one humor was thought to dominate, affecting both personality and the likely health problems that would be suffered.

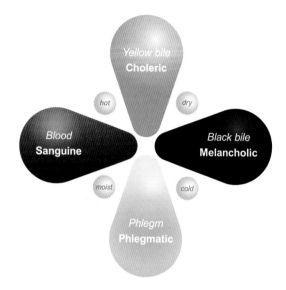

The four vital body fluids that needed to be kept in balance to maintain health were blood, phlegm, black bile, and yellow bile. These in turn related to the temperaments – sanguine, phlegmatic, melancholic, or choleric.

The melancholic nature was cold and dry, so typical illnesses could include constipation or digestive upsets with hot herbs used to purge the melancholic humor and restore balance. Herbs such as senna and Christmas rose (*Helleborus niger*), which is a drastic purgative, were also used for insanity and hysteria which were similarly linked with a surfeit of black bile and melancholy.

The phlegmatic nature was dominated by "cold and damp" with typical illnesses including catarrh and chest problems. Warm and drying herbs, such as thyme and hyssop, were used to restore balance and clear phlegm. In contrast, the choleric temperament was seen as "hot and dry" and associated with bad temper and liver disorders. Rhubarb root and other cool, moist plants such as violets were used to clear yellow bile.

The sanguine person, dominated by heat and damp, was the Galenical ideal: good humored and amusing but inclined to over-indulgence. Gout or diarrhea could be a problem, so cool and dry herbs, such as burdock and figwort, would be used to balance the system.

A SCIENCE OF LIFE

The term Ayurveda comes from two Indian words: *ayur,* or life, and *veda,* or knowledge. Ayurvedic medicine is thus sometimes described as a "knowledge of how to live," emphasizing that good health is the responsibility of the individual. In Ayurvedic medicine illness is seen in terms of imbalance with herbs and dietary controls used to restore equilibrium. The earliest Ayurvedic texts date from about 2500 BC, with successive invaders adding new herbal traditions: the Persians in 500 BC; the Moghuls in the fourteenth century, bringing the medicine of Galen and Avicenna (known as Unani medicine from *ionic* meaning Greek); and the British, who closed down the Ayurvedic schools in 1833 but luckily did not obliterate the ancient learning all together. Tibetan medicine has much in common with Ayurveda but can be vastly more complicated, having 15 subdivisions for the humors and placing strong emphasis on the effects of past lives – *karma* – on present health.

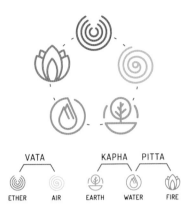

VATA   KAPHA   PITTA

ETHER   AIR   EARTH   WATER   FIRE

Ayurvedic Principles

As in ancient Greek and traditional Chinese medicine, the Ayurvedic model links the microcosm of the individual with the cosmos. At the heart of the system are the three primal forces: *prana* – the breath of life; *agni* – the spirit of light or fire, and *soma* – a manifestation of harmony, cohesiveness, and love. There are also five elements comprising all matter: earth, water, fire, air, and ether (a nebulous nothingness that fills all space and was known to the ancient Greeks).

The five universal elements are converted by the digestive fire (*agni*) into three humors that influence individual health and temperament and are sometimes called waste products of digestion. If digestion were perfect there would be no humoral imbalance, but because it is not, imbalance and ill health can follow. Air and ether yield *vata* (wind), fire produces the humor *pitta* (fire or bile), while earth and water combine to give *kapha* (phlegm). The dominant humor is also seen as controlling the character of the individual: a *vata*–type roughly conforms to Galen's melancholic personality, *pitta* matches the choleric type, and a *kapha* person is reminiscent of the phlegmatic. Food, drink, sensual gratification, light, fresh air, and spiritual activities are all used to "feed" the digestive fire and produce the correct mix of humors.

A health problem associated with excess phlegm, such as catarrh, edema, or water retention, for example, would be treated with warm, light and dry foods, fasting and avoiding cold drinks that would increase *kapha*. Herbal remedies might include hot spices such as cayenne, *pippali,* or cinnamon; bitters such as aloe or turmeric; pungent tonics such as saffron; and stimulating, mind-clearing herbs such as *gotu kola, guggul,* or myrrh, all designed to dry excess water or phlegm. In Ayurvedic theory, taste is important: pungent, bitter and astringent tastes can help to reduce *kapha*, so the diet should favor these over sweet, salty, or sour flavors. Treatment might also include massage with warm herbal oils, such as eucalyptus; burning pungent incense, such as frankincense; and encouraging the sufferer to wear bright, hot reds and yellows instead of cold blue or white.

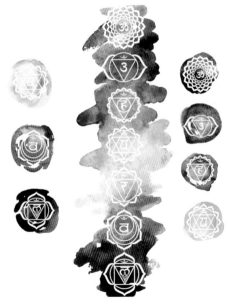

Crown chakra – Sahasrara Chakra – associated with the pineal gland
Herbs: gotu kola, nutmeg, valerian, wood betony

Brow chakra – Third eye or Ajna Chakra – associated with the pituitary gland
Herbs: elecampane, sandalwood, hibiscus, skullcap

Throat chakra – Visuhuddhi Chakra – associated with the thyroid glands
Herbs: cloves, licorice, vervain, wild celery

Heart chakra – Anahata Chakra – associated with the thymus gland and heart
Herbs: cardamom, saffron, rose, rue

Solar plexus chakra – Manipura Chakra – associated with the liver, gallbladder, and spleen
Herbs: self-heal, goldenseal, black pepper, lemon balm

Sacral plexus or Splenic chakra – Swadhistana Chakra – associated with the testes and ovaries
Herbs: coriander, fennel, *gokshura,* bearberry

Root or base chakra – Kundalini or Muladhara Chakra – associated with the womb, prostate, and adrenals
Herbs: *ashwagandha, haritaki, shatavari,* basil

TIBETAN HERBALISM

Before the Chinese invasion in 1959, Tibetan medicine was largely under the control of the lamas and closely linked with religion. Medical students memorized complex "tantras," which explained the cause and progression of disease, with the aid of "illustrated trees of medicine" with each leaf representing a cause of disease, type of humor, influence, or outcome (such as age of patient, his or her *karma,* season of the disease, and so on). Physicians used meditation and mantras to "energize" the remedy and increase its efficacy. Harvesting herbs was also carefully timed to use any helpful astrological influences.

CHINESE HERBAL MEDICINE

Traditional Chinese medicine is an ancient system of healing that can be traced back to about 2000 BC. The texts produced around that time are still studied and followed by practitioners and, while much has been added to the basic philosophy, very little has been taken out. In Chinese medicine, illness is seen as a sign of disharmony within the whole person, so the task of the traditional Chinese practitioner is always to restore harmony and balance. Herbs are central to treatment, aided by other therapies, such as acupuncture or specialist massage. Over the years, Chinese herbal traditions have become more familiar and are now used by many qualified practitioners.

ANCIENT CHINESE MEDICINE

The origins of Chinese herbalism are shrouded in myth. There are legendary characters, such as Shen Nong, the "divine cultivator," who identified many medicinal plants. Shen Nong was said to have "tasted the flavor of hundreds of herbs and drank the water from many springs and wells so that people might know which were sweet and which were bitter." He supposedly discovered tea drinking, too, when some leaves fell from a tea bush into a bowl of water boiling nearby. An important Chinese herbal (*Shen Nong Ben Cao Jing*) from around 200 BC is named after Shen Nong.

The founding father of Chinese medical theory is the "Yellow Emperor," who is reputed to have lived around 2500 BC. However, the classic text that bears his name, the *Huang Ti Nei Ching Su Wên,* or *Yellow Emperor's Canon of Internal Medicine*, is generally dated to around 1000 BC. It could well represent an older verbal tradition. As in the West, medicine at that time was inseparable from philosophy and religion, and the *Nei Ching* is an important Taoist text full of rich spiritual wisdom.

Historically, there were many different medical philosophies and techniques in China, with a mix of itinerant physicians, village herbalists, or native shaman. There were also the Taoist philosopher-doctors who produced the classic medical texts and would have been the first choice, in case of sickness, for the aristocracy.

MODERN CHINESE MEDICINE

By the nineteenth century, Western mission hospitals had begun to represent a real alternative to traditional practices. Chinese medicine survived, but only became a national medical system in the 1960s when Mao Tse Tung founded five colleges of traditional Chinese medicine. Today, older regional healing styles persist among traditional Korean, Vietnamese, and Japanese practitioners; classic styles are also followed by surviving Chinese medical families, many of whom have emigrated to Hong Kong, Singapore, or San Francisco.

THE PRINCIPLES OF CHINESE MEDICINE

As with early Greek philosophy, the Chinese tradition was based on a theory of elements, only in this case five, rather than the Greek four, which is used to explain every interaction between people and their environment. These elements – wood, fire, earth, metal, and water – are seen to be related and linked to the

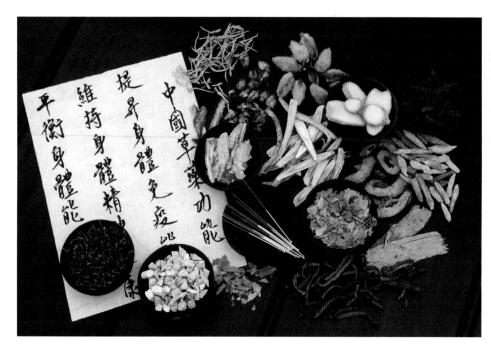

In traditional Chinese medicine, little has been taken out of the ancient texts, though much has been added.

annual cycle of the seasons, with wood encouraging fire, fire resolving to earth, earth yielding up metal, metal producing water (seen as condensation on a cold metal surface) and water giving birth to wood by encouraging the growth of vegetation.

Each element has a number of associations ranging from emotions and parts of the body to human sounds, the seasons, colors, and tastes, all underpinned by a simple logic. Wood, for example, relates to spring, germination, and the color green; fire to summer, heat, and the color red; and water to kidneys, winter, and the color black. For good health to prevail, the elements need to be in harmony; if one element becomes too dominant, illness may result.

Chinese practitioners often look for the cause of illness in a related element: weakness in the liver (wood), for example, may be due to deficiencies in the kidneys (water). A weak stomach (earth) might be caused by over-exuberant wood (liver) failing to be controlled by deficient metal (lungs).

YIN, YANG, AND QI

Complementing the basic model of the five elements is the Chinese doctrine of opposites: *yin* and *yang*. According to this belief, everything in the cosmos both contains and is balanced by its own opposite. *Yin* is seen as female, dark, and cold, while *yang* is characterized as male, light, and warmth. The usual sexual stereotypes of "female" and "male" should not really be associated with these terms because both *yin* and *yang* characteristics are present in all things and need to be held in balance to maintain health. Many ills are attributed to a deficiency or excess of either factor.

Different parts of the body are also described as predominantly *yin* or *yang*: body fluids and blood are mainly *yin*, for example, while *qi*, the vital energy, tends to be *yang*. *Qi* is regarded as flowing in a network of channels, or meridians, through the body and can be stimulated using acupuncture.

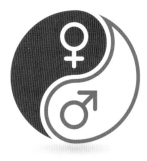

THE FIVE TASTES

Chinese medicine also identifies five tastes that can be characterized as hot or cold: pungent and sweet tastes are more likely to be heating while sour, bitter, and salty tastes tend to be more cooling. Some herbs combine several different tastes which affects these properties: *wu wei zhi* (schisandra fruits) translates as "five taste seeds" and encapsulate all the flavors. These characteristics also influence which part of the body the herb will affect. Hot things rise, for example, so herbs that are pungent or sweet tend to affect the upper and exterior parts of the body, while cold things sink, so sour, bitter, or salty herbs are more effective for the lower half of the body and the interior. In the treatment of arthritis, for example, the Chinese will often use *qiang huo* (*Notopterygium forbesii*) for pains in the shoulders and arms while *du huo* (*Angelica pubescens*) is preferred if hips or knees are affected. Both herbs would be used together to cover the whole body if needed.

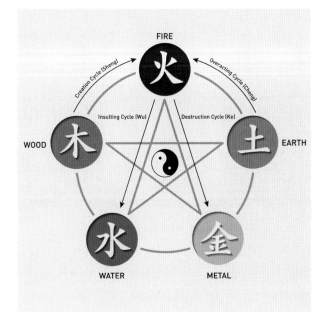

Pungent tastes are also dispersing and mobilizing so they move energy (*qi*) and blood and dispel stagnation. Sour tastes are contracting, sweet is nutritious and tonifying, while salty is softening. Bitter tastes are used to redirect the flow of *qi* downward so could be relevant in some types of coughs or vomiting.

PRESCRIBING HERBS

The Chinese usually prescribe herbs in standard formula (there are several thousand in regular use) and these may be adjusted slightly depending on the specific condition of the patient. The formula might include just two herbs or as many as twenty and the interaction between the different plants is just as significant as their individual properties. The result is often a potent brew that can have a dramatic therapeutic effect, but generally defies any simple, rational scientific explanation.

Herbs are generally given as pills, powders or, most usually, in the form of decoctions known as "*tang*" or "soup," which patients brew up at home for an hour or so in a special earthenware crock kept for the purpose. Sometimes the herbs may be cooked with rice to produce a cereal-like therapeutic meal.

In traditional Chinese herbals, the characteristics of a plant always include taste, dominant temperature, and generally an indication of the organ and channels it affects. These are sometimes obviously related: Chinese gold thread (*huang lian*, *Coptis chinensis*), for example, is a very bitter herb. It is cold and linked to the heart – characteristics that can be traced directly to the five-element model. It may be used in conditions associated with too much heat in the heart, which in traditional Chinese medicine would lead to insomnia, palpitations, and hot flushes.

Bai shao yao (white peony, *Paeonia lactiflora*) is sour and widely used for liver problems – both of which are aspects of the element wood – while many nutritious herbs, such as rice or oats, and major tonics, such as ginseng, are characterized as sweet and are good for the stomach and spleen.

The five elements in the Chinese model are related, with fire giving rise to earth, which yields metal, etc. The diagonal relationships in the diagram indicate how earth "controls" water, metal "controls" wood, etc. Relating this to health and disease explains why over-exuberant liver (wood) might over-control the spleen and stomach (earth), or that weak kidneys (water) both causes weakness in the liver (wood) and fails to control the heart (fire), leading to problems with both these organ systems as well.

	Wood	Fire	Earth	Metal	Water
Season	Spring	Summer	Indian Summer	Autumn	Winter
Environment	Wind	Heat	Dampness	Dryness	Cold
Development	Germination	Growth	Transformation	Reaping	Storing Color
	Blue/Green	Red	Yellow	White	Black
Solid organ	Liver	Heart	Spleen	Lungs	Kidneys
Hollow organ	Gallbladder	Small Intestine	Stomach	Large Intestine	Urinary bladder
Taste	Sour	Bitter	Sweet	Pungent	Salty
Emotions	Anger	Joy	Worry	Grief	Fear
Sense organs	Eyes	Tongue	Mouth	Nose	Ears
Part	Nails	Complexion	Lips	Body Hair	Hair
Tissue	Tendons	Blood Vessels	Muscles	Skin	Bones
Fluid	Tears	Sweat	Lymph	Mucus	Saliva
Storage of:	Soul	Consciousness	Intention	Vitality	Determination

CHARACTERISTICS OF *yin* AND *yang*

In traditional Chinese medicine, *yin* and *yang* need to be in balance to ensure good health. Imbalance leads to ill health and syndromes can be classified in terms of lack or surfeit of either yin or yang.

Yin	Yang
Negative	Positive
Female	Male
Passive	Active
Water	Fire
Coldness	Warmth/Heat
Dimness	Brightness
Downwards	Upwards
Stillness	Motion
Lower	Upper
Interior	Exterior
Deficiency	Excess
Slowness	Rapidity
Substance/matter	Functional/energy
Even numbers	Odd numbers
Right side	Left side
Inhibition	Excitement
Blood	Qi
Lower part of the body	Upper part of the body
Interior of the body	Exterior of the body

OUT OF THE DARK AGES

After the fall of Rome, European herbal traditions were not totally submerged by the ensuing "dark ages." The "barbarians" brought with them their own herbal healing customs to add to the Roman practices that survived and, with the spread of Christianity, there was considerable exchange of both actual medicines and tried and tested remedies. Throughout the medieval period the Church played a significant role both in cultivating physic gardens and introducing new herbs. With the advent of the printing press, classical knowledge spread from the confines of the cloister to complement the folk medicine and household herbal remedies passed through the generations.

EXPANSION OF HERBALISM IN EUROPE

Europe's oldest surviving herbal written in the vernacular, the Anglo-Saxon *Leech Book of Bald*, dates from the first half of the tenth century and includes remedies sent by the Patriarch of Jerusalem to King Alfred. Numerous remedies are described for ailments caused by "flying venom" and "elfshot," which were terms used to describe a wide range of sudden or wasting illnesses. Among the most popular herbs in Saxon times were wood betony, vervain, mugwort, plantain, and yarrow taken in many internal remedies but more often worn as amulets to ward off the evil eye.

Although medical schools spread through Europe – the most famous at Salerno was founded in the early tenth century and taught the Hippocratic principles of good diet, exercise and fresh air – healing and herbalism were largely in the hands of the Church, with all monasteries growing medicinal herbs and ministering to the sick as part of Christian duty. Healing was as much a matter of prayer as medicine, and early herbals frequently combine religious incantations with infusions concluding that with "God's help" the patient would be cured.

HEALTH CARE EVOLVES

As learning moved away from the cloister, emphasis was gradually again given to the healing skills and disciplines once taught at the Salerno school. By the 1530s, Paracelsus (born Philippus Theophrastus Bombastus von Hohenheim near Zürich in 1493) was revolutionizing European attitudes to health care. As much an alchemist as physician, he insisted in lecturing in German instead of the usual Latin. He regarded most apothecaries and physicians as crooked conspirators intent on milking the public. Condemning the complex and often lethal purgatives and emetics they prescribed, he urged a return to simpler medicines inspired by the Doctrine of Signatures.

Paracelsus was followed by physicians such as William Turner who wrote in English so that "the apothecaries and old wives that gather herbs" would understand which plants physicians really meant by their Latin prescriptions and would not put "many a good man by ignorance in jeopardy of his life." Nicholas Culpeper (1616–1654) was later to adopt a similar view earning the wrath of the College of Physicians by translating their *Pharmacopoeia* into English so that ordinary people could find medicines in the hedgerows instead of paying vastly inflated apothecary's bills.

HERBAL WARFARE

The battles between herb wives, apothecaries, and physicians raged through the seventeenth and eighteenth centuries, as medicine became more firmly under the control of the academic physicians with their university training, while dispensing was strictly regulated by the apothecaries. The emphasis was on expensive and complex nostrums using ingredients such as mercury and antimony.

By the time that the great herbals of Gerard (1597), Parkinson (1640), and Culpeper (1653) appeared, numerous new herbs were being imported from the East Indies and North America. Plants such as nasturtium (*Tropaeolum majus*), nutmeg, and yucca began to appear in the herbals, often accompanied by imaginative applications and claims for their medicinal properties. Tea is a classic example proclaimed as a cure-all in the seventeenth century and now regarded by many as no more than a popular drink.

DOCTRINE OF SIGNATURES

This theory maintained that the outward appearance of a plant gave an indication of the ailments it would cure. At times the theory was surprisingly accurate and similar theories still prevail in Africa and parts of the far East.

The knobbly roots of lesser celandine (*Ranunculus ficaria*), for example, were taken to resemble piles (hemorrhoids) for which the herb was (and still is) used. Yellow-flowered plants were associated with jaundice, so herbs such as toadflax (*Linaria vulgaris*), greater celandine (*Chelidonium majus*), and dandelion were all used for liver disorders.

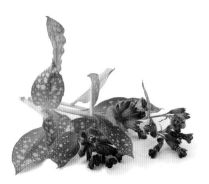
Lungwort (*Pulmonaria officinalis*)

The tiny oil sacks in the leaves of St. John's wort looked like holes while extracts from it are blood-red – both signs that it will be a good wound herb – while the leaves of lungwort (*Pulmonaria officinalis*) were taken to resemble diseased lungs, so the plant was used for bronchitis and tuberculosis. The round leaves of lady's mantle were compared by some to the cervix, making this an excellent herb for the womb, while both nutmeg and walnuts were compared with the brain and deemed helpful for strengthening mental activity.

NORTH AMERICAN TRADITIONS

The first European settlers arriving in North America brought with them the familiar healing plants from home: heartsease and plantain, which became known as "white man's foot" because it was soon found growing wherever the settlers penetrated. They also absorbed some Native American healing traditions, discovering new herbs such as boneset, echinacea, goldenseal, and pleurisy root (*Asclepias tuberosa*). Several of the American tribes also made great use of sauna-like sweat houses, and the idea of heat as a healing technique was adopted by Samuel Thomson and his followers. This melding of traditions bore fruit in the Physiomedical and Eclectic schools, which were later imported into Europe and have had a lasting effect on herbal practices in Britain.

RITUAL HERBALISM

Native American herbalism was shamanistic – it centered on the activities of the medicine man, or shaman. Through the use of drums and rattles and the smoking of mixtures of tobacco or peyote, the shaman would enter a trance-like state that enabled him to spirit-travel and seek out the soul of the sick person in order to rescue and heal it. Today, shaman in South America still use extracts from a vine – known in Colombia as *yage* and in Peru and Ecuador as *ayahuasca* – in the same way. Siberian shamans were once able to travel by taking fly agaric toadstool while European witches were able to "fly" with the help of deadly nightshade, henbane, thorn apple, or mandrake.

The Native Americans also made ritual use of the medicine wheel and assigned animal totems to the four cardinal directions. They equated these with different personality types, spiritual energies, diseases, and plant medicines. Typically, for example, the South could be symbolized by the coyote and the energies of growth and compassion, while the eagle and the powers of wisdom and enlightenment were symbols of the East. In his spirit-travels the medicine man would head in these symbolic directions to seek the soul of the sick person. Several Indian tribes also made great use of sweat houses – creating a sauna-like environment where the sick person would be encouraged to sweat to rid the body of toxins or bacteria.

THE PHYSIOMEDICAL MOVEMENT

Before the land battles with the plains tribes decimated the indigenous population, the early pioneers and Native Americans shared much of their herbal lore with each other. An early enthusiast for native lore was Samuel Thomson, who founded the Physiomedical movement. Born in New Hampshire in 1769, Thomson learned his craft as a child from Widow Benton, a "root and herb doctor" who combined Native American skills with the traditional role of "herb wife."

Thomson believed that parents were responsible for both their own and their children's health and patented "Thomson's Improved System of Botanic Practice of Medicine," a mixture of handbooks and patent remedies that swept America in the early nineteenth century. Thomson's principal theory was that "all disease is caused by cold," which in the bitter New England winters may well have been accurate. By the late 1830s Thomson claimed three million followers to his "system."

ECLECTICISM

Other "botanic" systems followed, with the Eclectic school founded by Dr. Wooster Beech in the 1830s. Like the Thomsonians, the Eclectics used herbal remedies and Native American healing practices, but combined more orthodox medical techniques in their analysis of disease. At its peak, Eclecticism claimed more than 20,000 qualified practitioners in the USA and was a serious rival to "regular" medicine. The challenge only ended in 1907 when, following a review of medical training schools, philanthropists Andrew Carnegie and John D Rockefeller decided to give financial support solely to the orthodox medical schools.

Thomsonian physiomedicalism was brought to Britain in 1838 by Dr. Albert Isaiah Coffin who set up a similar "system" of patent remedies and do-it-yourself guides to diagnosis. Wooster Beech followed in the 1850s to preach his Eclectic message, and the movement took hold in working class areas of the country, remaining popular, especially in the North, until well into the 1930s.

In 1864, the various UK groups merged to form the National Association of Medical Herbalists. The association continues to thrive today as the National Institute of Medical Herbalists, the oldest formalized body of specialist herbal practitioners in Europe.

PHYSIOMEDICALIST PHILOSOPHY

Central to the physiomedical view was the belief that it is possible to strengthen the body's "vital force" by keeping both tissues and nervous state in balance. The key therapeutic treatment involved "relaxing" or "astringing" tissues and "sedating" or "stimulating" nerves. Suitable herbs, classified as either stimulating or sedating, relaxing or astringent, were used to achieve this balance. Irritable bowel syndrome, for example, might be treated with chamomile to sedate the nervous system and relax the digestive tissues, followed by an astringent, such as agrimony, and a stimulant, such as ginger, to encourage the vital force and restore internal energy levels once more.

Among the most popular physiomedical herbs were relaxant plants like Indian tobacco; cayenne as a stimulant; black root (*Leptandra virginica*) used as a relaxant for the liver; fringe tree bark (*Chionanthus virginica*), which was both relaxing and stimulating for the liver and gallbladder; true unicorn root (*Aletris farinosa*) a uterine stimulant; black cohosh (*Actaea racemosa*) both stimulating and relaxing for the nervous system; and blue cohosh (*Caulophyllum thalactroides*) used as a stimulating relaxant for the female reproductive organs.

FROM PLANTS TO PILLS

Although extracts, such as essential oils, have been prepared from various plants for centuries, traditional herbalism has always preferred "whole" plants and used combinations of herbs to modify effects. The move to isolate and identify the individual active ingredients, and then use these as single drugs, began in the eighteenth century and many thousands are now known. These chemicals can display quite different properties from the herb. Initially these new drugs could only be obtained as plant extracts, but later the chemical structures of many extracts were identified and the drugs are now made synthetically. In the transition from the use of crude plants to clinical pills, modern medicine has lost the art of combining herbs to modify toxicity and of using whole plants, which themselves contain chemical ingredients that can reduce the risk of side effects.

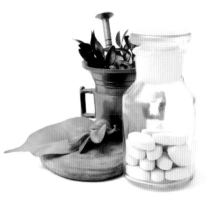

In the transition from the use of crude plants to clinical pills, medicine has lost the art of combining herbs to modify toxicity.

HERBS IN MODERN MEDICINE

One of the first modern drugs to be isolated from plant material was morphine, first identified in 1803 by Friedrich Wilhelm Serturner in Germany. He extracted white crystals from crude opium poppy. Similar techniques soon produced aconitine from monkshood, emetine from ipecacuanha, atropine from deadly nightshade, and quinine from Peruvian bark. All these compounds are categorized as alkaloids and are extremely potent, but could only be obtained from the raw plants until scientists were able to synthesize them.

The breakthrough came in 1852, when salicin, identified as one of the active ingredients in willow bark, was synthesized for the first time. This was later modified to be less of a gastric irritant and acetylsalicylic acid was launched as aspirin in 1899 by the drug company Bayer.

Now, plant extracts fill pharmacists' shelves. There are many ephedrine preparations from *ma huang* (*Ephedra sinica*), for example, both prescription and over-the-counter, which are mainly used for coughs, catarrh, hay fever or asthma. Pilocarpine, obtained from jaborandi, is used for treating glaucoma; vincristine, from the Madagascar periwinkle, is used for leukemia, while strophanthin from *Strophanthus kombé*, found in tropical Africa and use to tip poison arrows, is taken for severe heart problems.

Extracted chemicals can often be extremely potent and can cause effects that were unknown when the whole plant was used. Indian snakeroot, *Rauwolfia serpentina*, for example, has been used for centuries in Ayurvedic medicine for a range of ailments including snakebites, anxiety, headaches, fevers and abdominal pains. Mahatma Gandhi reputedly drank snakeroot tea at night if he felt over-stimulated. In the West, it was valued as a potent tranquilizer and used for high blood pressure; it was also prescribed in the treatment of schizophrenia and psychosis.

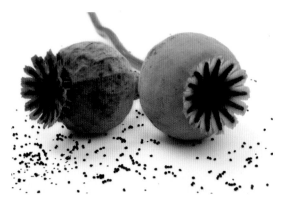

Extracted from opium poppy, morphine was one of the first modern drugs to be isolated from plant material.

In 1947, CIBA extracted the alkaloid reserpine from snakeroot and began marketing the drug Serpasil as a cure for hypertension. However, reserpine has unfortunate side effects that include severe depression and abnormal slowing of the heartbeat. By the 1960s the herb had been restricted to the status of a prescription-only drug in the UK and its use by herbalists is thus effectively banned. To this day, however, *Rauwolfia serpentina* remains widely used in other parts of Europe and Asia – taken by many as a soothing tranquillizer.

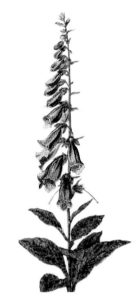

FOXGLOVE

According to tradition, a young physician, William Withering, persistently failed to bring about an improvement in a patient suffering from severe dropsy caused by heart failure. Suddenly, the patient started to recover and his relatives admitted administering an herbal brew based on an old Shropshire family recipe. In 1775, Dr. Withering obtained a copy of the recipe and began experimenting with the various herbs it contained, identifying foxglove as the most significant. In 1785 he published *An Account of the Foxglove and Some of its Medical Uses*, which detailed 200 cases of dropsy and/or heart failure that he had successfully treated with the herb, along with research notes on the parts of the plant producing the strongest effects and the optimum time to harvest.

Withering also realized that the therapeutic dose of foxglove is very close to that at which toxic side effects develop, so great care was needed in its administration. Further analysis followed and the cardiac glycosides digoxin and digitoxin were eventually extracted. These are still used in the treatment of heart conditions today.

MEDICINAL MEALS

Today's categorization of plants as herbs, vegetables, fruits, and even "weeds" is a recent invention. To the seventeenth-century cook, cabbage, carrots, and cucumbers were all "kitchen herbs," just as marigolds or marjoram were. We often forget, too, that the active constituents, such as alkaloids or saponins, in "herbs" are not confined to the plants we label as such: fruits and vegetables can be both therapeutic or, in excess, damaging. Past cultures have classified foods by temperature or taste, matched to the body's needs to maintain balance. Hippocrates noted that fresh foods "give more strength" because they are more alive, while Tibetan medicine regards frozen foods as colder and heavier than their fresh originals.

GALENICAL MENU MAKING

Galen and his followers labeled not only what we term "herbs" as hot or cold, dry or damp, but "foods" as well. In the Galenical system meat tended to be heating, fish was damp, fresh beans and apples cold and damp, wheat generally hot and damp and so on.

Food intake was considered to have a direct action on the four humors: blood, phlegm, yellow and black bile. For example, eating too many cold and damp foods would encourage the phlegmatic humor leading to catarrh. Too many hot, dry foods, on the other hand, encouraged the choleric humor (yellow bile) with resulting liver problems or skin disorders.

The medieval housewife would automatically balance the character of different ingredients, cooking fish with "hot and dry" fennel, or adding pepper to "cold and moist" beans, and she would have been quite appalled at the thought of serving strawberries in the middle of winter, as we are able to do now: this cold fruit would inevitably lead to stomach chills if eaten at such a time. Today we have lost sight of this sense of balance, eating foods regardless of climate.

BALANCING *Yin* AND *Yang* WITH DIET

A balanced diet in Chinese terms is not necessarily one with the right amounts of protein, vitamins, fats, or sugars, but one that balances the body's energies and ensures that the correct relationship between *yin* and *yang* is maintained.

Foods are classified according to the five-element model with five flavors: pungent, sweet, sour, bitter, and salty, and five temperatures: hot, cold, warm, cool, and neutral. Many foods are also related to particular organs and acupuncture meridians, just like Chinese herbs. Cool, bitter, and salty foods are more *yin* in character while hot, sweet, and pungent foods are more *yang*. Most fruits, for example, are considered very *yin* in character, similar to the cold and damp classification of Galenical medicine.

In a hot, dry climate, *yin* can be adversely affected, so eating an adequate quantity of fruit is one way of feeding this type of energy. A tourist from the cold north who heads for the tropics in the depth of winter is a fairly *yin* individual to start with, since he or she comes from a cold, damp climate. In the unfamiliar tropical temperature, such a person may be tempted to "cool off" by eating too many paw-paws, pomelos, mangoes, and melons, which pushes *yin* energies into excess and results in the cold-moist type of diarrhea that mars so many holidays.

Just as in the Galenical or the Ayurvedic systems, the Chinese may categorize people according to their physical constitution – those who are predominantly hot or cold, dry or damp. For example, a "hot" person, who opens windows and walks around in a T-shirt on a cold autumn day, may be thirsty and perhaps prone to boils, acne, hot flushes, or constipation. He or she should eat more cold, bitter foods (such as celery) and avoid pungent foods (like onions), which tend to be more heating and drying.

The idea of hot and cold foods still persists in the traditional cuisine of China and therapeutic restaurants, where diners can select dishes to balance their energy needs, are found throughout the Far East. The emphasis is always on eating particular food types to maintain balance and prevent disease. Foods are not intrinsically good or bad; what matters is how they affect each individual.

In the West, many fashionable "diets" run a great risk of imbalance, as the faddists eliminate entire categories of food from their diet, weakening some aspects of their vital energies and essence. Too little meat, for example, can weaken *yang* energies, while too much can put *yin* under pressure.

THE TASTE OF HEALTH IN AYURVEDA

In Ayurvedic medicine taste is all-important, and different foods can be categorized according to the six defined tastes. These are believed to act on the body to increase or decrease the three humors: *kapha* (phlegm), *pitta* (fire or bile) and *vata* (wind).

These humors are regarded as the waste products of digestion – consequently, if food intake is too heavily biased towards one or another of the humors, imbalance and illness will follow. A balanced diet should contain a good mixture of the six tastes, while in ill health particular tastes can be emphasized to restore balance. The correct combination of tastes is also considered so essential for growth and normal developments that special herbal pills containing all six tastes are regularly given to children.

Sweet or *madhura* tastes increase body secretions – particularly milk or semen – and reduce fire-related problems: burning sensations, toxins, etc. Sweet tastes should be avoided where a surfeit of dampness is causing the problem, such as in colds, chills and some rheumatic complaints.

Sour or *amla* tastes reduce air or wind (*vata*) while strengthening both dampness and fire in the system. Sour foods stimulate the digestion and are often recommended for digestive weakness or debility in the elderly. Too many sour foods, however, lead to muscle weakness inflammations and illnesses related to an excess of fire.

Salty or *lavana* tastes encourage fire and dampness: salt helps to retain fluids and also clean the body's ducts by attracting water and thus loosening toxic material. Salt tastes are therefore used as expectorants and for internal swellings.

· Pungent or *katu* tastes strengthen air and fire and reduce dampness. Pungent tastes are stimulating and warming so are used for such conditions as common colds and chills, lethargy, or depression. They are also a remedy for obesity and late-onset diabetes. Too many pungent foods, however, leads to an excess of air and fire, which can result in thirst, faintness, nervous exhaustion, burning sensations in the body, and other results of over-stimulation.

Astringent or *kasaya* tastes are light, cold, and drying – encouraging *vata* but decreasing fire and dampness. Astringent remedies are used for diarrhea, hemorrhages, wounds, and excessive menstruation or urination. Too many astringent foods can dry out a person, leading to constipation, dry mouth, stiff joints, wind, and debility.

Bitter or *tikta* taste is composed of air and ether so it encourages wind (*vata*) while reducing both fire and dampness. Its action involves stimulating the digestion to absorb mucus-forming kapha and also cleansing the ducts of the channels.

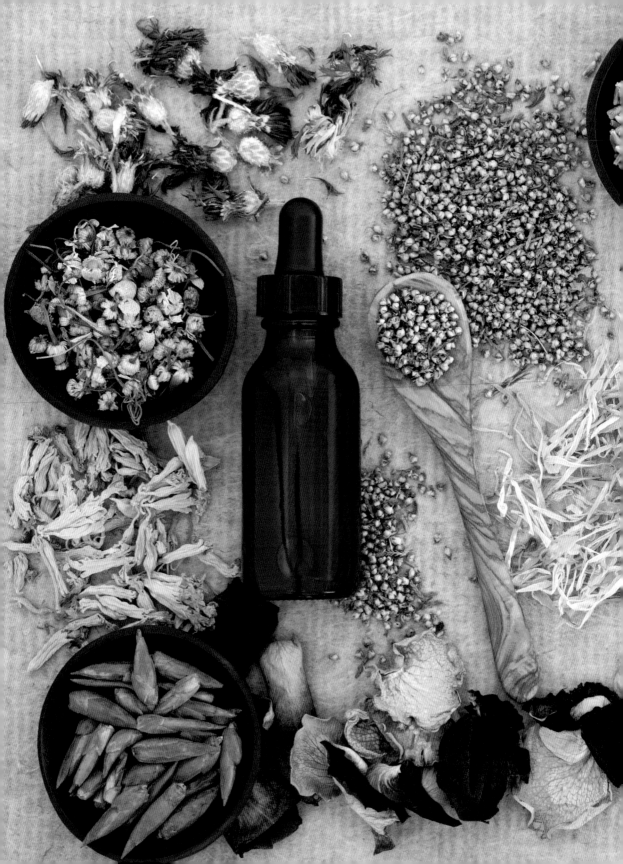

A–Z of Medicinal Herbs

This index includes a representative selection of the many thousands of plants with medicinal properties and shows the range of herbal remedies available. Each entry gives details of the parts used, actions, active ingredients, and "character" based on traditional Western, Chinese, or Ayurvedic classification. There are also suggested applications: before using these, refer to the ailment-by-ailment guides in Home Remedies (p. 152) or to Other Medicinal Herbs (p. 253). All preparations and dosages are standard (pp. 142–147) unless otherwise specified. Do not take essential oils internally unless directed by a heath care professional.

Achillea millefolium
Yarrow

The plant's Latin name is derived from the Greek hero Achilles and during the Trojan wars yarrow was reputedly used to treat wounds herb. A folk name – nosebleed – confirms its traditional first aid use as an emergency styptic to stop bleeding. Today, yarrow is valued mainly for its astringent, anti-catarrhal and diaphoretic action in colds and influenza and also for its effect on the circulation, digestive and urinary systems. The plant can usually be found growing in meadows.

Character: Cool and dry with a sweet, astringent but slightly bitter taste.

Constituents: Volatile oil (inc. proazulenes), isovalerianic acid, salicylic acid, asparagine, sterols, flavonoids, bitters, tannins, coumarins.

Actions
Aerial parts/flowers: astringent, diaphoretic, peripheral vasodilator, digestive stimulant, restorative for menstrual system, febrifuge.

PARTS USED

AERIAL PARTS
Used for all types of catarrhal conditions and as a bitter digestive tonic to stimulate bile flow. The herb contains asparagine, which is a diuretic and it can also be used for cystitis, urinary infections, etc. Yarrow also tonifies the blood vessels, stimulates the circulation, and can be used for high blood pressure. It is useful in a variety of menstrual disorders including heavy periods. Harvest during flowering early summer to late autumn.

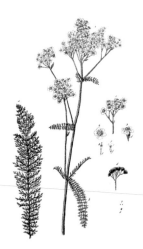

LEAVES
The leaves encourage clotting so can be used fresh for nosebleeds and minor wounds. However, inserting a leaf in the nostril may also start a nosebleed and this was once a treatment for migraines. Harvest throughout the growing season.

FLOWERS
Rich in chemicals called proazulenes, which are converted by steam into anti-allergenic and antispasmodic chamazulenes. The flowers are used for various allergic catarrhal problems, such as hay fever.

ESSENTIAL OIL
The dark blue oil, extracted by steam distillation of the flowers, is generally used as an anti-inflammatory. Extracts have also successfully been used as a mosquito repellent.

APPLICATIONS

Aerial parts

Infusions: Use to encourage sweating to reduce fevers. Combine with elderflowers and peppermint for colds and influenza. The infusion also makes a good appetite stimulant and digestive tonic.
Tinctures: Use a standard dose for cardiovascular problems, urinary disorders, or menstrual irregularities.
Compress: Use a pad soaked in infusion on dilute tincture to soothe varicose veins.

Leaves

Fresh: Single leaves, inserted in the nostrils can be used to stop nosebleeds: the feathery leaves encourage clotting.
Poultice: For emergency first aid bind washed fresh leaves to cuts and grazes.

Flowers

Steam inhalation: Use 1 tablespoon of fresh flowers in a bowl of boiling water for hay fever and mild asthma.

Infusion: Use externally as a wash for eczema or internally drink as tea for hay fever and upper respiratory catarrh.

Essential oil

Massage oil: Use 5–10 drops of yarrow oil in 25 ml of infused St John's wort oil for inflamed joints as in arthritis or tennis elbow.
Chest rub: Combine with essential oils of eucalyptus, peppermint, hyssop, or thyme in a carrier vegetable oil for chesty colds. Use no more than a total of 20 drops of essential oil in 25 ml of base (e.g. almond or sunflower oil).

CAUTIONS:
- In rare cases yarrow can cause an allergic reaction, usually in the form of skin rashes, and prolonged use can increase skin photosensitivity.
- Large doses should be avoided in pregnancy.

Actaeas racemosa
Black cohosh

Native Americans used black cohosh, also known as black snakeroot or squaw root, to treat rheumatism, yellow fever, snakebite, and kidney disorders, as well as numerous gynecological problems. Early settlers also used the herb for smallpox and by the early nineteenth century had entered the European herbal repertoire. Several oriental species (usually *A. foetida* or *A. dahurica*) are used in Chinese medicine as *sheng ma*, primarily regarded as a remedy for colds and measles.

Character: Pungent, sweet, slightly bitter, cold.

Constituents: Triterpene glycosides, cinnamic acid derivatives, chromone, isoflavones, tannins, salicylic acid.

Actions: Antispasmodic, antiarthritic, anti-inflammatory, ant-rheumatic, mild analgesic, relaxing nervine, sedative, relaxes blood vessels, promotes menstruation, diuretic, antitussive, reduce blood pressure, lowers blood sugar levels.

PARTS USED

ROOT & RHIZOME

A. racemosa
Black cohosh is widely used by Western herbalists for treating rheumatic problems, coughs and respiratory ailments, gynecological disorders, and as a sedative for nervous conditions. Recent German studies confirm that the herb effectively relieves menopausal symptoms, and it is now known to be strongly estrogenic. Traditionally the herb was used to prevent threatened miscarriage, although such use requires skill and experience.

Sheng ma / A. foetida or *A. dahurica*
The Chinese use the dried root of related species mainly to combat wind and heat evils and clear heat from the blood. *Sheng ma* is given for feverish colds, measles, headaches, and mouth ulcers. In very low doses (under 3 g) it is used to treat prolapse of the uterus or rectum.

APPLICATIONS

Root & rhizome

A. racemosa
Decoction: Use half a cup of standard decoction per dose for back pain, facial neuralgia, sciatica, and rheumatic pains. Combine with an equal amount of bogbean and valerian.
Tincture: Use 20 drops per dose with an equal amount of St. John's wort for relieving the hot flushes, night sweats, and emotional upsets associated with the menopause. The tincture can also be used with antirheumatic herbs in remedies for low back pain, osteoarthritis, sciatica and general muscle aches and pains.
Syrup: Combine with elecampane and licorice for whooping cough and bronchitis.

Capsules: Use 1 x 200 mg two or three times a day of powdered herb in capsules for back pains and rheumatic problems; combine with devil's claw.

Sheng ma / A. foetida or *A. dahurica*
Decoction: Use with red peony (*chi shao yao*), licorice, and *ge gen* for measles and feverish chills.
Tincture: Use with tonic herbs such as *huang qi*, ginseng, and *bai zhu* to strengthen spleen and stomach *qi*.

CAUTION:
* Excess can cause nausea and vomiting.
* The herb should be avoided in pregnancy.

Agrimonia spp.
Agrimony

Mainly valued today as a healing herb for the mucous membranes and for its astringent properties to stop bleeding, *A. eupatoria* has been used since Saxon times for wounds. In the fifteenth century, it was the prime ingredient of "arquebasade water" – a battlefield remedy for arquebus wounds. This healing power is now attributed to the herb's high silica content. A related variety (*A. pilosa*), known as *xian he cao* in China, is used in a similar way.

Character: Cool and drying with a bitter, astringent taste.

Constituents: Tannins, silica, essential oil, bitter principle, flavonoids, minerals, vitamins B and K.

Actions: Astringent, diuretic, tissue healer, hemostatic, stimulates bile flow, some antiviral activity reported; *A. pilosa* is also considered antiparasitic.

PARTS USED

A. eupatoria
LEAVES/AERIAL PARTS
A cooling astringent, the aerial parts can be used for various "hot" conditions to clear inflammations, phlegm, and toxins, and encourage healing. It is can be useful in diarrhea, hepatitis, gallbladder disease, cystitis, kidney infections or bronchitis. It is also a good styptic, helping to reduce bleeding in cuts. Topically it is good for skin ulceration and inflammations. The herb is gathered before and during the early part of flowering in summer.

A. pilosa
AERIAL PARTS
As well as stopping bleeding (both internally or externally), the Chinese variety also has antibacterial and antiparasitic actions and is used for *Trichomonas vaginalis* infections, tapeworms, dysentery, and malaria.

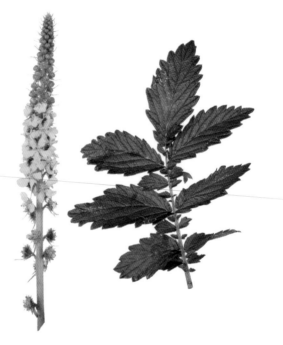

APPLICATIONS

A. eupatoria

Leaves and aerial parts
Infusion: Gentle, cooling astringent remedy ideal for diarrhea, especially in infants and children, and can be taken by breastfeeding mothers to dose babies. The infusion can also be used externally as a wash for wounds, sores, eczema (especially weeping/wet types), and varicose ulcers.
Gargle: A standard infusion can also be used as a gargle for sore throats and nasal catarrh.
Tincture: More potent and drying than the infusion and effective if the condition involves excess phlegm or mucus – useful for cystitis, gallbladder disease, urinary infections, bronchitis, heavy menstrual bleeding and haematuria.

Eyewash: A weak infusion (10 g to 500 ml of water) can be used in an eye bath for conjunctivitis.
Poultice: A poultice of the leaves can be used for migraines.

A. pilosa
Decoction: Used for bleeding disorders, including heavy uterine bleeding, haematuria (e.g. in cystitis), dysentery, and digestive parasites.
Douche: Use the decoction (cooled and strained) for *Trichomonas vaginalis* infections.
Compress: A compress soaked in the decoction can be used for boils and carbuncles.

CAUTIONS:
• Astringent herb so best avoided in constipation.

Alchemilla xanthoclora
Lady's mantle

Reminiscent of the Virgin's cloak in medieval paintings, the leaves with scalloped edges are reputed to give lady's mantle its name. Like many herbs with "lady" or "mother" as part of their common name, it is a valuable gynecological herb specifically for heavy menstrual bleeding and vaginal itching. Highly astringent and rich in tannins, it was one of the most popular wound herbs on the battlefields of the fifteenth and sixteenth centuries.

Character: Cool and dry with an astringent and bitter taste.

Constituents: Tannins, salicylic acid, saponins, phytosterols, volatile oil, bitter principle.

Action: Astringent, menstrual regulator, digestive tonic, anti-inflammatory, wound herb.

PARTS USED

AERIAL PARTS
The astringent aerial parts are good for gastro-enteritis and diarrhea. As well as helping to control heavy periods they can also be used for menstrual pains, to regulate the cycle, and for vaginal discharges. The herb is useful in inflammation and infections. Water extracts have recently been shown to be highly antioxidant. Harvest while flowering in the summer.

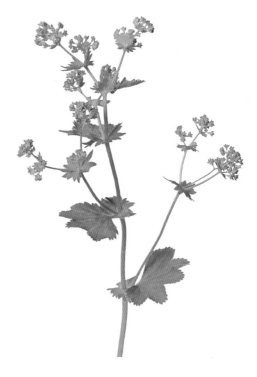

APPLICATIONS

Aerial parts

Infusion: Use for diarrhea or gastro-enteritis: take up to five times daily for acute symptoms.

Wash: Apply the infusion externally as a wash for weeping eczema or sores.

Gargle: Use the infusion for sore throats, laryngitis or as a mouthwash for mouth ulcers.

Douche: Use the infusion for vaginal discharges or itching.

Tincture: Convenient for regular use for menstrual irregularities or menopausal problems.

Cream: An effective cream for vaginal itching can be made using lady's mantle and rosewater with emulsifying ointment or another base. Typically combine 50 g of ointment base with around 20 ml rosewater and 15 ml of lady's mantle infusion or tincture (exact quantities will depend on the type of base and its absorbency) and use night and morning.

Pessaries: The tincture can be used in pessaries for vaginal discharges and itching. Use 20 drops of standard tincture in 20 g of cocoa butter to make 12–16 pessaries (depending on mold size).

CAUTIONS:
• Should be avoided in pregnancy as it is a uterine stimulant.

Allium sativa
Garlic

Prized as a medicinal herb for at least 5,000 years, garlic has long been known to reduce blood cholesterol levels after a fatty meal. Even orthodox medicine acknowledges that the plant reduces the risk of further heart attacks in cardiac patients; it is also a stimulant for the immune system and antibiotic. Garlic's distinctive odour is largely due to sulphur-containing compounds, including allicin, which account for most of its medicinal properties: commercially "deodorized" preparations are thus significantly less effective.

Character: Very hot and dry with a pungent taste.

Constituents: Volatile oil with sulphur-containing compounds – notably allicin, alliin and ajoene; enzymes, B vitamins, minerals, flavonoids.

Actions: Antibiotic, expectorant, diaphoretic, hypotensive, anti-thrombotic, reduces cholesterol levels, hypoglycemic, antihistaminic, antiparasitic.

Parts Used

Cloves
The cloves are widely used for infections, especially chest problems, digestive disorders, including dysentery and gastroenteritis, and fungal infections. They are a good long-term remedy for cardiovascular problems, excessive cholesterol levels, atherosclerosis, and the risk of thromboses. Garlic is a very heating herb with diaphoretic action, dilating the peripheral circulation and reducing blood pressure. It also helps to regulate blood sugar levels, so can be helpful in late-onset diabetes and may act as a preventative for cancer. Topically, the fresh cloves are effective for skin infections and acne. In China, where it is known as *da suan*, garlic is also used to treat hookworms, pinworms, and ringworm.

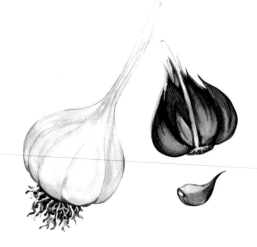

Applications

Fresh cloves: Rub on acne pustules or mash and used to draw corns. The mashed cloves can be used on warts and verrucae. Add the cloves regularly to the diet as a prophylactic against infection, to reduce blood cholesterol levels, and to improve the quality of the cardiovascular system. Additional crushed cloves (3–6 daily in acute conditions) can be eaten for severe digestive disorders (gastro-enteritis, dysentery, worms) and infections.

Juice: Drink for digestive disorders and infections or to combat atherosclerosis.

Tincture: Can be used as an alternative to the juice.

"Pearls": Many types are available commercially – the more deodorized, the less effective the preparation will be.

Powder: Garlic powder can be made into capsules as a rather aromatic alternative to commercial "pearls." Clinical trials suggest that 2 g of powder daily can be effective as a preventative for further heart attacks in those who have already suffered one attack. Daily capsules can also combat infections including candidiasis.

Maceration: Steep 3–4 garlic cloves in water or milk overnight and next day drink the liquor for intestinal parasites.

CAUTIONS:
- Garlic is very heating and can act as a stomach irritant. Combining it with carminatives like coriander, anise, fennel, lemon balm, etc., can help especially in cooking.
- Garlic oil can be a skin irritant. It should be avoided if the condition involves hot, dry symptoms and can deplete body fluids.
- While culinary quantities are generally safe, garlic should not be taken in therapeutic doses during pregnancy and lactation.

Aloe vera
Aloe

The aloe originates from tropical Africa where related species are used as an antidote to poison arrow wounds. It was known to the Greeks and Romans who used the juice for wounds: one of Pliny's many recommendations was to rub leaves on "ulcerated male genitals and chaps of the anus." Aloe was a favorite purgative throughout the Middle Ages. In China, similar uses developed – although the sap alone is used – while in India the sap is highly regarded as a cooling tonic. Aloe reached the West Indies in the sixteenth century and is widely cultivated there.

Character: Leaf: bitter, hot, moist. Gel: salty, cool, moist.

Constituents: Anthraquinone glycosides, resins, polysaccharides, sterols, saponins, chromones.

Actions: Purgative, cholagogue, wound healer, tonic, demulcent, antifungal, styptic, sedative, anthelmintic, reputed rejuvenate and anti-aging, reduces blood sugar and cholesterol levels.

PARTS USED

LEAVES
A strong purgative, the leaves are good for chronic, stubborn constipation. They stimulate bile flow and digestion and can be useful for poor appetite. Extracts of the leaves were once used on children's fingers to stop them biting their nails. Aloes can be grown as houseplants in temperate climates.

GEL OR SAP
The thick mucilaginous sap is an ideal home first-aid cure for burns, wounds and sunburn. It is also useful for any dry skin condition and can be used for treating fungal infections such as ringworm and athlete's foot. Extracts of the gel have been successfully used on mouth ulcers while US research suggests it may be active against breast and liver cancers and HIV. In Ayurveda, the gel is regarded as an important tonic for liver, blood, and female reproductive organs. It is known as *lu hui* in China and *kumari* in Sanskrit.

APPLICATIONS

Leaves

Powder: Use 100–500 mg of powder per dose or in capsules as a purgative for stubborn constipation and to stimulate bile flow.

Tincture: Use 1–3 ml of a standard tincture per dose as an appetite stimulant or for constipation. The taste is unpleasant.

Gel

Fresh herb: Apply the split leaf directly to burns, wounds, dry skin, fungal infections, insect bites, etc. Up to 2 teaspoons of the sap can be taken in a glass of water or fruit juice three times daily as a tonic.

Inhalant: Use the gel in a steam inhalant or vaporizer for bronchial congestion.

Tonic wine: Fermented aloe gel with honey and spices is known as *kumaryasava* in India and is used as a tonic for anemia, poor digestive function, and liver disorders.

Ointment: Collect a large quantity of gel and boil down to a thick paste. Store in clean jars and use as the fresh leaves.

CAUTIONS:
- Avoid in pregnancy.
- Aloe should not be taken internally by young children.
- High doses of the leaves may cause vomiting.

Alpinia spp.
Galangal

Originally from Southeast Asia, galangal (*A. galanga*) is important in both Chinese and Ayurvedic medicine. It is known as *kulanjian* in Hindi and is used as a popular stomach remedy. The dried rhizomes were brought to Europe by Arab traders from the ninth century and were a favorite with Hildegard of Bingen who used galangal for a wide range of heart disorders. Lesser galangal (*A. officinarum*) is used in similar ways as a digestive remedy in India and is known as *gao liang jiang* in China.

Character: Pungent, hot, dry.

Constituents: Essential oil (including cineole, eugenol, pinene), sesquiterpene lactones (including galangol), flavonoids.

Actions: Carminative, digestive tonic, promotes sweating, prevents vomiting, stimulant, antifungal.

Parts Used

Dried Rhizome

A. galanga
Galangal is used in India for digestive and respiratory problems and is classified as an aphrodisiac tonic. German studies, based on the work of Hildegard of Bingen, have confirmed that the herb is also effective at easing heart pains, dizziness, and fatigue, and it can be given for the symptoms of chronic heart disorders like angina pectoris.

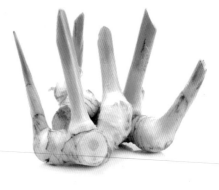

A. officinarum
The Chinese use lesser galangal (*gao liang jiang*) as a warming remedy for stomach and spleen, to relieve cold and pain, and to move *qi*. It is used for indigestion, gastro-enteritis, stomach pains, colds, and chills.

Fresh Rhizome

A. galanga
Galangal, used in Thai and Middle Eastern cooking, is commonly found in Western supermarkets. The root can be used much like fresh ginger in warming decoctions for colds, chills, and travel sickness.

Applications

Fresh rhizome

A. galanga
Decoction: Use 1–2 slices per mug for minor digestive problems and chills.

Dried rhizome

A. galanga
Powder/capsules: Take 1–2 x 200 mg capsules for digestive upsets, stomach cramps, indigestion and flatulence.
Tincture: Use 10 drops per dose as a circulatory and heart tonic; use 2–3 drops on the tongue as required for angina pectoris attacks, dizziness and palpitations.

A. officinarum
Decoction: Use for chills, minor stomach pains and indigestion.
Capsules: Take one or two 200 mg capsules before travelling to combat motion sickness.
Tincture: Take 2–10 drops per dose for nausea, stomach chills or indigestion.

CAUTION:
- Heart problems such as angina pectoris need professional treatment.
- Do not use galangal to replace prescribed medication without consulting your health care professional.

Althaea officinalis
Marshmallow

Taking its botanical name from a Greek word, *altho*, meaning "to heal," marshmallow has been used since ancient Egyptian times. The root, rich in sugars, is very mucilaginous and a soothing demulcent. The leaves are not as mucilaginous as the root and are used as an expectorant and soothing remedy for the urinary system. Both leaves and root have been used as a vegetable. All the mallow family have similar properties, with varieties like garden hollyhocks and common mallow occasionally used medicinally as well.

Character: Cool and moist with a sweet taste.

Constituents
Root: Mucilage, polysaccharides, asparagine, tannins.
Leaves: Mucilage, flavonoids, coumarin, salicylic and other phenolic acids.

Actions
Root: demulcent, expectorant, diuretic, wound herb.
Leaves: expectorant, diuretic, demulcent.
Flowers: expectorant.

PARTS USED

ROOT
Externally the root is used for wounds, burns, boils, and skin ulceration. Internally it is taken for inflammations of the mucous membranes – such as gastritis, enteritis, oesophagitis, peptic ulceration – to ease the symptoms of hiatus hernia, and in urinary inflammations such as cystitis. Harvest in the autumn or winter.

LEAVES
Mainly used to soothe and heal bronchial and urinary disorders including conditions such as bronchitis, irritating coughs, cystitis, and urethritis. Harvest after flowering in late summer.

FLOWERS
Although rarely available commercially, they can be gathered from home-grown plants and are mainly used to make expectorant syrups for coughs. Garden hollyhock flowers can be used as an alternative. Harvest in summer.

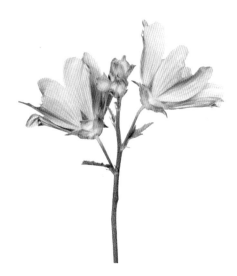

APPLICATIONS

Roots

Tincture: Used for inflammations of the mucous membrane in digestive and urinary systems.
Maceration: 25 g of root to 500 ml of cold water and allowed to stand overnight. This can be very thick and mucilaginous and may need further dilution but is a good soothing brew for oesophagitis, gastric ulceration, or cystitis.
Poultice: Use the root or a paste of the powdered root mixed with water for skin inflammations and ulceration.
Ointment: For wounds, skin ulceration, or to help draw splinters, melt 50 g anhydrous lanolin, 50 g beeswax, and 300 g soft paraffin together over water bath. Add 100 g of marshmallow root powder and heat for an hour. When this mixture has cooled to room temperature, stir in 100 g of powdered slippery elm bark to form a thick mixture.

Compress: Compresses soaked in the tincture or decoction can be used externally as the poultice.

Leaves

Infusion: Mainly used for bronchial or urinary disorders: use standard doses.
Tincture: Used as the infusion. For coughs, it can be combined with herbs like white horehound or hyssop, while for urinary complaints combine with yarrow and buchu, for example.

Flowers

Syrup: A cough syrup can be made by combining a standard infusion of the flowers (25 g to 500 ml) with 500 g of honey or sugar.
Infusion: Can be combined with coltsfoot, sweet violet and corn poppy flowers to make the French "*tisane des quartre fleurs*" used as an expectorant and anti-catarrhal tea.

Ammi visnaga
Khella

Since ancient times, khella seeds have been used in Arab and Middle Eastern medicine as a smooth muscle relaxant to ease colic and asthma. Pliny reports that the plant was used in a similar way to cumin, and Hippocrates referred to it as "royal cumin," because he believed its effects to be superior to cumin. The use of khella spread to Europe from North Africa with the Moors, and it was a popular remedy for whitening teeth in parts of Spain. A close relative *A. majus* (bishop's weed) is used in similar ways and was called *ameos* or *ammi* in Elizabethan times.

Character: Hot, dry, pungent.

Constituents: Furanochromones and coumarins (including khellin), borneol, linalool, flavonoids, sterols.

Actions: Antispasmodic, relaxant, anti-asthmatic, diuretic, relaxes the coronary arteries.

PARTS USED

SEEDS
A. visnaga
These are the source of two important drugs – chromoglycate, used to treat asthma, and amiodarone, used to normalize heartbeat.

A. majus
The seeds of bishop's weed are used as a diuretic and a treatment for skin problems such as vitiligo and psoriasis.

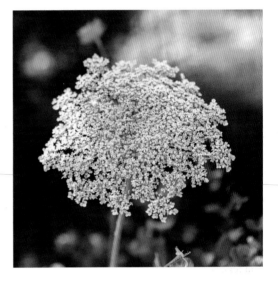

APPLICATIONS

Seeds

A. visnaga
Infusions: Use a weak infusion for asthma, bronchial spasms or bronchitis.
Tinctures: Use 20 drops in a little water per dose to relieve colic, urinary spasms and gall bladder pain. The same mixture can also help in asthma.
Steam inhalant: Put 1 teaspoon of seeds into a basin of boiling water and use as a steam inhalant to relieve mild asthma attacks, bronchial spasms, hay fever, and colic.
Capsules: Use 1-2 x 200 mg capsules up to three times daily to combat mild asthma attacks or to improve the blood supply to the heart in angina pectoris.

Syrup: Use a syrup made from the infusion for bronchitis or whooping cough.

A. majus
Cream: Apply regularly to patches of psoriasis or vitiligo.

CAUTIONS
- The use of khella is restricted in some countries, including Australia.
- Long-term use or high doses may lead to nausea and insomnia.
- Stop use immediately if allergic reactions occur.
- Avoid in diabetes and high blood pressure.

Angelica spp.
Angelica

The liqueur, Benedictine, derives its distinctive flavor from *A. archangelica*, a tall biennial. The candied stalks and roots were traditionally taken as a tonic to combat infection and improve energy levels. Several other species are used in Eastern medicine, including *A. polyphorma* var. *sinensis* (*dang gui*), one of the most important of the great Chinese tonic herbs used in many patent remedies as a nourishing blood tonic and to regulate the menstrual cycle. Many over-the-counter preparations based on *dang gui* are available in the West.

> **Character:** Sweet, pungent and warm; generally drying.
>
> **Constituents:** Volatile oil, bitter iridoids, resin, coumarins, valerianic acid, tannins, bergapten; vitamins A and B also reported in Chinese spp.
>
> **Action:** *A. archangelica*. *Root*: antispasmodic, diaphoretic, expectorant, carminative, diuretic. *Leaves*: carminative, topical anti-inflammatory. *Essential oil*: digestive tonic, antirheumatic.
>
> *A. polyphorma* var. *sinensis*: *Root*: blood tonic, circulatory stimulant, laxative.

PARTS USED

A. archangelica

LEAVES

Mainly used for indigestion and bronchial problems, the leaves are generally considered less heating and more gentle than the root. Harvest in summer.

ROOT

Used for digestive and bronchial problems, to stimulate the appetite and liver, to relieve rheumatism and arthritis and promote sweating in chills and influenza. As a uterine stimulant, angelica has been used in prolonged labor or retention of the placenta. Harvest in the autumn of its first year.

A. polyphorma var. *sinensis*

ROOT

Dang gui is valuable in anemia, menstrual pain, or as a general tonic after childbirth. It clears liver stagnation (of both energy and toxins), has been used to treat liver cirrhosis, and can relieve constipation especially in the elderly.

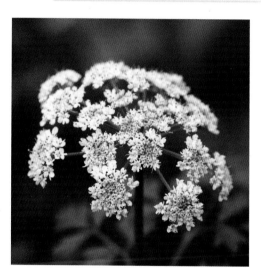

APPLICATIONS

A. archangelica

Leaves

Infusion: Use in standard doses for indigestion.
Compress: Use the infusion or diluted tincture for pleurisy.
Tincture: Up to 3 ml, three times daily as a simple for bronchitis or flatulent digestion.
Cream: Anti-inflammatory cream for skin irritations and dermatitis.

Roots

Tincture: Take for bronchial catarrh, chesty coughs, digestive disorders or as a liver stimulant.
Maceration: The root steeped in water overnight can be used as an alternative to the tincture and in similar ways.

Compress: Soak a pad in the diluted tincture or decoction and apply to painful or rheumatism or arthritic joints.

A. polyphorma var. *sinensis*

Root

Decoction: Used for anemia, menstrual irregularities, menstrual pain or weakness after childbirth; also for constipation in the elderly.
Tincture: Use as the decoction.

CAUTIONS

- Large or regular doses of all the angelicas should be avoided in pregnancy and diabetes.
- All varieties are heating and can be contraindicated in hot conditions.

Apium graveolens
Celery

A familiar and popular vegetable, celery is also an important medicinal herb. In Eastern medicine, it is characterized as bitter-sweet making it a moist and cooling food and thus good for balancing hot, drying, spicy chili dishes, for example. The whole plant is gently stimulating, nourishing, and restorative for debilitated conditions. In the past, celery was grown as a vegetable for winter and early spring; because of its antitoxic properties it was a good cleansing tonic after the stagnation of winter. A homoeopathic extract of the seeds is widely used in France to relieve retention of urine.

Character: Slightly cool and moist with a bitter-sweet taste.

Constituents: Volatile oil, glycosides, furanocoumarins, flavonoids.

Actions: Antirheumatic, sedative, urinary antiseptic, diuretic, carminative, hypotensive, some antifungal activity reported.

PARTS USED

SEEDS
Mainly used as a diuretic, these can help clear uric acid and other toxins from the system making them especially useful for gout, where uric acid crystals collect in the joints, and arthritis. Slightly bitter, they act as a mild digestive stimulant. Harvest after the plant flowers in its second year.

ROOT
Rarely used today, the root is also an effective diuretic and has been used for urinary stones and gravel. It also acts as bitter digestive and liver stimulant. Harvest after flowering.

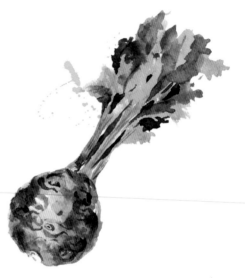

STALKS
This shares the other medicinal properties of other parts of the plant to a lesser extent. Eating fresh stalks can help stimulate milk flow after childbirth. Although wild celery is more effective, commercially grown vegetables can also be used.

ESSENTIAL OIL
Distilled from the seeds and is more potent therapeutically. Use with care.

APPLICATIONS

Seeds
Infusion: A useful tea for joint inflammations (specifically rheumatoid arthritis and gout) can be made from 2 teaspoons of celery seed and 1 teaspoon of *lignum vitae* (*Guaiacum officinale*) per cup of boiling water.
Tincture: Combined with root and used as below.

Root
Tincture: Used mainly as a diuretic in hypertension and urinary disorders or as a component in arthritic remedies. Also used as a kidney energy stimulant and cleanser. A mixed tincture made from seed and root can is also used.

Essential oil
Massage oil: Use up to 20 drops in a teaspoon of olive or almond oils as a massage for arthritic inflamed joints.
Footbath: For very painful gout in the feet or toe joint use 15 drops of oil in a bowl of warm water to soak the feet.

Stalks
Juice: The whole fresh plant (seeds, root, stalks, leaves) can be juiced and used internally for joint and urinary tract inflammations such as rheumatoid arthritis, cystitis, or urethritis. The juice is also nourishing for debilitated conditions and nervous exhaustion.

CAUTIONS
- Traces of bergapten in the seeds could increase photo-sensitivity if the extracted oil is used externally in bright sunshine.
- The oil and large doses of the seeds should be avoided in pregnancy as apiol can act as a uterine stimulant.
- Do not use commercially supplied seeds intended for cultivation as these are often treated with fungicides.
- Internal use of the essential oil is not recommended for home use.

Arctium lappa
Burdock

Once widely used in over-the-counter cleansing remedies, burdock is familiar for its hooked fruits, or burs, which enthusiastically attach themselves to clothing. This property is reflected in the herb's botanical name, from the Greek *arctos*, or bear, suggesting rough coated fruits, and *lappa*, to seize. Burdock was a traditional blood purifier, often combined in folk brews such as dandelion and burdock wine, and it was once popular for indigestion. In Japan, the roots, known as *gobo*, are eaten as a vegetable while in China the seeds, *niu bang zi*, are used to dispel the "wind and heat evils"; they also have been used to lower the blood sugar levels.

Character
Seeds: cold with a pungent and bitter taste.
Root/Leaves: cool and drying, bitter but the root is also slightly sweet to the taste.

Constituents: *Leaf/root*: bitter glycosides, flavonoids, tannins, volatile oil, antibiotic polyacetylenes, resin, mucilage, inulin, alkaloids, essential oil. *Seeds*: essential fatty acids, vitamins A and B2.

Action: *Root*: alterative, mild laxative, diuretic, diaphoretic, antirheumatic, antiseptic, antibiotic. *Leaves*: aperient, diuretic. *Seeds*: febrifuge, anti-inflammatory, antibacterial, hypoglycemic.

PARTS USED

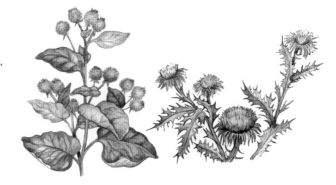

ROOT

Western herbalists consider the root the most important part of burdock and use it as a cleansing, eliminative remedy whenever there is a build-up of toxins leading to skin problems, digestive sluggishness, or arthritic pains. The plant is also hypoglycemic so can be used to regulate glucose metabolism in late-onset, non-insulin-dependent diabetes.

It is often used in combination with yellow dock (*Rumex crispus*) for skin disorders and the slightly bitter taste helps stimulate the digestion. Harvest in the autumn.

LEAVES

Generally considered less effective than the root, but can be used in very similar ways. They are particularly useful for stomach problems including indigestion and general digestive weakness. The leaves are gathered before and during the early part of flowering.

SEEDS

These were used by the American eclectics for skin diseases and as a diuretic. In Chinese medicine they are regarded as suitable for the common cold that is characterized by sore throat and unproductive cough.

APPLICATIONS

Roots

Decoction: Cleansing remedy for many skin disorders especially persistent boils, sores and dry, scaling eczema. Can also be used as a face wash for acne and fungal skin infections such as athlete's foot or ringworm.
Tincture: In combination with specific arthritic or digestive herbs to detoxify the system or stimulate the digestion; also for urinary stones and gravel.
Poultice: For skin sores and leg ulcers.

Leaves

Infusion: For indigestion in wineglass doses before meals and as a mild digestive stimulant.
Poultice: For bruises and skin inflammations (including acne).
Infused oil: A hot infused oil can be used for treating varicose ulcers.

Seeds

Decoction: For feverish colds with sore throat and cough works well combined with honeysuckle flowers and forsythia berries. Use with heartsease for skin eruptions.

Artemisia spp.
Wormwood & Mugwort

Wormwood (*A. absinthium*) and mugwort (*A. vulgaris*) are highly regarded medicinal herbs in both Eastern and Western cultures. The Anglo-Saxons listed mugwort as one of the "nine sacred herbs" given to the world by the god Woden. It was also reputedly planted alongside roads by the Romans who liked to put sprigs in their sandals to prevent aching feet on long journeys. Both herbs are bitter digestive remedies while as wormwood's name implies it is also used to expel parasitic worms. Extracts of a Chinese variety, *qing hao* (*A. annua*), are increasingly used as an antimalaria remedy in many parts of the world.

Character: Bitter, pungent, and drying. Generally considered quite cold, although *A. annua* is more warming in character.

Constituents: Volatile oil (inc. sesquiterpene lactones and azulenes), bitter principle, flavonoids, tannins, silica, antibiotic polyacetylenes, inulin, hydroxycoumarins.

Actions: Bitter digestive tonics and uterine stimulants. *A. absinthium* anthelmintics; *A. vulgaris* is also a stimulating nervine, menstrual regulator, and antirheumatic.

PARTS USED

LEAVES AND FLOWERING TOPS

A. absinthum
These contain anti-inflammatory azulenes and potent anthelmintics like absinthin and santonin to combat parasitic worms, while the polyacetylenes are antibiotic. As a very bitter herb, wormwood is a good digestive remedy to stimulate the appetite and liver function. It is also a uterine stimulant traditionally used during childbirth. It contains thujone, which can be addictive and gave the drink "absinthe" its notorious reputation. Harvest during flowering in late summer.

A. vulgaris
As a gentle nervine and menstrual regulator, mugwort can be helpful at the menopause. It can be used for scanty or delayed menstruation as well as for stopping excessive and prolonged menstrual flow. In the East, a local variety of mugwort leaf (*A. vulgaris* var. *indicus* or *ai ye*) is used as moxa – the sticks of dried herb that are burned at the end of acupuncture needles (moxibustion) for "cold" conditions like arthritis while treatment at a point just below the naval is also used for certain sorts of menstrual pain. Harvest while flowering in summer.

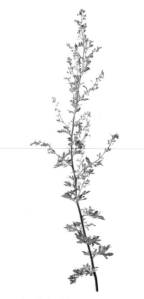

A. absinthium

APPLICATIONS

A. absinthum

Infusion: For hepatitis, jaundice, sluggish digestion, poor appetite, and gastritis. As an anthelmintic use is similar to southernwood.
Compress: A pad soaked in the infusion soothes bruises and insect bites.
Wash: The infusion can be used externally for skin infections such as scabies and mange.
Tincture: Similar applications to the infusion but do not exceed 3 ml daily.
Wine: Many bitter aperitifs (like vermouth) contain wormwood to act as a digestive stimulant before meals.
Powders: Doses up to 10 g daily can be used to clear severe parasitic infestations but treatment should not be attempted without professional advice.

A. vulgaris

Infusion: For menopausal syndrome.
Tincture: Used for many types of menstrual disorders including scanty menstruation, prolonged bleeding, or menstrual pains. In childbirth used for prolonged labor and retained placenta. A good bitter stimulant in liver stagnation and sluggish digestion.
Decoction: Combine with dry ginger to make a warming tea for menstrual pain.

CAUTIONS
- All *Artemisia* spp. should be avoided during pregnancy and breastfeeding. They are uterine stimulants and may cause fetal abnormalities.
- Take for short periods only.

Asparagus spp.
Asparagus

A popular seasonal vegetable in the West, asparagus (*A. officinalis*) has also been used as a medicinal herb since ancient times. Pliny called it "one of the most beneficial foods to the stomach," adding that it also "improves the vision, moves the bowels . . . is aphrodisiac, very useful as a diuretic and relieves pain in the loins and kidneys." In India, a related species (*A. racemosus*) is one of Ayurveda's most important tonics, *shatavari*. The name literally means "she who possess a hundred husbands" and is said to reflect the potent rejuvenating effect the herb has on the female reproductive organs.

Character: Bitter, sweet, cool.

Constituents: Steroidal glycosides (asparagosides), bitters, flavonoids, asparagine.

Actions
A. officinalis: diuretic, bitter digestive stimulant, mild laxative, sedative, source of folic acid and selenium.
A. racemosus: tonic, demulcent, antibacterial, antitussive, expectorant, antitumor.

PARTS USED

DRIED ROOT

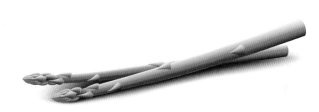

Shatavari/A. racemosus
Shatavari is the most important of Ayurveda's women's tonics. It is used for any debility associated with the sexual organs including infertility, menopausal problems, and following hysterectomy. It is also regarded as a soothing demulcent for the digestive and respiratory systems.

Tian men dong/A. racemosus
The Chinese call the tuberous roots of both *A. racemosus* and *A. cochinchinensis, tian men dong*, which literally means "lush winter aerial plant." It is used to nourish *yin* and clear heat so is given for symptoms of kidney energy weakness, such as night sweats and impotence, as well as to replenish body fluids, as in dry coughs, dry throat, or constipation.

A. officinalis
Asparagus root is mainly used as a soothing diuretic and cleansing remedy for urinary tract inflammations or rheumatic problems.

SHOOTS

A. officinalis
Although the shoots are not as effective a diuretic as the root, they are still a very palatable way of taking medicine for mild cases of cystitis, fluid retention associated with the menstrual cycle, or slight edema.

APPLICATIONS

Dried root

Tian men dong/A. racemosus
Decoction: Use with ginseng and *sheng di huang* for lingering coughs and debility following influenza.

Shatavari/A. racemosus
Powder: Take up to 3 g of the powder daily in warm milk as a tonic for the female reproductive system.
Tincture: Use the tincture with an equal amount of almond oil, well-shaken, as a rub for stiff joints and muscle spasm.

A. officinalis
Juice: Take 10 ml three times a day of the fresh root juiced in a food processor, as a diuretic.

Shoots

A. officinalis
Fresh shoots: Eat 3–4 young shoots at meals once or twice a day for cystitis or swollen ankles.

CAUTION
* Traditionally, *tian men dong* is avoided in cases of diarrhea and coughs caused by common colds.

Avena sativa
Oats

Oats are the traditional staple of Northern Europe: a warm, sweet food that for centuries helped to combat our cold, damp climate. Porridge made from oatmeal (the crushed grain) is still an excellent way to start the day with a nutritious and uplifting food. Medicinally the whole plant (known as oatstraw) is used and is gathered when the grains are ripe. The herb is a good restorative nerve tonic, ideal for depression and *qi* deficiency. More recently, research has shown that oat bran (and to a lesser extent oatmeal) can help reduce cholesterol levels when these are abnormally high.

Character: Warm and moist with a sweet taste.

Constituents: Saponins, flavonoids, many minerals, alkaloids, steroidal compounds, vitamins B1, B2, D, E, carotene, wheat protein (gluten), starch, fat.

Actions: *Oatstraw:* antidepressant, restorative nerve tonic, diaphoretic.
Seeds: antidepressant, restorative nerve tonic, nutritive.
Bran: antithrombotic, reduces cholesterol levels.
Fresh plant: antirheumatic in homoeopathic tincture.

Parts Used

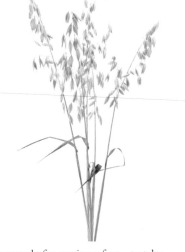

Oatstraw (whole plant)
An excellent tonic for the whole system, which can be used for both physical and nervous debility. Ideal for mental depression. Oats can also be used for thyroid and estrogen deficiency and can be supportive in degenerative diseases like multiple sclerosis and for colds – especially if recurrent or persistent. The crop is harvested when the grains are ripe and the whole plant dried and chopped.

Seeds
The grains have very similar properties to the whole plant and can be used for the same conditions. Harvested in late summer and milled to produce oatmeal, which is also useful externally for skin problems.

Bran
Recent research has shown that oat bran is particularly effective at reducing serum cholesterol levels. It is produced from the coarse husk of the grains separated from oatmeal during the milling process.

Bach Flower Remedy – Wild Oats
As the name perhaps suggests, Dr. Edward Bach recommended his Wild Oats flower remedy for sowing a few – to take when one is uncertain of the future or at one of the great crossroads of life, such as choosing a career or for dissatisfaction with the present.

Applications

Oatstraw (whole plant)

Fluid Extract: Use doses of 2–3 ml as a sedative and antidepressant in anxiety, insomnia, etc. Combines well with vervain. The tincture can be used in a similar way. Also as a nutritive addition to remedies for colds and chills encouraging sweating.
Decoction: The whole dried plant is used in a standard decoction as the fluid extract. The decocted liquid can also be used as a healing wash for skin conditions.

Oatmeal (ground seeds)

Poultice: For skin conditions (due to the high silica content) such as eczema, herpes (cold sores) or shingles.

CAUTIONS:
• For those sensitive to gluten (e.g., as in coeliac disease) decoctions or tinctures should be allowed to settle and then the clear liquid only decanted for use.

Azadirachta indica
Neem

Neem is traditionally used in Ayurvedic medicine as a cooling remedy for fevers and is an important insecticide. The plant is also known as bead tree from the hard nuts once used in making rosaries. The timber is highly prized for its insecticidal properties and is used for making worm-resistant furniture. In parts of Africa neem hedges have also been introduced to provide a readily available source of insecticide. The seed oil is traditionally used as a contraceptive and modern studies suggest that it has spermicidal properties.

Character: Bitter, pungent, cooling.

Constituents: Meliacins, triterpenoid bitters, tannins, flavonoids.

Actions: Anti-inflammatory, antifungal, bitter tonic, expels worms, prevents vomiting, cleansing, reduces fevers.

PARTS USED

BARK
Remedies including the bark are used in Ayurvedic medicine for malaria, tuberculosis, diabetes, tumors, arthritis, and rheumatic problems. The herb is believed to encourage the *vata* humor while reducing *pitta* and *kapha*, so is also taken for obesity and diabetes.

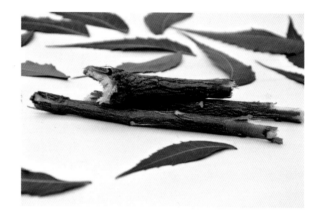

TWIGS
Traditionally neem twigs are sharpened and used as toothpicks.

SEEDS/SEED OIL
Neem oil, extracted from the seeds, is a traditional treatment for leprosy. Modern research suggests the oil is strongly antibacterial. The crushed seeds are made into a paste for treating piles.

LEAVES
Neem leaves are often sold in Indian food markets. Infusions are used in folk medicine for malaria and parasitic worms. The juice, made by crushing the fresh leaves, is also used in ointments and pastes for eczema and ringworm.

APPLICATIONS

Bark

Wash: Use a strong decoction as a wash for skin infestations such as lice and scabies – use 50 g of bark to 750 ml of water.
Tincture: Combine with other anti-inflammatory and cleansing herbs for arthritis and rheumatism.
Decoction: Use for feverish conditions.

Leaves

Infusion: Use the infusion as a hair rinse for lice and nits: add 5–10 drops of tea tree oil per cup.

Poultice: The crushed leaves made into a paste or poultice can be used on ringworm or eczema. Alternatively use a compress soaked in the infusion.

Seed oil

Lotion: Add 5–10 drops of the oil to 100 ml of distilled witch hazel as a lotion for ringworm and athlete's foot.

CAUTION:
- Neem should not be given to the elderly, very young, or debilitated.

Borago officinalis
Borage

The great herbalist, John Gerard, writing in 1597, quotes the old tag "*ego borago gaudia semper ago*" (I borage, always bring courage). Modern research has given a new slant to the saying, as the plant is now known to stimulate the adrenal glands, encouraging the production of adrenaline – the "fight or flight" hormone – which gears the body into action in stressful situations. The herb's pretty blue flowers have been added to salads since Elizabethan times to "make the mind glad" – a practice that modern cooks can also follow.

Character: Cold and moist with a slightly sweet taste.

Constituents: *Aerial parts/leaves*: saponins, mucilage, tannins, vitamin C, calcium, potassium. *Seeds*: essential fatty acids including cis-linoleic and gamma-linolenic acids.

Actions: *Leaves*: Adrenal stimulant, galactagogue, diuretic, febrifuge, antirheumatic, diaphoretic, expectorant.
Juice: Antidepressant, topical anti-pruritic, demulcent and anti-inflammatory.
Seeds: Important source of essential fatty acids.

Parts Used

Leaves
The fleshy, rather course leaves of borage can be used as an adrenal tonic for stress or to counter the lingering effects of steroid therapy. The saponin content means that they also have an expectorant action and are useful for dry, rasping coughs or the early feverish stages of pleurisy or whooping cough. Harvest throughout the growing season – they can also be chopped and eaten in salads.

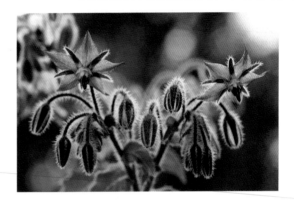

Juice
Pulping the fresh leaves yields a thick mucilaginous juice, which is particularly useful for nervous depression or grief. And although the leaves themselves can feel rough and irritating to the touch, the juice makes a soothing lotion for any dry, itching skin condition.

Flowers
Nowadays these are occasionally used in salads or to decorate that very English summer drink, Pimm's. Traditionally, they were added to wine to "maketh men merrie" and were also used in cough syrups.

Seeds and seed oil
Recently, the important essential fatty acids, cis-linoleic and gamma-linolenic, have been identified in the seed oil and this is now used as an alternative to evening primrose oil for eczema and rheumatic or menstrual disorders. The oil can be used externally for eczema or is available commercially in capsules generally marketed as "starflower" oil.

Applications

Leaves

Tincture: Use 2–5 ml three times daily as a post-steroid therapy tonic and for the effects of stress.

Infusion: A standard infusion can be used for the early stages of lung disorders (especially pleurisy) or for feverish colds. In lactating mothers, borage tea can be used with fennel to stimulate milk flow.

Juice: Use 10 ml three times daily for depression, grief, or excessive anxiety.

Lotion: Dilute fresh or bottled juice 50:50 with water as a lotion for irritated, dry skin. It can also be helpful for nervous rashes.

Seeds

Capsules: Use 500 mg in capsule form daily as a supplement in cases of eczema or rheumatoid arthritis. Can also be helpful in some cases of menstrual irregularities, irritable bowel syndrome or, like evening primrose oil, as emergency first aid for hangovers (use 1 g the "morning after").

Flowers

Syrup: Make a standard infusion and sweeten with honey or sugar (500 g to 500 ml of infusion) as an expectorant for coughs. Can be combined with mullein or marshmallow flowers.

Brassica oleracea
Cabbage

Cultivated in the West since at least 400 BC, cabbage is a valuable medicine. It has been used since Dioscorides's time as a digestive remedy, joint tonic, and for skin problems and fevers; raw cabbage was also eaten by overindulgent Romans to prevent drunkenness. Cabbage, known as colewort, was a standby in folk medicine for all sorts of family ills.

Character: Slightly sweet and salty, drying, and cool.

Constituents: Minerals, vitamins A, B1, B2, and C, amino acids, fats.

Actions: Anti-inflammatory, antibacterial, antirheumatic, tissue proliferant and healing, liver decongestant.

PARTS USED

LEAVES

Externally it can be used on wounds, ulcers, inflammations and arthritic joints, neuralgia, and a range of skin conditions, especially acne. In folk medicine the leaves have been taken internally for almost every ailment including digestive disorders, lung complaints, migraines, fluid retention, and all manner of aches and pains. Recent clinical trials have demonstrated its effectiveness for stomach ulcers.

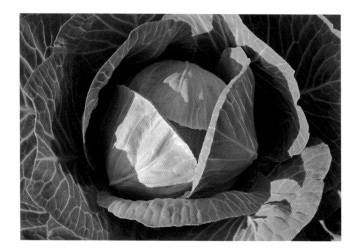

APPLICATIONS

Leaves

Fresh leaves: Use directly on arthritic or sprained joints by stripping out the central rib of the leaf and beating gently to soften it slightly, then bind onto the joint with an elasticated bandage. A similar leaf can be inserted between breast and bra cup for mastitis and to relieve engorged breasts. Fresh cabbage leaves can also be rubbed on insect bites and placed on varicose ulcers for 3–4 hours or overnight.

Lotion: For acne mix 250 g of fresh leaves and 250 ml of distilled witch hazel in a blender. Strain and add two drops of lemon juice oil to the mixture and use night and morning.

Decoction: Boil 60 g of cabbage leaves in 500 ml water for an hour and use in wine glass doses internally for colitis.

Syrup: Use the standard decoction or red or green cabbage and sweeten with 250 g of honey, use in 10 ml doses for chesty coughs, asthma, and bronchitis

Juice: Process fresh cabbage leaves in a juicer with a little water and drink up to 1 liter of it daily to repair gastric or duodenal ulceration. Treatment generally needs to be continued for at least three weeks. Chamomile or fennel seed tea can be taken as well to counteract any excessive flatulence.

Calendula officinalis
Pot marigold

The golden flowers of pot marigolds are a favorite among herbalists: Macer's twelfth-century herbal recommended simply looking at the plant to "drawyth owt of ye heed wikked hirores [humors]," improve the eyesight, and generally make the viewer feel more cheerful and clear-headed. In Culpeper's day marigold was used to "strengthen the heart" and was highly regarded as a remedy for smallpox and measles. Today it is widely used in patent homoeopathic remedies.

Character: Slightly bitter and pungent, drying, and gently cooling.

Constituents: Saponins, flavonoids, mucilage, essential oil bitter principle, resin, steroidal compounds.

Actions: Astringent, antiseptic, antifungal, anti-inflammatory, wound herb, menstrual regulator, cholagogue.

PARTS USED

PETALS OR FLOWER HEADS
Marigolds have a long flowering season, often from early summer to October or November. The petals can be gathered at any time and should be dried quickly but without artificial warmth – commercially dried specimens usually include the flower heads although the petals alone are better. Use externally for a wide range of skin problems and inflammations; use internally for many gynecological conditions, feverish or toxic conditions, and to move liver energies.

LEAVES
Although no longer specifically used, the leaves were once used in poultices for hot, gouty swellings.

ESSENTIAL OIL
Marigold oil is sometimes produced commercially but can be difficult to obtain; it is an effective antifungal for vaginal thrush and can also be added to skin remedies. A good substitute is infused marigold oil made from the cold infusion method.

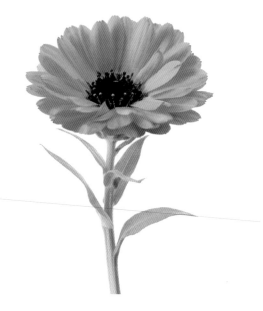

APPLICATIONS

Petals

Infusion: Use a standard infusion for gastritis and oesophagitis. Also for menopausal problems and menstrual pain.

Tincture: Use in standard 5 ml doses for stagnant liver problems including gall-bladder disorders and sluggish digestion. Also for menstrual problems, particularly irregular or painful periods. Combine with herbs like chasteberry for premenstrual disorders. Combine with cleavers and red clover for lymphatic disorders such as glandular fever. Generally, 90% alcohol is used for making marigold tincture.

Mouthwash: Use a standard infusion for mouth ulcers and gum disease.

Compress: Apply a pad soaked in the infusion to slow-healing wounds or varicose ulcer. The infusion can be used as a wash for similar conditions.

Cream: Use for any problem involving inflammation or dry skin – wounds, dry eczema, sore nipples in breast feeding, minor burns and scalds, sunburn, etc.

Infused oil: Use on chilblains, hemorrhoids, broken capillaries. Can be used as a base for massage oils for rheumatism.

Essential oil

Pessaries: For vaginal thrush, add 10 drops of marigold oil and 10 drops of tea tree oil with 15 g of melted cocoa butter. Pour into pessary molds and allow to set. Use 1–2 times daily.

Bath: Add 5–10 drops of oil to bath water for nervous anxiety, irritability, or depression. Combines well with basil.

CAUTIONS:
- Do not confuse this plant, or its essential oil, with preparations made from the French marigold – *Tagetes patula* – and related species, which can be used as weed killers, insecticides, and for warts.

Camellia sinensis
Tea

Known in China as *cha*, tea has become such a familiar drink that we forget it is also a potent medicinal herb. The Chinese have been drinking tea since around 3000 BC and regard it as a good stimulant, an astringent for clearing phlegm, and a digestive remedy. The three types of tea – green, black, and oolong – are made from the leaves of the same species. Far Eastern research shows that some green teas appear to reduce the risk of stomach cancer.

Character: Bitter-sweet taste and drying – green and oolong teas are cooling; black tea is warming.

Constituents: Alkaloids (inc. caffeine and theobromine), tannins (polyphenols), catechins, volatile oil, fluoride (in some varieties).

Actions: Stimulant, astringent, some varieties reduce cholesterol levels, antitumor properties reported in green teas.

Parts Used

Leaves

The young fresh leaves and leaf buds are pan fried to destroy enzymes and then rolled or dried to make green tea. For oolong tea, the fresh leaves are wilted in sunlight, bruised slightly and then partly fermented. Black tea is a fully fermented variety.

Green tea: Rich in fluoride, green tea can be used to combat tooth decay: two cups of Gunpowder (a popular type of green tea) contains the body's entire daily requirement of fluoride. Green teas are antioxidant and have been shown to combat both stomach and skin cancers and boost the immune system.

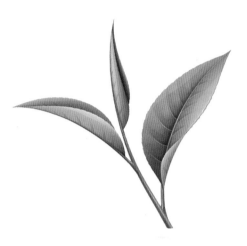

Oolong tea: Some types, such as *pu erh*, are particularly effective at reducing cholesterol levels after a fatty meal. Japanese research also suggests that oolong tea can reduce high blood pressure and limit the risk of atherosclerosis.

Black tea: Widely drunk in Europe, India and North America, black tea is rich in tannins and highly astringent which makes it a good remedy for diarrhea. Russian researchers have also shown that black tea increases the rate at which strontium-90 is excreted from the body after exposure to radiation.

Applications

Green tea

Infusion: After meals to improve dental hygiene and limit the risk of caries.

Poultice: Damp green or black tea leaves can be used on insect bites to reduce itching and inflammation.

Compress: A pad soaked in weak green tea (which is more astringent than black) makes an emergency first aid treatment to ease bleeding from cuts and grazes.

Oolong tea

Infusion: After fatty meals to reduce cholesterol levels and as a prophylactic for arterial disease.

Black tea

Infusion: A strong infusion (2 teaspoons per cup of boiling water) of ordinary tea (without milk or sugar) for diarrhea. Antibacterial action (especially against *Streptococcus* and *Staphylococcus* spp.) also makes this remedy suitable for food poisoning and dysentery. A similar infusion of strong black tea is a favorite Cantonese remedy for hangovers.

Poultice: Used tea bags can be used as poultices for tired eyes.

Wash: A weak infusion can be used as a soothing wash for sunburn.

CAUTIONS:

- High levels of caffeine-like alkaloids can lead to increased heart rate. Intake should be limited (no more than two cups daily) by those already suffering from irregular heartbeat. Pregnant women and nursing mothers should also limit intake because of the alkaloid content.

- Bitter taste can stimulate gastric acid production so excessive consumption is also best avoided by those with stomach ulcers.

Capsella bursa-pastoris
Shepherd's purse

More often considered an invasive garden weed than a medicinal herb, shepherd's purse has its place in both Eastern and Western practices. The heart-shaped seed pods resemble the leather pouches once carried by shepherds, hence the common name; another is mother's hearts – a reminder that this is a useful herb for gynecological conditions. Shepherd's purse is mainly used as a styptic to reduce bleeding. In China the seeds are said to improve eyesight.

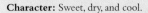

Character: Sweet, dry, and cool.

Constituents: Saponins, mustard oil, flavonoids, resin, monoamines, choline, acetylcholine, sitosterol, vitamins A, B and C.

Actions: Astringent, uterine relaxant, styptic, urinary antiseptic, circulatory stimulant, hypotensive.

PARTS USED

WHOLE PLANT
Shepherd's purse is eaten as a salad herb in many parts of the world. In Europe, it is used to stop both internal and external bleeding and it has a specific action on the uterus. In China, where it is known as *ji cai*, the sweet taste is considered good for the spleen. It is also used to treat a number of eye disorders including glaucoma and corneal problems. Harvest throughout the year.

FLOWERS
Not generally separated from the plant in Western medicine, the flowers are used in Chinese folk medicine for dysentery and uterine bleeding.

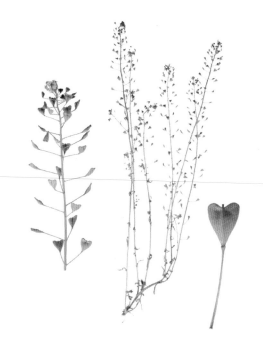

APPLICATIONS

Whole herb

Tincture: Up to 10 ml doses three times a day for heavy uterine bleeding, cystitis (especially if the case is severe and there is blood in the urine), or chronic diarrhea.

Infusion: A strong infusion (twice the standard mix) of fresh or recently dried herb is best. Use as with the tincture. A hot infusion can also be sipped during labor to stimulate contractions.

Decoction: Chinese medicine generally favors decocting the herb (30 g of herb to 500 ml water and reducing to about 150 ml) for uterine bleeding and diarrhea, as well as feverish and infectious conditions.

Poultice: The fresh herb can be applied to bleeding wounds as an emergency styptic in first aid.

Compress: A pad soaked in the infusion or diluted tincture can be used for cuts and grazes. Small cotton wool swabs soaked in the tincture can be inserted in the nostril for nosebleeds.

CAUTIONS:
• Avoid in pregnancy unless taken during labor as it is a uterine stimulant.

• For any sudden change in uterine bleeding or cases of hematuria seek professional advice before attempting self-medication.

Capsicum frutescens
Cayenne

Chilies arrived in Britain from India in 1548 and were known as Ginnie pepper; by 1597 Gerard described them as "extreme hot and dry, even in the fourth degree" and recommended the herb for scrofula, a prevalent lymphatic throat and skin infection known as the King's Evil. Cayenne was a popular herb with the nineteenth-century physiomedicalists who used it to warm the system, increase sweating, and as a circulatory and nerve stimulant for chills, rheumatism, and depression.

Character: Very hot, pungent, and drying.

Constituents: Alkaloids, fatty acids, flavonoids, vitamins A, B1, and C, volatile oil, sugars. carotene pigment.

Actions: Circulatory stimulant, diaphoretic, gastric stimulant, carminative, antiseptic, antibacterial.
Topically: Counter-irritant, rubefacient.

Parts Used

Fruit
A potent stimulant for the whole system that increases blood flow, tonifies the nervous system, and stimulates *yang* energies. It increases sweating and is antibacterial, so is an ideal remedy for colds and chills. It is also a good digestive remedy, helping to stimulate the appetite and relieve indigestion. As a stimulant for the circulation, cayenne is ideally taken internally for cold fingers and toes, while an ointment of the herb can also be used on unbroken chilblains. It is also good for various throat problems including laryngitis, tonsillitis, and hoarseness. The herb is widely available as a culinary flavoring in powdered, fresh, or dried forms. It can be grown as an annual vegetable crop and picked when the fruits ripen in the late summer.

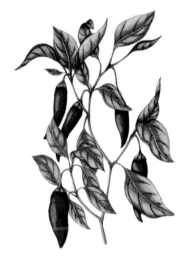

Infused oil
Although the fresh plant can be burning and irritating to the skin, when used in infused oils and ointment its action is mediated and it makes a good rubefacient (encouraging blood flow to an area) for rheumatism and other cold conditions.

Applications

Fruit

Infusion: Use half a teaspoon of herb per cup of boiling water and then dilute a tablespoon of this infusion with more hot water and sip as required. Ideal for colds and chills, cold hands and feet, shock, or depression. Use 2–3 drops of the undiluted infusions to stimulate digestive function.

Compress: A pad soaked in the infusion or diluted tincture can be used for rheumatic pains, sprains, or bruising.

Tincture: Use 5–10 drops in hot water as a circulatory stimulant and tonic. Can be combined with nervines like vervain and oats in depression.

Gargle: Use 5–10 drops of tincture to half a tumbler of warm water for sore throats or laryngitis; this is especially useful in debilitated and deficient conditions.

Infused oil: This can be used both as a warming massage for rheumatism, lumbago, arthritis, and similar conditions and to move blood. A little applied to the skin around a varicose ulcer (not on the ulcer) can encourage blood flow away from the congested area. Use 25 g of cayenne powder to 500 ml of sunflower oil and heat over a water-bath for 2 hours.

Ointment: Both this and the infused oil can be used on chilblains – as long as the skin is not broken.

CAUTIONS:
* Avoid using the seeds which can be toxic.
* Excessive consumption can lead to gastro-enteritis and liver damage.
* Avoid during pregnancy and breastfeeding.
* Compresses left on the skin for long periods can cause blistering. Caution is needed with very sensitive skins.

Cinnamomum zeylanicum
Cinnamon

A popular culinary spice, added to puddings, mulled wine and as a tea-time treat in cinnamon toast, cinnamon is pungent and warming, used for all sorts of "cold" conditions, from common colds and stomach chills to arthritis and rheumatism. In the West, we generally use the bark of *C. zeylanicum*, which is sold rolled as cinnamon sticks. The Chinese prefer their native variety *C. cassia*, which has similar properties. They use both bark (*rou gui*) and twigs (*gui zhi*). Traditionally, the bark was believed best suited for the torso, while the twigs would reach the far peripheries to warm fingers and toes. Recent research has highlighted hypoglycemic properties useful in treating diabetes.

Character: Pungent and sweet – the bark is very hot but the twigs are less so.

Constituents: Volatile oil, tannins, mucilage, gum, sugars, coumarins.

Action: *Bark*: carminative, warming digestive remedy, diaphoretic, antispasmodic, antiseptic, tonic.
Essential oil: antibacterial and antifungal.

PARTS USED

INNER BARK

C. zeylanicum

In the West, the inner bark is used mainly for digestive upsets: indigestion, general sluggishness, colic, and diarrhea. Alcoholic extracts have also been used against the *Heliobacter pylorii* bacterium now believed to cause stomach ulcers.

C. cassia,

In Chinese medicine *rou gui* is considered very warming and tonifying for the kidneys and is used for various conditions, including asthma and menopausal syndrome, that can be linked to weak kidney *qi*. Cinnamon bark can also be used for "cold" conditions.

TWIGS

C. cassia

Gui zhi can be used as a circulatory stimulant useful for cold hands and feet. Like the bark, they encourage sweating and can be used for any "cold" condition.

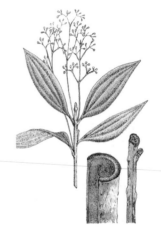

ESSENTIAL OIL

C. zeylanicum

Distilled from the bark, this is a potent antibacterial which is used internally in many parts of the world for chronic infections. Externally it makes a warming rub for abdominal colic and for chest infections and can also be used for insect bites.

APPLICATIONS

Inner bark

Decoction: Use for chronic diarrhea, kidney weakness, or conditions related to weakened kidney energy (*qi*). Can be used for cold conditions if the twigs are not available.
Tincture: Dilute with hot water for colds and chills.
Powder/Capsules: Use for cold conditions affecting the kidney and digestion.

Twigs
C. cassia
Decoction: Ideal for colds, stomach chills, etc. Combines well with ginger.
Tincture: Dilute with hot water and use as the decoction.
Compress: Use a pad soaked in the decoction or diluted tincture for arthritic and rheumatic pain.

Essential oil
C. zeylanicum
Steam inhalant: Use 5 drops of cinnamon oil in boiling water as an inhalant for coughs and respiratory irritation. Combines well with 2–3 drops of eucalyptus, thyme and/or lavender.
Massage: Use 10 ml in 25 ml of vegetable oil as a massage for abdominal colic, stomach chills, or diarrhea.

CAUTIONS:
- Avoid in pregnancy (especially the essential oil).
- Do not take essential oils internally without professional guidance. Cinnamon oil can irritate the mucous membranes and should be used in gelatin capsules internally.
- Use only with care in overheated or feverish conditions.

Citrus spp.
Bitter orange and tangerine

A valuable medicinal herb, oranges originated in China and by the Middle Ages were a favorite with Arabian physicians. In the sixteenth century, an Italian princess (Anna-Marie de Nerola) reputedly discovered an oil extracted from the flowers, which she used to scent her gloves. Today, neroli oil, as it is known, is one of the most expensive essential oils – far too precious to lavish on gloves. The Chinese remain the greatest enthusiasts of medicinal oranges: the bitter or Seville orange (*C. aurantium*), used in marmalade, and the tangerine/satsuma group (*C. reticulata*) are mainly used.

Character: Bitter orange/*C. aurantium*: Sour, bitter tasting and slightly cold. Tangerine peel/*C. reticulata*: Warm with a pungent, bitter taste.

Constituents: Volatile oil, vitamins A, B and C, flavonoids, bitters.

Action: Bitter orange *C. aurantium*: *Fruits:* carminative, hypertensive, diuretic, expectorant, energy tonic. *Essential oil:* Neroli – sedative, tonic, antiseptic, antispasmodic; Bergamot orange *C. bergamia*: *Essential oil:* bergamot – antibacterial, carminative, antispasmodic, sedative, expectorant, vermifuge. Tangerine *C. reticulata*: *Peel:* diuretic, digestive remedy, expectorant.

PARTS USED

TANGERINE PEEL (*C. reticulata*)
The Chinese use two forms – the green (*qing pi*) from unripe fruit and a well-dried "old" type – *chen pi* – from ripe tangerines or satsumas. Both are used to move stagnant energy (*qi*) from different parts of the body and are carminative for the digestive system. *Chen pi* is also used as an expectorant for coughs especially when there is a lot of thin watery phlegm. The peel can be collected from fresh and ripe fruit and dried.

BITTER ORANGE FRUITS (*C. aurantium*)
In China, the unripe and ripe fruits are also collected separately. They are both carminative and help move stagnant energy. Like bitter herbs they are digestive stimulants. Unripe bitter orange (*zhi shi*) is more potent than the ripe fruit (*zhi ke*) although both are cooling, expectorants best used where the phlegm is thick and yellow.

BERGAMOT ORANGE PEEL OIL (*C. bergamia*) – bergamot
In Italian folk medicine, the oil is used for intestinal worms in children and also for fevers and infections. Although potentially irritating, if well-diluted it can be helpful for a range of skin conditions and has been used as an analgesic for headaches.

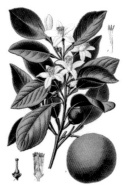

BITTER ORANGE FLOWER OIL (*C. aurantium*) – neroli
True neroli, like bergamot, comes from the bitter orange, although sweet orange blossoms (*C. sinensis*) are used to make an inferior orange oil. Neroli is antidepressant and calming. In aromatherapy, it is used in insomnia, anxiety, and hysterical states, and also to slow and calm the heart in palpitations.

APPLICATIONS

*Bitter orange/*C. aurantium
Decoction: Use for indigestion and constipation. Can also be combined with *dang gui* for menstrual pains.
Tincture: In drop doses for shock.

*Tangerine peel/*C. reticulata
Decoction: Use either the immature or old peel for indigestion and abdominal bloating; *chen pi* can be used for coughs or combined with other expectorant herbs such as hyssop, mulberry or elecampane. A small piece is traditionally added to tonic herbal mixtures (such as ginseng, *he shou wu*, or *dang gui*, etc.) to modify the action.
Tincture: Use as decoction.
Syrup: Combine with coltsfoot or other cough syrups.

*Bergamot oil/*C. bergamia
Baths: 5–10 drops in a hip bath for vaginal itching or infections.
Ointments: In very small amounts (no more than 1 ml of bergamot oil to 100 ml of ointment base) for skin conditions including psoriasis and acne. Also as an insecticide for scabies.

Mouthwash: 2–3 drops to a glass of warm water as a mouthwash for bad breath due to oral bacteria. Do not swallow the mouthwash.

*Neroli oil/*C. aurantium
Creams: Add 1–2 drops to skin cream.
Massage: 1–2 drops can be added to massage rubs for nervous conditions, and digestive upsets.
Orange flower water: A by-product of steam distillation good as a soothing carminative or for fear and shock; add 5–10 ml to baby's feeding for colic or sleeplessness.

CAUTIONS:
- If preparing your own *chen pi* from commercially bought tangerines try to use organically grown fruit to minimize pesticide contamination.
- Bergamot oil increases photosensitivity of the skin – it should never be applied in bright sunshine; potentially irritant.
- Essential oils should not be taken internally without professional advice.
- Bitter orange should be used with caution in pregnancy.

Commiphora molmol
Myrrh

An oleo-gum resin collected from the stems of bushy shrubs growing in Arabia and Somalia, myrrh has been regarded as one of the treasures of the East for millennia. Ancient Egyptian women burned pellets of it (mixed with cinnamon and frankincense) to rid their homes of fleas. In folk tradition, it was used for muscular pains and in rheumatic plasters. Called *mo yao* in China, it has been used since at least the Tang Dynasty (600 AD) primarily as a wound herb and blood stimulant.

Character: Hot and dry with an acrid, bitter taste.

Constituents: Volatile oil, resin, gums.

Actions: Antifungal, antiseptic, astringent, immune stimulant, bitter, expectorant, circulatory stimulant, anti-catarrhal.

PARTS USED

RESIN

This is collected by cutting the branches of the myrrh bush, which then exudes a thick, pale yellow liquid. As it dries this liquid hardens to a reddish-brown solid which can then be dissolved in tinctures and oils ready for use. A strong astringent, myrrh has been used as a wound herb in the past and makes an excellent gargle for sore throats and mouth ulcers. It is an effective antifungal and has also been used on intestinal parasites. Recent research suggests it can lower serum cholesterol levels and may help prevent atherosclerosis. In China *mo yao* is used to "move" blood and relieve painful swellings. Myrrh tastes particularly unpleasant.

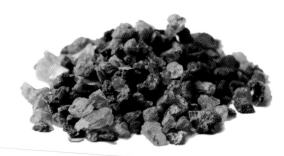

OIL

Distilled from the resin, myrrh oil has been used since Ancient Greek times to heal wounds. It is generally considered *yang* in character but is anti-inflammatory rather than heating. It makes a good expectorant and is used in chest rubs for bronchitis and coughs with thick phlegm.

APPLICATIONS

Resin

Tincture: Use for all sorts of infectious and feverish conditions – from head colds to glandular fever. It is ideal for upper respiratory catarrh and can also be added to expectorant mixtures – especially for excessive, thick phlegm. Use up to 5 ml of tincture per day in 1–2 ml doses – well diluted with water. The diluted tincture can also be used as a douche for vaginal thrush.

Mouthwash/gargle: Use 1–2 ml of tincture in half a tumbler of water as a gargle or mouthwash. Combines well with sage, rosemary or purple coneflower.

Decoction: In China myrrh is added to decoctions (usually in doses of 3–12 g) with abdominal pains. It is combined with safflower for menstrual pains.

Essential oil

Lotion: The diluted oil (no more than 2 ml in 100 ml of water) can be used externally on wounds and chronic ulcers and is both antiseptic and astringent. It can also be used in lotions for hemorrhoids.

Pessaries: Use for vaginal thrush. Add 10 drops of myrrh oil to 30 g of melted cocoa butter and allow to set in a pessary mold (enough for 24 pessaries). Can be combined with thyme or tea tree oil.

Chest rub: Use 2 drops in 5 ml of almond or sunflower oils for bronchitis or colds with thick phlegm.

CAUTIONS:
• Avoid in pregnancy.

Crataegus spp.
Hawthorn

Traditionally valued for its astringency, hawthorn was used in diarrhea, for heavy menstrual bleeding, or as a first aid remedy to draw splinters. Over the past century, the plant's considerable tonic action on the heart has been identified and today it is one of our most popular herbs for cardiac problems. The species generally used in the West are *C. oxycantha* and *C. monogyna*, whereas in China the berries of *C. pinnatifida* are taken to improve the digestion and stimulate the circulation, relieving both food and blood stagnation.

Character: *Berries*: sour, slightly sweet and warm; *Flowers*: cooler and more astringent.

Constituents: Flavonoid glycosides, procyanidins, saponins, tannins, minerals.

Actions: Peripheral vasodilator, cardiac tonic, astringent.

Parts Used

Flowering tops
C. oxycantha and *C. monogyna*
The flowering tops are widely used as a heart tonic. Their precise action is still being researched, but it seems that it improves the coronary circulation reducing the risk of angina attacks and this in turn helps to normalize blood pressures. More recently high doses of hawthorn given by injection (in Germany) have been successfully used for highly irregular heartbeats. Harvest in early summer.

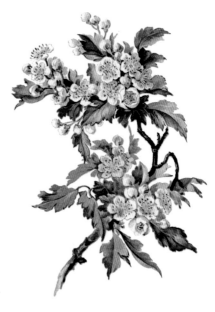

Berries
C. oxycantha and *C. monogyna*
Research suggests that the berries contain fewer of the significant cardiac-influencing constituents than the flowering tops, although both are used by Western herbalists. The berries can also be used in more traditional ways – as an astringent for diarrhea or in remedies for heavy menstrual bleeding.

C. pinnatifida – *shan zha*
Chinese hawthorn berries are mainly used for symptoms of "food stagnation" – this can include abdominal bloating, indigestion, and flatulence – helping to stimulate the digestion. *Shan zha* is said to "move" blood and is used for relieving stagnation especially after childbirth. Partially charred hawthorn berries are a regular standby for diarrhea.

Applications

Flowering top

C. oxycantha and *C. monogyna*
Infusion: Use a standard infusion as a general tonic for heart problems and to improve peripheral circulation. Combines well with linden flowers, yarrow or *ju hua* within a general strategy for hypertension.
Tincture: Use a standard tincture as the infusion in angina, hypertension, and related disorders with other suitable herbs.

Berries

C. oxycantha and *C. monogyna*
Juice: Use juice from the fresh berries as a cardiac tonic, for diarrhea, poor digestion, or as a digestive tonic.

Decoction: Use 30 g of berries to 500 ml of water and decoct for 15 minutes (short decoction). Use for diarrhea, or with *ju hua* and *gou qi zi* for hypertension.

Shan zha / *C. pinnatifida*
Capsules: Use the powdered berries with *san qi* powder for abdominal pain due to blood stagnation or for the pain of angina.
Decoction: Use 10–20 g with *zhe ke* for abdominal bloating or combine with *dan shen* and *dang gui* for period and post-partum pain.

Dendranthema x grandiflorum
Ju hua

Florist's chrysanthemums have been used in Chinese medicine since the days of Shen Nong (c. 2500 BC) and are specifically associated with the liver and eyes. The leaves have been used medicinally since around 500 AD and the stems and root are used in folk medicine. In China, the herb is drunk as a tonic in chrysanthemum wine and is sold as a cooling tea in ready-made cartons like fruit juice. The flowers were first introduced into Europe in the seventeenth century, but it took another 100 years for them to become a familiar garden ornamental.

Character: *Flowers*: pungent, sweet, biter, cool. *Leaves*: hot, wet, neutral. *Stems*: sweet, bitter, cool.

Constituents: Essential oil (including camphor carvone and borneol), alkaloids (including stachydrine and adenine), sesquiterpene lactones, flavonoids.

Actions: Cooling, anti-inflammatory, antimicrobial, reduces fevers, promotes sweating antiseptic, lowers blood pressure, dilates coronary artery and stimulates blood flow.

PARTS USED

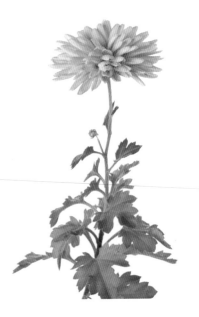

FLOWER HEADS
In China, the flower heads are always steamed before drying to reduce their inherent bitterness. They are used to clear wind and heat, which may be causing feverish colds, as well as to cool and calm the liver, clear toxins, and soothe eye inflammations. Modern research has also shown that *ju hua* can reduce raised blood pressure, especially when associated with headaches and dizziness. As a relaxant for the coronary arteries it can also relieve the pain of angina pectoris.

LEAVES
The leaves (*ju hua ye*) are more heating than the flowers but are also strongly antimicrobial. They are used for boils, sores and blurred vision. The fresh leaves are mainly used in juices, decoctions, or poultices, or they can simply be eaten fresh as a salad.

STEMS
The young stems (*ju hua miao*) are used in China to clear liver fire, which can be a cause of vertigo, and to treat eye problems.

APPLICATIONS

Flower heads

Infusion: Take regular cups to ease eye strain and headaches associated with over-work, stress, irritability and emotional upsets.

Decoction: Use with an equal amount of *jin yin hua* in a standard decoction to help reduce high blood pressure. *Ju hua* can also be combined with mulberry leaf, mint, and apricot seeds for common colds and coughs.

Tincture: Use up to 50 drops per dose for headaches and irritability.

Powder: Add half a teaspoon of powder to a small glass of rice wine to relieve vertigo.

Poultice: Use a few of the once-infused flowers on gauze as eye pads to relieve the pain of eye strain, conjunctivitis, and other red or painful eye conditions.

Pillows: Sleep on a pillow stuffed with flowers to relieve colds and headaches.

Leaves

Poultice: Use the crushed fresh leaves soaked in a little warm water or alcohol as a poultice for boils, acne pustules, and skin sores.

Decoction: Take a regular decoction of dried leaves to relieve symptoms of vertigo or dizziness.

CAUTION:
• *Ju hua* is traditionally avoided in diarrhea and debility.

Dioscorea spp.
Yam

Used to make the original contraceptive pills when synthetic hormone production was not a commercial proposition, Mexican wild yam (*D. villosa*) contains hormonal substances very similar to progesterone. It also relaxes smooth muscle – hence another of its common names: colic root. Many other yams are used as a starting material to produce the hydrocortisones for orthodox eczema creams. Several related species are used in Chinese medicine: D. *hypoglauca* (*bei xie*) is used for urinary disorders, while *D. opposita* (*shan yao*) is an important tonic for the spleen and stomach.

Character: Neutral and generally drying. Most varieties are bitter tasting but *D. opposita* is sweet.

Constituents: Alkaloids, steroidal saponins, tannins, phytosterols, starch.

Actions
D. villosa: Relaxant for smooth muscle, antispasmodic, cholagogue, anti-inflammatory, diaphoretic.
D. opposita: Expectorant, digestive stimulant, kidney tonic.
D. hypoglauca: antibacterial, anti-inflammatory, soothes urinary tract.

PARTS USED

RHIZOME
D. villosa
Mexican wild yam is an important muscle relaxant and antispasmodic used for colicky pains. It can also be taken for acute rheumatic conditions.

D. opposita
The Chinese yam, *shan yao*, is an important tonic herb in Chinese medicine. Its main action is on the kidneys, lungs, and stomach, and it is included in remedies for asthma, menopausal syndrome, urinary disorders, and weak kidney energies.

D. hypoglauca
In China, *bei xie*, or seven-lobed yam, is used mainly for urinary tract infections such as cystitis. Antibacterial and anti-inflammatory, it has also been used for rheumatoid arthritis. Extracts of *bei xie* are used in the synthesis of contraceptive pills.

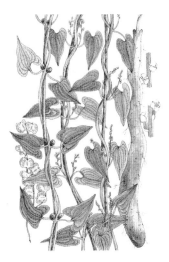

APPLICATIONS

D. villosa
Decoction: Use a standard decoction for the colicky pains associated with irritable bowel syndrome (spastic bowel) or diverticulosis. Can also be used for menstrual pains or drunk frequently once labor has started. Decoct with willow bark for arthritic pains.
Tincture: Take regular drop doses for labor or post-partum pains. Can be combined with arthritic remedies, such as celery seed, angelica, meadowsweet, bog bean, or willow, for the acute stages of rheumatoid arthritis.

D. opposita
Decoction: Combine with herbs such as *shu di huang, shan zhu yu, fu ling, gou qi zi*, and licorice for menopausal symptoms associated with kidney *yin* deficiency.

Tincture: Use standard doses for dry asthmatic coughs – can combine with elecampane, hyssop, and *ma huang.*

D. hypoglauca
Decoction: Use around 10–15 g with other herbs – such as *fu ling,* sweet flag, and licorice – for urinary infections and prostatitis, or with *huai niu xi* for rheumatic pains.
Tincture: Use up to 10 ml daily for urinary infections or in combination with other herbs for inflammatory arthritic conditions.

CAUTIONS:
• Avoid high doses of *D. opposita* or *D. hypoglauca* in pregnancy or if trying to conceive.

Echinacea spp.
Echinacea or purple coneflower

The Native Americans used echinacea to treat snakebite, fevers, and for healing old, stubborn wounds. The early settlers soon adopted the plant as a home remedy for colds and influenza, and it became popular with the nineteenth-century Eclectics. In the past fifty years, it has achieved worldwide fame as a potent immunostimulant and antibiotic and has also been used in AIDS therapy. Cultivated purple coneflower is usually *E. purpurea*, although *E. angustifolia* is considered more potent by some practitioners.

Character: Cool, dry, and mainly pungent.

Constituents: Volatile oil, glycosides, amides, antibiotic polyacetylenes, inulin.

Actions: Antibiotic, immune stimulant, anti-allergenic, lymphatic tonic.

PARTS USED

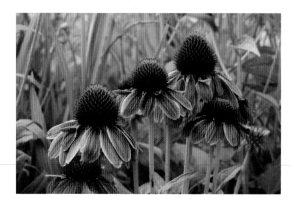

ROOT
Generally used in tinctures or powder for almost any type of infection or inflammation; it can be especially useful for recurring kidney infections as well as more common catarrh and colds. Harvest after flowering, wash, chop and dry.

LEAVES
These are less commonly used, although German research in the 1990s demonstrated that aerial parts of *E. purpurea* can be as effective an antibiotic as the root.

APPLICATIONS

Root

Tincture: Use small, frequent doses (2–5 ml) every 2–3 hours for influenza, chills, and urinary tract infections during the first couple of days of acute symptoms. For more chronic conditions use standard doses and combine with other suitable herbs – such as with buchu and couch grass for kidney infections; white deadnettle and saw palmetto for prostate problems; or cleavers for lymphatic enlargement and glandular fever. Can also be used in large doses (10 ml) for food or animal poisoning (including snakebites).

Decoction: Take 10 ml doses of a standard decoction every 1–2 hours for the acute stage of infections. Combines well with hemp agrimony.

Powder: Use powdered root as a dust for infected skin conditions like boils, erysipelas, or weeping infected eczema. Combine with marshmallow powder for boils.

Gargle: Use 10 ml of the tincture in a glass of warm water as a gargle for sore throats.

Capsules: Take three 200 mg capsules up to three times daily at the onset of acute infections (such as colds, influenza, kidney, or urinary tract infections).

Wash: Use the decoction or dilute tincture as a wash for infected, putrid wounds. Bathe affected area frequently.

Leaf

Infusion: Take a glass of a standard infusion 3–4 times daily for common colds.

CAUTIONS:
- High doses can occasionally cause nausea and dizziness.
- Allergic reaction to echinacea is extremely rare but has been reported.

Ephedra sinica
Ma huang

The *Ephedra* species belong to the Gnetopsida group of plants—an oddity among botanical families and one that would seem to be a relic of distant prehistory.

In China, *ma huang* has been used as an anti-asthmatic for at least 5,000 years. The alkaloid ephedrine, extracted from the plant, was first identified by Chinese scientists in 1924; two years later, the pharmaceutical company Merck produced a synthetic version still used to treat asthma. The Indian variety, *E. gerardiana*, known as *somlata*, is thought to have been the prime ingredient of *soma*, a potent tonic and elixir of youth praised in the *Rigveda*.

Character
Twigs: Pungent, bitter, and warm.
Root: Pungent and neutral.

Constituents: Alkaloids (inc. ephedrine), saponins, volatile oil.

Action
Twigs: Antispasmodic, febrifuge, diaphoretic, diuretic, antibacterial and antiviral properties identified in the essential oil.
Root: Anti-hydrotic.

PARTS USED

E. sinica

TWIGS

These relieve bronchial spasm in asthma and appear to have anti-allergenic properties useful in hay fever and nettle rash. In China, they are used for common colds, especially those that are linked to "wind cold" and characterized by chills, headaches, shifting aches and pains, and chesty coughs.

ROOT

Known as *ma huang gen* in China, the root is specifically used for night sweats and excessive sweating, which in traditional Chinese medicine can be associated with a deficiency of *yin* energy. This property is in marked contrast to the twigs, which, as a diaphoretic, actually promote sweating.

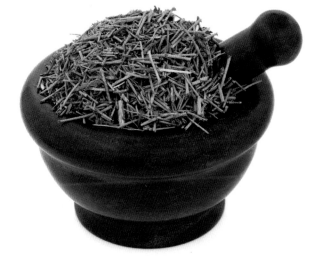

APPLICATIONS

E. sinica

Twigs

Tincture: In the UK, the maximum permitted dose is 2.5 ml of a 1:4 tincture three times daily. This is used for asthma, hay fever, or severe chills. Combine with cowslip root and thyme tinctures for bronchial asthma, whooping cough, emphysema, and other severe chest conditions: 20 drops three times daily.

Decoction: In China, up to 6 g of the twigs may be used per dose, although maximum legal dose in the UK is one-tenth that: 600 mg. Use for common colds, coughs, asthma, hay fever, etc. Also as a diuretic in kidney weakness.

Root

Decoction: Used in debility where *yin* or *qi* weakness is leading to uncontrolled sweating.

CAUTIONS:
- Not to be used by patients taking monoamine oxidase inhibitors as antidepressants.
- Should also be avoided in severe hypertension, glaucoma, and coronary thrombosis.
- Restricted in the UK under the 1968 Medicine Act for use by practitioners only.

Equisetum arvensis
Horsetail

A prehistoric botanical relic, horsetail is a close relative of the trees that grew 270 million years ago during the Carboniferous period, and which are the source of our modern coal seams. Its brittle jointed stems are extremely rich in silica, and since the time of the Ancient Greeks horsetail has been used for wounds. It is now considered an invasive weed. The Chinese use a related species, *E. hiemale*, or *mu zei*.

Character: Cold and dry with a slightly bitter taste.

Constituents: Silica, alkaloids (inc. nicotine), saponins, flavonoids, bitter principles, minerals (inc. potassium, manganese, magnesium), phytosterols, tannins.

Action: Astringent, styptic, diuretic, anti-inflammatory, tissue healer.

PARTS USED

AERIAL PARTS
E. arvensis
The astringent, healing stems check bleeding in wounds, nosebleeds, heavy periods, and blood in the urine. A strong diuretic for urinary tract and prostate disorders, horsetail is also healing for the urinary mucosa, and can be useful in bed-wetting and as a cooling astringent for catarrh. Its other main area of activity is in lung disease where it can repair long-standing, deep-seated damage, as in tuberculosis and emphysema.

E. hiemale
These are mainly used to cool fevers and as a specific for eye inflammations, conjunctivitis, cataracts, and corneal disorders.

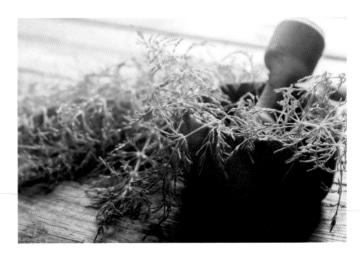

APPLICATIONS

E. arvensis

Juice: This is the best form of horsetail to use: 5–10 ml three times daily for urinary disorders or to repair long-standing damage to the lungs.

Decoction: This must be simmered for at least three hours to extract the main constituents. Use as an astringent for heavy periods or for internal healing in gastric ulceration, inflammations of the urinary tract, prostate problems or lung disorders. Can also be helpful for skin conditions such as acne and eczema,

Powder: Can be made into a paste and used on leg ulcers, wounds, sores, chilblains, etc.

Mouthwash/gargle: Use the diluted decoction for mouth and gum infections or throat inflammations.

Tincture: Generally not as effective as the decoction. Best made by preserving the decoction with alcohol. Use as the juice or decoction.

Capsules: Powdered horsetail can be taken in capsule form, which can be more convenient than juices or decoctions.

CAUTIONS:
- Seek professional guidance in all cases of blood in the urine or for sudden changes in menstrual flow leading to heavy bleeding.

Eucalyptus globulus
Eucalyptus

A traditional Aboriginal fever remedy, eucalyptus was introduced to the West in the nineteenth century by the director of the Melbourne botanical gardens, and cultivation spread in southern Europe and North America. The properties of oils from different species vary slightly, but all are very antiseptic. Russian research has suggested that some species are effective against the influenza virus, while others are antimalarial or highly active against a wide range of bacteria.

Character: Cool and moist, pungent and bitter.

Constituents: Volatile oil, tannins, aldehydes, bitter resin.

Actions: Antiseptic, antispasmodic, stimulant, febrifuge, hypoglycemic, anthelmintic.

PARTS USED

ESSENTIAL OIL
Made by steam distillation of the leaves, the oil is one of the most antiseptic essences in the herbal repertoire, used in a wide range of infections such as influenza, measles, diphtheria, typhoid, and scarlet fever. It is available commercially, although infused oil, which has a similar though less potent action, can be made at home.

LEAVES
In traditional Aboriginal medicine these were used in poultices for any type of wound or inflammation and various decoctions were also taken internally – although this is not recommended for home use today. Today it is used in lozenges and capsules for chest and catarrhal problems.

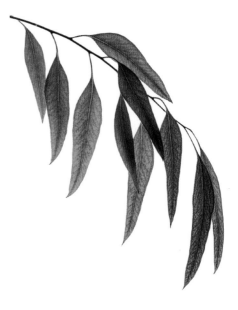

APPLICATIONS

Essential oil
Chest rub: Use 10 drops of eucalyptus oil in 25 ml of almond oil (or similar) as a chest rub for colds, bronchitis, asthma and other infections.

Gargle: 5 drops well mixed in a glass of water can be used as a gargle for throat infections.

Compress: A pad soaked in a solution of 2 ml of oil well dispersed in 100 ml water can be applied to inflammations, painful joints and burns.

Oil: The essential oil diluted in a vegetable oil or ointment base (approx. 5–10 drops of essential oil in 10 ml of carrier) can be used topically for cold sores (*Herpes simplex*).

Massage oil: Combines well with rosemary as a massage rub for rheumatic and arthritic pain.

Steam inhalation: Use 10 drops in a hot water as a steam inhalation for any chest infections. Combines well with 1 drop of peppermint oil.

Leaves
Steam inhalation: Boiling water poured over a few leaves releases the oil and makes an effective steam inhalation for chest infections, or catarrh.

Fumigant: Burning leaves on an open fire similarly fills the room with antiseptic vapors – useful for flea infestations.

Capsules: Powdered leaves are available in commercial capsules (200–250 g) for treating respiratory infections and bronchitis; use only as directed on the package.

CAUTIONS:
- Eucalyptus should not be taken internally unless under professional guidance.
- Use with caution for small children.

Eupatorium spp.
Gravel Root, Boneset, Hemp Agrimony

A favorite with native Americans, gravel root (*E. purpureum*) was known as Joe Pye weed after a New England medicine man who used it to cure typhus. Boneset (*E. perfoliatum*) was also used by the settlers for "breakbone fever" – an influenza-like infection characterized by severe pain – and is now used as an antiviral for flu. Interest in a related European variety, hemp agrimony (*E. cannabium*), has revived in recent years as various immunostimulant properties have been identified in the herb.

Character: Bitter and pungent, drying, and cool or cold depending on species.

Constituents: Tannins, bitters, volatile oils, flavonoids, sesquiterpene lactones.

Actions: *E. cannabium*: febrifuge, diuretic, antiscorbutic, laxative, tonic, cholagogue, expectorant, diaphoretic, antirheumatic, immune stimulant.

E. perfoliatum: diaphoretic, peripheral vasodilator, laxative, cholagogue, antispasmodic, expectorant.

E. purpureum: soothing diuretic, antirheumatic, emmenagogue.

PARTS USED

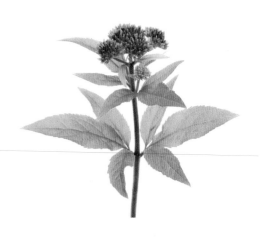

AERIAL PARTS
E. cannabium
Considered a remedy for feverish colds, the aerial parts were also used externally for putrid sores. Recent research has identified a bitter compound called eupatoriopicrin believed to have an antitumor action, and there is also an immunostimulant action that increases resistance in viral infections. Harvest while flowering in late summer.

Root: In Europe, the root is used as an expectorant and – in higher doses – as a purgative.

E. perfoliatum
Mainly used for feverish colds, but it also has a stimulating and cooling effect on the liver so is useful for hepatitis, jaundice, or to stimulate the appetite in convalescence.

ROOT
E. purpureum
Gravel root, as the name implies, describes this plant's main action: as a diuretic useful for clearing urinary stones. It is also taken for prostate problems, some types of menstrual pain, and to ease childbirth. Harvest in autumn.

APPLICATIONS

E. cannabium

Aerial parts

Tincture: For feverish colds and influenza. Take 5 drops at frequent intervals. Also can be added to anti-catarrhal mixtures such as elderflower and ground ivy.

Infusion: Drink a standard infusion for rheumatic pains and arthritis. A stronger infusion is purgative for liver stagnation and some types of constipation; it can be useful for constipation in the elderly.

E. perfoliatum

Aerial parts

Infusion: Drink frequent doses of standard infusion (every half hour or so) during the acute phase of influenza and severe colds – best taken lukewarm. The very hot infusion is more stimulating for the liver and digestive system. Small doses are best in convalescence.

Tincture: Very similar in action to the infusion.

E. purpureum

Root

Decoction: Use for menstrual pains or sip during labor. Also has a cleansing effect for persistent urinary infections.

Tincture: Use 2–3 ml three times daily for urinary disorders, including cystitis and gravel, or discharges associated with infection. Combine with white deadnettle for prostate problems.

CAUTIONS:
• Avoid gravel root in pregnancy.

Filipendula ulmaria
Meadowsweet

A popular Elizabethan strewing herb, meadowsweet was also used to flavor wine and taken to ease fevers and pain. Anti-inflammatory chemicals called salicylates were first extracted from it in the early nineteenth century. In 1899, the German pharmaceutical company Bayer succeeded in synthesizing acetylsalicylic acid, a similar chemical. They called this new wonder drug aspirin, after *Spiraea ulmaria*, the old botanical name for meadowsweet.

Character: Cold and astringent but can be both moist and drying.

Constituents: Salicylates, flavonoids, tannins, volatile oil, citric acid, mucilage.

Actions: Anti-inflammatory, antirheumatic, soothing digestive remedy, diuretic, diaphoretic.

PARTS USED

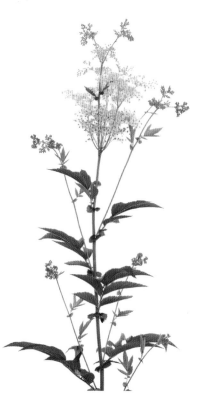

AERIAL PARTS
Cooling to reduce both fevers and inflammations, meadowsweet also contains mucilages and tannins, which protect the digestive tract and modify the action of salicylic acid. Long use of aspirin can often damage the gastric mucosa leading to ulceration and bleeding but meadowsweet does not show these side effects and is a gentle digestive remedy for acidity and some types of diarrhea. Harvest while flowering in the summer.

FLOWERS
Russian research suggests that the flowers can be effective in treating cervical dysplasia.

APPLICATIONS

Aerial parts

Infusion: Use a standard infusion for feverish colds, children's stomach upsets, or for rheumatic pains.

Tincture: Generally has a stronger action than the infusion: can be added to remedies for gastric ulceration or excess acidity, such as licorice and sweet flag, and is also used for arthritis with herbs like angelica, bogbean, willow, or devil's claw.

Compress: A pad soaked in the dilute tincture can be applied to painful arthritic joints, for rheumatism or neuralgia.

Eye bath: The cooled infusion can be used in an eye bath for conjunctivitis and other eye complaints.

CAUTIONS:
- Avoid in cases of salicylate sensitivity.

Foeniculum officinalis
Fennel

The Romans believed that serpents sucked the juice of fennel to improve their eyesight, and Pliny recommends it for "dimness of human vision." The plant was also regarded as an early slimming aid, and its Greek name, *marathron*, is reputedly derived from a verb meaning "to grow thin." In the past, chewing the seeds was a favorite way to stop gastric rumbles during lengthy sermons in church on Sundays.

Character: Warming and dry with a pungent but sweet taste.

Constituents: Volatile oil (inc. estragole, anethole), essential fatty acids, flavonoids (inc. rutin), vitamins, minerals.

Actions: Carminative, circulatory stimulant, anti-inflammatory, galactagogue, mild expectorant, diuretic.

PARTS USED

SEEDS
Carminative for the digestive system, the seeds are also to promote milk flow in breastfeeding, while if the nursing mother drinks fennel tea the baby will get a colic remedy with meals. In Chinese medicine, fennel seeds (*hui xiang*) are considered tonifying for the spleen and kidney and are used for urinary and reproductive disharmonies. Gather in late autumn when ripe.

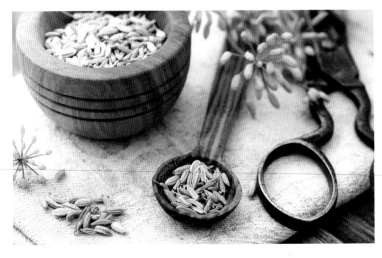

ROOT
The root is not as effective as the seeds, but was once used in similar ways. It can be gathered in late autumn when the bulbous stems are collected as a vegetable.

ESSENTIAL OIL
Distilled from the seeds, the oil is mainly used as a carminative for digestive problems. It is also a mild expectorant and sometimes used in chest rubs for coughs and respiratory complaints.

APPLICATIONS

Seeds

Infusion: A useful and palatable digestive remedy ideal for drinking after meals for flatulence, indigestion, colic, and other digestive upsets. Can also be taken by nursing mothers to increase milk flow.

Mouthwash: For gum disorders and loose teeth.

Decoction: Used in Chinese medicine for abdominal pain, colic, and stomach chills.

Tincture: Used mainly for digestive problems. Often combined with laxatives to prevent griping. Reputedly reduces the toxic effects of alcohol on the body.

Gargle: Use the infusion as a gargle for laryngitis or sore throats.

Root

Decoction: Used mainly for urinary problems such as gravel, or disorders associated with high uric acid content.

Essential oil

Chest rub: Can be combined with thyme and eucalyptus oil in a vegetable oil base (total 25 drops of essential oil to 25 ml of carrier) for bronchitis and other chest complaints.

CAUTIONS:
- Essential oils should not be taken internally without professional advice.
- Uterine stimulant: avoid high doses in pregnancy, although small amounts used in cooking are safe.

Fragaria vesca
Strawberries

The berries, leaves, and root of the wild or alpine strawberry have all been used medicinally in the past. The root was once a popular household remedy for diarrhea and the stalks were used for wounds. The berries were also considered very cooling, or as Gerard put it: to "quench thirst, cooleth heate of the stomicke and inflammation of the liver," although he also warned that although eating them in winter or on a "cold stomicke" was risking an increase in phlegmatic humor and digestive upsets.

Character: Cool and moist with a sweet and sour taste.

Constituents: Tannins, mucilage, sugars, fruit acids, salicylates, minerals, vitamins B, C, and E.

Actions: Astringent, wound herb, diuretic, laxative, liver tonic, cleansing.

Parts Used

Leaves
A gentle astringent for diarrhea and digestive upsets, the leaves are also a cleansing diuretic for rheumatism, gout, and arthritis. Wild strawberry plants can be found from late spring to autumn and the leaves used fresh or dried.

Berries
A popular cosmetic remedy for centuries, strawberries were used in face packs to whiten the complexion and remove freckles. They also make an emergency treatment for mild sunburn and are a good liver tonic. Strawberry juice shows antibacterial properties and was used in typhoid epidemics. Rich in sugars and mucilage, strawberries are also laxative.

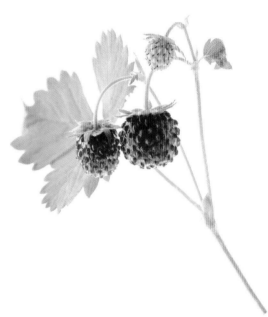

Applications

Leaves

Infusion: Use a standard infusion for diarrhea. Combine with meadowsweet and St. John's wort for mild arthritic pains.

Berries

Poultice: Crushed berries can be used on sunburn or to soothe skin inflammations.

Wine: The berries steeped in wine were a traditional remedy for "reviving the spirits and making the hart merrie."

Fresh fruit: Eat strawberries for gastritis and as a liver tonic – good in convalescence after hepatitis.

Fucus vesiculosis
Bladderwrack

Several varieties of seaweed have been used therapeutically in different cultures. In the eighteenth century, iodine was first isolated by distilling the long ribbons or thalli of bladderwrack, which became the main source of the element for more than fifty years. A preparation made by reducing the herb to a charcoal was used to treat goiter caused by thyroid deficiency related to lack of iodine. In the 1860s it was claimed that bladderwrack could counter obesity by increasing the metabolic rate, and since then the herb has featured in numerous slimming remedies.

Character: Salty, cool, and moist.

Constituents: Mucilage, iodine and other minerals, mannitol, volatile oil.

Actions: Metabolic stimulant, nutritive, thyroid tonic, antirheumatic, anti-inflammatory.

PARTS USED

THALLI

As a gentle metabolic stimulant, the thalli are useful in debility and convalescence. They also show antirheumatic properties used both internally and in topical oils and creams. Bladderwrack is rich in iodine, which, if lacking from the diet, can lead to thyroid deficiency. It is also a good nutritive source of many trace elements. The plant is commonly called kelp, although this is also the name given to various *Laminaria* spp. of seaweed, which can lead to confusion. It should be collected at sea in a healthy, live state, rather than gathered from beaches.

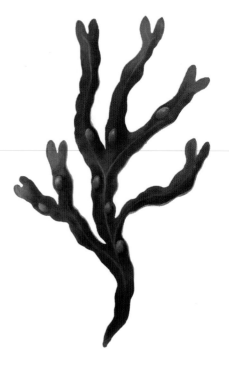

APPLICATIONS

Thalli

Tincture: Use standard doses as a thyroid stimulant in cases of deficiency or as a gentle metabolic stimulant for those with a sluggish constitution. Combine with arthritic remedies – such as willow, meadowsweet, or bogbean – for chronic inflammatory conditions like rheumatoid arthritis.

Tablets/capsules: Available commercially – use 3–6 tablets/capsules daily as a metabolic stimulant. Can help reduce obesity related to thyroid under-activity.

Infused oil: Use 500 g of dried bladderwrack to 500 ml of vegetable oil. Macerate overnight and then heat on a water-bath for two hours. Strain. Use the oil for arthritic joint pains or rheumatism – add a few drops of rosemary or thyme oil if available.

Infusion: Use a standard infusion as the tincture or as part of a weight-reducing program, especially if obesity is linked to slow metabolism.

CAUTIONS:
* Like many sea creatures, bladderwrack is at risk from heavy metal pollution. It should not be collected where the levels of cadmium, mercury, and similar pollutants are high.

* Avoid if you suffer from hyperthyroidism.

Galium aparine
Cleavers

Cleavers, also known as goosegrass (because geese like to eat it), is regarded by gardeners as a vigorous weed that twines through hedges and shrubs producing long sticky stems and burr-like seeds. The young shoots are among the first of the annual weeds to appear in spring and make an excellent cleansing tonic at that time of year – a remedy still widely used in many parts of Europe.

Character: Cold, slightly dry, and salty.

Constituents: Coumarins, tannins, glycosides, citric acid.

Actions: Diuretic, lymphatic cleanser, mild astringent.

Parts Used

Whole herb
Best used fresh, when the herb is a potent diuretic and lymphatic cleanser, effective in many cases involving swollen or enlarged lymph nodes. It is often described as a blood purifier or depurative, and is used for skin problems and other conditions where the body is failing to rid itself of toxins. It can also be used as a vegetable – gently sweated in the pan like spinach. Harvest throughout the growing season.

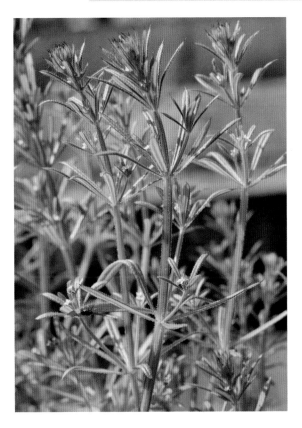

Applications

Whole plant

Juice: Juice or pulp the fresh plant to make an effective diuretic and lymphatic cleanser for a range of conditions including glandular fever, tonsillitis, and prostate disorders. Prepare daily and take in tablespoon doses.

Infusion: Generally less strong than the juice, used for urinary problems like cystitis and grave or as a cooling drink in fevers.

Tincture: Use as the tincture or combine with other lymphatic and detoxifying herbs like poke root or *lian qiao*.

Compress: A pad soaked in the infusion can be useful for burns, grazes, ulcers, and other skin inflammations.

Cream: Cleavers cream can be helpful for psoriasis if used regularly.

Hair rinse: The infusion can be used as a hair rinse for dandruff or scaling scalp problems.

Gentiana spp.
Gentian

Character: Very bitter and cold, astringent and drying.

Constituents: Bitter glycosides, alkaloids, flavonoids.

Actions: Bitter, tonic, appetite and gastric stimulant, anti-inflammatory, used in fever management.

The gentians reputedly take their name from a king of Illyria, who, according to Pliny, first discovered their ability to reduce fevers. In medieval times, gentian was an ingredient of the alchemical brew *"theriac,"* a cure-all made to a highly secret recipe – "a misterie" according to Gerard – that was used as an antidote to poisons and as an elixir of life. *G. lutea* is the main variety used in the West, while the Chinese use both the large-leaved varieties, usually *G. macrophylla* or *G. dahurica* (*qin jiao*) and *G. scabra* (*long dan cao*).

PARTS USED

ROOT

G. lutea

A strong digestive stimulant, the root is effective for conditions involving poor appetite or sluggish digestion. It is also used in fever management to both cool the system and ensure that digestive function is maintained so stomach contents do not stagnate. Harvest in the late summer and autumn.

G. macrophylla and *G. scabra*

Bitter remedies, these roots are used for digestive and feverish conditions. In Chinese medicine, they are usually described as clearing "heat and damp" and may be prescribed for some types of hypertension related to heat in the liver or for urinary infections and rheumatic disorders.

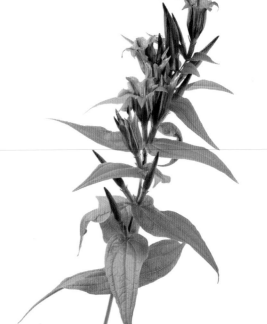

G. macrophylla

APPLICATIONS

G. lutea

Tincture: Use up to 2 ml, three times a day, of a standard tincture as a digestive stimulant. Can be helpful in liver disease, including hepatitis, and gallbladder inflammations and where jaundice is a symptom. Drop doses can allay cravings for sweet foods.

Decoction: Use 10 g to 500 ml of water and decoct for 20 minutes. Take a standard dose before meals for abdominal distension or feelings of fullness and stomach pains.

G. scabra Long dan cao

Decoction: Used in combination with other Chinese herbs for liver disorders, hypertension, and urinary infections. *Long Dan Xie Gan Wan* is a standard formula available in tablet form to clear heat from the liver and gall-bladder where symptoms can include sore eyes, headaches, and constipation.

G. macrophylla Qin jiao

Decoction: Used in combination with other Chinese herbs for rheumatic pains, fevers, and allergic inflammations. Often used with *du huo* and cinnamon.

Ginkgo biloba
Ginkgo

Dating back at least 200 million years and extinct in the wild for centuries, the ginkgo or "maidenhair tree" survived as a sacred plant growing in temple gardens in Japan and Eastern China. The tree, a deciduous conifer with separate male and female forms, was introduced in Europe in 1730 and became a favorite ornamental in city parks and gardens. Since the 1980s, Western medical interest in the plant has grown dramatically as its potent actions on the cardiovascular system have been identified.

Character: Sweet, bitter, astringent, and neutral.

Constituents: *Leaves*: Flavonoid glycosides, bioflavones, sitosterol, lactones, anthocyanin; *Seeds*: Fatty acids, minerals, bioflavones.

Actions: *Leaves*: Vasodilator, circulatory stimulant. *Seeds*: Astringent, antifungal, antibacterial.

PARTS USED

LEAVES
Part of the herbal repertoire since the 1980s, the leaves are now used for various circulatory diseases, including Raynaud's, and are particularly effective at improving the blood flow to the brain as in cerebral arteriosclerosis in the elderly. Research has also shown that ginkgolide (a glycoside) can be as effective as standard pharmaceutical drugs in treating severely irregular heartbeats. The leaves also used for venous disorders including varicose veins, hemorrhoids, and leg ulcers, while recent studies have suggested that it can help to reduce the symptoms of dementia in Alzheimer's disease. Gather fresh leaves in summer.

SEEDS
In China, the seeds, called *bai gou*, are considered to act on the lung and kidney acupuncture meridians and are traditionally used for asthmatic disorders and chesty coughs with thick phlegm. They also have a tonifying effect on the urinary system and are also used for incontinence and excessive urination. The seeds are of course only found on the female plants.

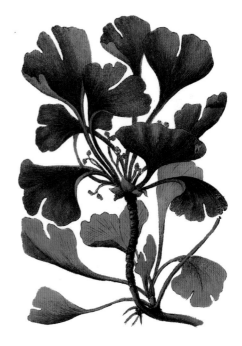

APPLICATIONS

Leaves

Fluid extract: An extract of the fresh leaves is marketed in Europe as Tebonin and is used for treating cerebral arteriosclerosis in the elderly and for diseases of the peripheral circulation.

Tincture: This can usefully be combined with other herbs for the cardiovascular systems such as periwinkle and linden flowers for circulatory problems or melilot for venous disorders.

Seeds (bai gou)

Decoction: The seeds are combined with herbs like ma huang, coltsfoot, and mulberry leaves for treating asthma and severe or persistent coughs. Usually no more than 3–4 seeds will be added to the decoction (enough for three doses).

CAUTIONS:
- High doses of the seeds can lead to skin disorders and headaches.
- Cases of contact dermatitis with the fruit pulp (not used medicinally) have been recorded.
- Long term and excessive use may increase bleeding time and cause spontaneous hemorrhage.

Glycyrrhiza spp.
Licorice

Licorice has been used medicinally since at least 500 BC and today still has a place in official pharmacopoeia as a "drug" for stomach ulceration. *G. glabra* originates in the Mediterranean region and Middle East, but has been cultivated in Europe since at least the sixteenth century. In China, *G. uralensis* or *gan cao* is used: it is called the "great detoxifier" and is thought to drive poisons from the system and eliminate harmful side effects of other herbs. It is also an important tonic, often called "the grandfather of herbs."

Character: Very sweet, neutral, and moist.

Constituents: Saponins, glycosides (inc. glycyrrhizin), estrogenic substances, asparagine, coumarins, flavonoids, sterols, choline (amines), volatile oil.

Actions: Anti-inflammatory, antiarthritic, tonic stimulant for adrenal cortex, lowers cholesterol levels, soothing for gastric mucosa, possibly anti-allergenic, antipyretic, expectorant.

PARTS USED

ROOT
G. glabra
Licorice contains a substance called glycyrrhizin which is 50 times sweeter than sucrose and encourages the production of hormones like hydrocortisone. This helps to explain its anti-inflammatory action in conditions such as rheumatoid arthritis and also its role in re-stimulating the adrenal cortex after steroid therapy. It produces a protective mucus coating for the stomach which can help heal ulceration and is also a potent expectorant for dry coughs or asthma.

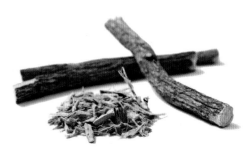

G. uralensis
An energy tonic, particularly for the spleen and stomach encouraging growth and vigor, the root is added to many Chinese herbal formulas to balance other herbs. It is used for asthmatic coughs as an antispasmodic and ulcer remedy and to cool hot conditions. The dried root can be chewed like candy and is popularly given to children to encourage muscle growth.

JUICE STICKS
G. glabra
The solidified extract is sold in sticks and forms the basis of many proprietary laxative preparations as licorice stimulates bile flow and has a gentle action in constipation.

APPLICATIONS

Root

G. glabra
Tincture: Used for lung disorders, gastric inflammation, or to encourage adrenal function after steroid therapy. Also used as an anti-inflammatory in arthritic and allergic conditions. Helps to disguise the flavor of other medicines.
Fluid extract: Slowly dissolving the juice sticks by macerating in cold water produces a strong extract which can be conveniently used as the decoction or in syrups. For stomach ulceration, pieces of juice stick can be dissolved in chamomile tea.
Decoction: Useful for reducing stomach acidity in cases of ulceration.
Syrup: Combine the decoction with honey to make a soothing and expectorant cough syrup. Combines well with thyme, hyssop, or elecampane. Useful for asthma, bronchitis, etc.
Wash: Use the dilute tincture for skin inflammations and itching.

G. uralensis
Decoction: Combine with ginseng as a daily tonic drink.
Tonic wine: Macerating piece of Chinese licorice root in gin or vodka for a few weeks produces a tonic wine to be drunk in small doses after meals.

CAUTIONS:
- Avoid in hypertension as licorice is believed to cause fluid retention.
- Should not be used by people taking digoxin-based drugs.
- Excessive use of licorice-containing sweets and chewing gums has been linked to hypertension and abnormally high blood potassium levels.

Hamamelis virginiana
Witch Hazel

The healing properties of Virginian witch hazel were highly valued by various Native American peoples: the Menominees rubbed the decoction into their legs to keep them supple during sports, while the Potawatomis put witch hazel twigs into sweat baths to relieve sore muscles. The herb was adopted by settlers and listed in the *US National Formulary* until 1955. Distilled witch hazel is widely available today and is well known in domestic first aid.

Character: Cool, dry, bitter, pungent, astringent.

Constituents: Tannins, flavonoids (including kaempferol and quercetin), saponins, bitters, volatile oil (including eugenol and safrole), choline, Gallic acid.

Actions: Astringent, stops internal and external bleeding, anti-inflammatory.

PARTS USED

LEAVES & TWIGS
The leaves are less astringent than the bark and tend to be used in poultices or taken in infusions. Powdered leaves in capsules are sold commercially to combat varicose veins. Distilled witch hazel is produced by combining the wigs with leaves in a steam extraction process.

BARK
The bark is used in commercial tinctures, ointments, and fluid extracts rather than for distilled witch hazel production. Like leaf and twig extracts it is mainly used to stop bleeding, ease irritation, and treat varicose veins and hemorrhoids.

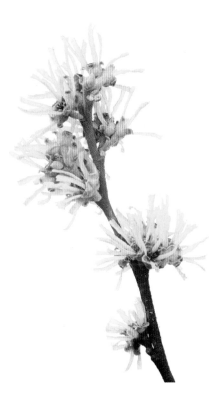

APPLICATIONS

Leaves

Infusion: Take for diarrhea or bleeding piles. A daily cup can also help combat capillary fragility associated with steroidal therapy.

Mouthwash/gargle: Use the infusion for sore throats, mouth ulcers, tonsillitis, pharyngitis, and spongy or bleeding gums.

Wash: Use the infusion to bathe varicose veins, bruises, grazes, irritant skin rashes, and areas of capillary fragility.

Distillate: Commercially available distilled witch hazel can be used as a wash, like the infusion, or to soak a cotton swab as a nasal plug for nosebleeds or applied to cuts and grazes to stop bleeding.

Eye pads: Use a cotton swab soaked in an infusion or distilled witch hazel to relieve tired eyes.

Twigs

Decoction: Use as an infusion of the leaves.

Bark

Tincture: The dilute tincture can be used externally as a substitute for distilled witch hazel.

Ointment: Use on piles or irritant varicose veins.

Cream: Use for minor, cuts and grazes or bruising.

Harpagophytum procumbens
Devil's claw

Native to the Kalahari Desert in southern Africa, devil's claw was introduced to the West after a Boer farmer noticed native Bushmen gathering the roots to treat digestive upsets and rheumatism. The plant was sent to Germany for investigation, and by the late 1950s its anti-inflammatory and antirheumatic properties were well established. The name devil's claw derives from the characteristic claw-shaped fruits produced in the autumn, which are reputedly used as mouse traps in Madagascar. Today the herb is widely used to treat arthritis and rheumatism.

Character: Bitter, astringent, cooling.

Constituents: Iridoid glycosides (including harpagide, harpagoside and procumbide), phenols, carbohydrates, flavonoids (including kaempferol and luteolin), phytosterols.

Actions: Anti-inflammatory, antirheumatic, analgesic, sedative, diuretic, digestive stimulant.

PARTS USED

TUBER

The tubers of devil's claw, rather than the whole root structure, are used medicinally, although some commercial preparations combine the entire root mix thereby diluting the overall therapeutic effect. Researchers have also found that constant use of the herb for at least six weeks significantly improves the movement of arthritic joints and reduces swelling. Devil's claw can also be used as a bitter digestive stimulant for a range of liver and gallbladder disorders.

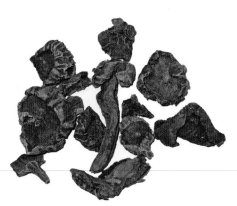

APPLICATIONS

Tuber

Decoction: Take a cup before meals to stimulate the digestion in cases of liver congestion, poor appetite, or mild gall bladder disorders.

Tincture: Take 20-30 drops per dose for at least six weeks for osteoarthritis or rheumatic pains.

Wash: Use the decoction as a wash for irritated and inflamed piles and varicose veins.

Cream: Apply to arthritic and rheumatic aches and pains three or four times a day. Add a few drops of rosemary to improve pain relief. The same mix can be used on sprained or strained joints and muscles.

Capsules/Tablets: Take 2-3 x 200 mg capsules three times daily for arthritic and rheumatic pains as a maintenance dose in chronic conditions. Increase to 4 capsules per dose during any flare-up in symptoms. Check dosages of commercially available tablets and use an equivalent amount.

Powder: Use to dust open wounds to encourage healing.

CAUTIONS

- Devil's claw is believed to stimulate uterine contractions and should be avoided in pregnancy.

- It should also be avoided in cases of gastric or duodenal ulcer.

Humulus lupulus
Hops

Used in brewing in Europe since at least the eleventh century, hops were never included in traditional English ale. Initially their use was thought to encourage the melancholic humor and too many hops in German-style beer was, as Gerard records, "ill for the head." Hops were believed, however, to purge excess choleric and sanguine humors, and beer was regarded as a more "physicall drinke to keep the body in health" than the traditional English ale. Hops contain a high proportion of estrogen-like compounds and, as a result, too much beer can lead to a loss of libido in men.

Character: Cold and dry with a bitter but slightly pungent taste.

Constituents: Volatile oil, valerianic acid, estrogenic substances, tannins, bitter, flavonoids.

Action: Sedative, anaphrodisiac, restoring tonic for nervous system, bitter digestive stimulant, diuretic.

PARTS USED

STROBILES

The flowers on the female plants, known as strobiles, are used medicinally.

The character of the plant changes significantly with age as the constituents oxidize. The strobiles are best used fresh for insomnia, and dried hops used in pillows for sleeplessness should be replaced every few months because dried hops more than six months old can be stimulating.

LUPULIN

The small yellow glands from freshly dried hop strobiles are removed and sold commercially as lupulin or *Pharmacopoeia*. This is a brownish-yellow powder and was official in the British and US *Pharmacopoeia* until the 1940s. It is still available from pharmacists in parts of Europe, and is generally dispensed in pills or sachets.

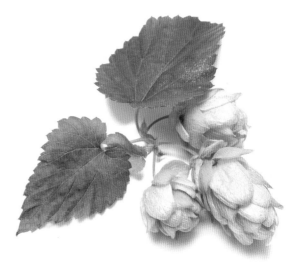

APPLICATIONS

Strobiles

Tincture: Use up to 2 ml three times a day as a sedative for nervous tension and anxiety. It can also be combined with digestive remedies – marshmallow, plantain, chamomile, peppermint, etc. – for irritable bowel syndrome. As an astringent it can be especially useful for mucus colitis; use 30 drops on a sugar lump for nervous stomachs. Hops can also be used for some sexual problems (such as premature ejaculation).

Infusion: Use a tea of fresh hops for insomnia with 2 teaspoons of fresh flowers per cup of boiling water, infused for five minutes. Freshly dried hops can also be used but older plant material may be less effective. Freeze-dried material, if available, is better than conventionally dried herb.

Wash: Use an infusion of fresh or freshly dried hops as a wash for chronic ulcers, skin eruptions, and wounds. Alternatively use a pad soaked in infusion or dilute tincture as a compress on varicose ulcers.

Compress: Use a pad soaked in the infusion or dilute tincture on varicose veins.

Capsules: Available commercially; take two before meals as an appetite stimulant. Do not use continuously for more than a few days.

CAUTIONS:

- The growing plant can also cause contact dermatitis.
- Hops should be avoided in depression as it acts as a mild depressant on the higher nerve centers. Do not exceed stated doses.
- The estrogen-like effect may disrupt the menstrual cycles in women working in hop fields.

Hydrastis canadensis
Goldenseal

A traditional healing herb of the North American Indians that has entered the Western herbal repertoire: goldenseal was used by the Cherokee for local inflammations, indigestion, and to improve the appetite, while the Iroquois used it for whooping cough, liver disorders, fevers, and heart problems. It was introduced into Europe in 1760. During the nineteenth century, the herb was a favorite with Thomsonian and Eclectic practitioners and was listed in the United States *Pharmacopoeia* until 1926 and the US *National Formulary* until 1955.

Character: Bitter and astringent, dry and predominantly cold.

Constituents: Alkaloids, volatile oil, resin.

Actions: Astringent, tonic, digestive and bile stimulant, anti-catarrhal, laxative, healing to gastric mucosa, hypertensive.

PARTS USED

RHIZOME

An excellent drying, anti-catarrhal remedy for the mucosa – gastric, upper respiratory tract, vagina – useful for conditions like mucus colitis, nasal inflammations, or ear infections. It is good for gynecological problems and can help reduce menopausal symptoms, ease swollen painful breasts, heavy periods, menstrual pain, and PMS symptoms linked with stagnation, and has also been used for difficult or stalled labor.

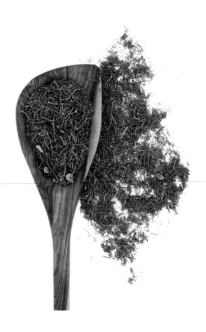

APPLICATIONS

Tincture: Up to 0.5–2 ml three times a day: larger doses are more laxative. Use for any catarrhal condition: nasal catarrh, mucus colitis, gastroenteritis, vaginal discharge. Also as a liver tonic for sluggish digestion and for digestive problems associated with food sensitivity and alcohol excess. Use with licorice for gastric ulceration, and add to remedies for PMS or heavy menstrual bleeding.

Mouthwash: Use the dilute tincture (2–3 ml in a tumbler of warm water) for mouth ulcers, and gum disease. Can also be used as a gargle for sore throats and catarrhal conditions.

Powder: Use the powder as snuff for nasal catarrh. The powder mixed in water can be used as the tincture.

Capsules: Use 1 x 200 mg capsule three times daily for catarrh and infections (gastric or respiratory). Combine with chaste-tree berry powder for symptomatic relief of hot flushes and night sweats at the menopause. Combine with eyebright for symptomatic relief of hay fever.

Douche: Use the dilute tincture as a douche for vaginal discharges and infections (including thrush). Can help vaginal itching (use 5 ml of goldenseal in 100 ml rosewater).

Ear drops: Use a 1 ml of goldenseal tincture in 10 ml of water as ear drops for glue ear, catarrhal congestions, "blocked" sensation in the ears.

Wash: Use the dilute tincture (5 ml of goldenseal in 100 ml rosewater) to bathe irritant skin inflammations, eczema, measles, etc.

CAUTIONS:
- Uterine stimulant so avoid in pregnancy.
- Hypertensive so should be avoided in cases of high blood pressure.
- Do not use ear drops of any sort if there is a risk that the ear drum has perforated.
- Goldenseal is now seriously endangered in the wild; avoid buying wild-crafted material and use barberry as an alternative in digestive complaints.

Hypericum perforatum
St. John's wort

It is said that St. John's wort supposedly takes its name from the Knights of St. John of Jerusalem who used it as a wound herb on Crusade battlefields. It was also used to ward off evil spirits, and the insane were often compelled to drink St. John's wort infusions in an attempt to cure their madness. Old herbals often refer to tutsan (*H. androsaemum*) – from the French *toutsain*, or "all heal" – which was also used for injuries, ulcers, and inflammations but was taken internally to "purge choleric humors." Although tutsan later fell into disuse as a medicinal herb, St. John's wort became credited with similar properties.

Character: Bittersweet, cool, and drying.

Constituents: Glycosides, flavonoids (inc. rutin), volatile oils, tannins, resins.

Actions: Astringent, analgesic, anti-inflammatory, sedative, restoring tonic for the nervous system.

PARTS USED

AERIAL PARTS
Now recognized as a potent antidepressant and as effective as many orthodox drugs, the herb also makes a good restorative nerve tonic ideal for anxiety and irritability and can be especially effective for menopausal problems. It is good for long-standing nervous exhaustion. As an antiviral it has been used in AIDS and HIV treatments. St. John's wort can help relieve a variety of nerve pains – used both internally and externally – including sciatica and neuralgia.

FLOWERING TOPS
Used to prepare St. John's wort oil, a blood-red infused oil made by steeping the flowers in sunflower oil in the sun for a few weeks. This can be used topically for burns, inflammations (of skin, muscles, and connective tissues), and neuralgia. Harvest while flowering in mid- to late summer.

APPLICATIONS

Aerial parts

Infusion: Use for depression, anxiety or emotional upsets associated with the menopause or premenstrual syndrome; also helpful in colds and infections combined with herbs such as elderflower.

Tincture: Use standard doses for at least two months for long-standing nervous tension leading to exhaustion and depression. Drop doses (5–10 drops) at night can be useful for childhood bed-wetting.

Wash: Use the infusion to bathe wounds, skin sores and bruises.

Flowering tops

Infused oil: Use St. John's wort oil on burns, muscle or joint inflammations (including conditions like tennis elbow), neuralgia, and sciatica. For burns, add a few drops of lavender oil; for joint inflammations add 4–10 drops of chamomile or yarrow oil to 10 ml of the infused oil to increase efficacy.

Cream: Use for localized nerve pains, such as sciatica, sprains, and cramps. Can also help to relieve breast engorgement during lactation. Can also be used as an antiseptic and styptic on grazes, sores, ulcers, etc.

CAUTIONS:
- Can cause dermatitis if pruning or gathering the plant in moist but sunny conditions.
- Seek professional advice before using St. John's wort if taking prescription drugs.
- In very rare cases cataracts and nerve hypersensitivity have been linked to long-term or excessive use of St. John's wort. It is also said to increase photosensitivity, but there is little clinical evidence for this.

Hyssopus officinalis
Hyssop

Prescribed by Hippocrates for pleurisy, hyssop, with rue, was recommended by Dioscorides for asthma and catarrh. Its name derives from the Greek *azob*, or "a holy herb," although the hyssop mentioned in the Bible seems more likely to have been a local variety of marjoram. Hyssop is one of the more important of the 130 herbs used to flavor Chartreuse liqueur.

Character: Bitter, pungent and dry, slightly warming.

Constituents: Volatile oil, flavonoids, tannins, bitter substance (marrubin).

Action: Expectorant, carminative, peripheral vasodilator, diaphoretic, anti-catarrhal; topically anti-inflammatory, antiviral for *Herpes simplex*.

Parts Used

Aerial parts
Mainly used as an expectorant in bronchitis, chesty colds, and asthma, the aerial parts ease flatulence and soothe griping pains and were once popularly combined with figs for constipation. They also promote sweating in chills and influenza. Harvest during flowering in summer.

Flowers
In the past these were collected separately from the leaves and used to make cough syrups often in combination with other flowers such as mullein and marshmallow.

Essential oil
This increases alertness and is used as an uplifting and gently relaxing nerve tonic suitable for nervous exhaustion linked with over-work and anxiety or for depression. It is especially helpful for easing feelings of both grief and guilt.

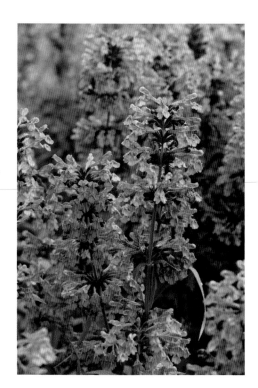

Applications

Aerial parts

Infusion: Drink hot during the early stages of colds or influenza. It also makes a soothing carminative for digestive upsets and nervous tummies.

Tincture: Can be combined with other expectorants – such as licorice, coltsfoot, and anise – for bronchitis and stubborn coughs.

Syrup: Use an infusion of the whole herb (or the flowers only if you have them) and preserve with honey or sugar: 500 ml of infusion to 500 g honey. Can be combined with coltsfoot and mullein flowers or licorice for stubborn coughs and lung weakness.

Essential oil

Baths: 5–10 drops in the bath for nervous exhaustion, melancholy, or sorrows.

Chest rub: 10 drops in 20 ml of carrier oil for bronchitis and chesty colds. Combines well the essential oils of thyme and eucalyptus.

CAUTIONS:
- The essential oil contains the ketone pino-camphone, which in high doses can cause convulsions (although low doses of the herb were used for petit mal).
- The essential oil should not be taken internally.

Inula spp.
Elecampane

One of the most important herbs for the Greeks and Romans, elecampane (*I. helenium*) was regarded almost as a cure-all for ailments as diverse as dropsy, menstrual disorders, digestive upsets, and sciatica. The Anglo-Saxons used the herb as a tonic, for skin diseases, and leprosy. By the nineteenth century its uses had become limited to skin disease, neuralgia, liver problems, and severe coughs. Today it used almost solely for respiratory problems. In China *I. japonica* is used.

Character: Bitter – the flowers and also slightly salty and the root slightly sweet, warm and dry.

Constituents: Mucilage, bitter principle, volatile oil (inc. azulenes), inulin, sterols, possible alkaloids.

Actions: Tonic, stimulating expectorant, diaphoretic, antibacterial, antifungal, antiparasitic.

PARTS USED

ROOT
I. helenium
An excellent tonic, especially for debility following influenza or bronchitis, the root is a good stimulating expectorant to shift stubborn phlegm and is good for childhood coughs and congestion. It contains inulin which has been used as a sugar substitute in diabetes. Harvest in the autumn, wash and chop into small pieces before drying.

FLOWERS
I. japonica
In Chinese, the flowers – *xuan fu hua* – are recommended for asthma and bronchitis with excessive phlegm and also for vomiting and acid reflux. Chinese research has demonstrated mild antibacterial properties and also a stimulant effect on the nervous system, digestion, and adrenal cortex.

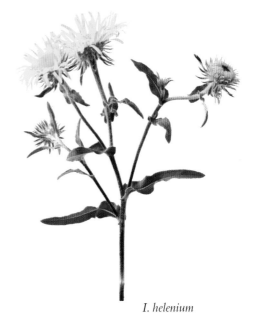

I. helenium

APPLICATIONS
I. helenium

Root
Decoction: Use a standard decoction for bronchitis, asthma and upper respiratory catarrh. Can also ease hay fever symptoms. Take regularly as a general tonic or for long-standing chronic respiratory complaints. Can be combined with white horehound, hyssop, or licorice. Also acts as a digestive tonic and liver stimulant.
Tincture: Use as a tonic in debility and chronic respiratory complaints. Combine with vervain for liver stagnation or with calumba or *chen pi* for digestive weakness.
Syrup: Mix the decoction sugar or honey as a cough syrup. Can be combined with thyme and licorice for bronchitis and emphysema.

Wash: Use the decoction or diluted tincture for eczema, rashes, varicose ulcers, etc.
I. japonica

Flowers
Syrup: Sweeten 500 ml of a standard infusion of the flower heads with 500 g of honey and use in 10–20 ml doses for coughs.
Decoction: Use a standard decoction for nausea, vomiting or coughs characterized by copious phlegm. Alternatively decoct 10 g with 10 g each of fresh ginger root and *ban xia* and 5 g of licorice root and use the mixture for excess phlegm in the stomach with nausea, abdominal distension, flatulence, and vomiting of mucus/sputum.

CAUTIONS:
• May cause allergic skin reactions.

Jasminum spp.
Jasmine

The highly aromatic climbing plant, common jasmine (*J. officinale*) was brought to Europe in the sixteenth century and rapidly gained popularity with the French perfumers. The scented oil is extracted using *enfleurage*, a technique involving layering the flowers with wax between glass sheets. A close relative, royal jasmine or *jati* (*J. grandiflorum*) is an important Ayurvedic tonic and cleansing remedy. Jasmine tea, popular in China, is scented using Arabian jasmine (*J. sambac*) which originated in the Persian Gulf.

Character: Bitter, pungent, astringent, cooling.

Constituents: Alkaloids (including jasminine), essential oil (iaphrncluding benzyl alcohol, linalool, and linyl acetate), salicylic acid.

Actions: *Flowers:* Aphrodisiac, astringent, bitter, relaxing nervine, sedative, mild analgesic, encourages milk production. *Essential oil:* Antidepressant, antiseptic, antispasmodic, aphrodisiac. encourages milk flow, sedative, uterine tonic, encourages parturition.

Parts Used

Flowers
J. grandiflorum

In Ayurveda, *jati* are regarded as a *sattvic* tonic, encouraging principles of light, perception, and harmony associated with *sattva*, one of the three basic qualities of health. Their sattvic nature also emphasizes love and compassion. For women they are a mild aphrodisiac and cleansing for the uterus. *Jati* is also used to reduce fevers and strengthen the immune system.

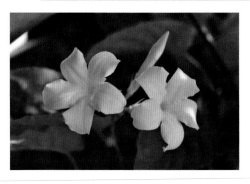

J. officinale

The flowers are rarely used as most commercial production is geared to the essential oil trade so they can be difficult to obtain. They are very similar, but significantly less potent, than the oil – worth adding to relaxing infusions if you have a garden plant available.

Essential oil
J. officinale

Jasmine oil is extremely expensive so is often adulterated with synthetic chemicals and only the very best grades should be used medicinally. In aromatherapy it is included in massage rubs for menstrual pain, anxiety and depression, impotence and frigidity, and for abdominal massage during childbirth to encourage parturition and ease labor pains. It is also added to chest rubs for coughs and breathing difficulties.

Flowers/Jasmine Tea
J. sambac

Arabian jasmine has been used for scenting Chinese teas since at least 300 AD. Traditionally the flowers, known as *mo li*, were left next to heat-dried green tea for several hours to absorb the scent. Modern commercial producers generally mix the petals in with the tea instead.

Applications

Essential oil

J. officinale

Massage oil: Add 1–2 drops to massage rubs for anxiety, insomnia, or depression. For problems with impotence or frigidity mutual massage between partners using 1–2 drops of jasmine oil in a teaspoon of almond oil before love making can help.

Flowers

J. grandiflorum

Infusion: Take for infections, fevers, or urinary inflammations. Combine a few flowers with lemon balm or skullcap for a calming tea at the end of a stressful day.

Wash: Use an infusion to bathe cuts and grazes and stop bleeding.

Compress: Use a compress soaked in the cool infusion or dilute tincture and applied to the forehead for sunstroke or heat stroke, headaches or emotional upsets.

Flowers/jasmine tea

J. sambac

Infusion: Traditionally used as a soothing and warming remedy to help relieve diarrhea.

Juglans spp.
Walnut & Butternut

According to legend, when the gods walked upon the earth they lived on walnuts, hence the name *Juglans* or *Jovis glans*, Jupiter's nuts. The tree has been grown for its nuts in Europe since Roman times; these yield an oil containing essential fatty acids, such as alpha-linolenic, which are vital for healthy cell function and prostaglandin development. The butternut or white walnut (*J. cinerea*) from eastern North America is a useful laxative.

Character: Bitter and astringent, mostly warm and drying, although the fresh rind is cooling.

Constituents: Quinones, oils, tannins; nuts contain essential fatty acids including cis-linoleic and alpha-linolenic.

Actions
J. cinerea: Purgative, astringent, cholagogue.
J. regia: Astringent, anthelmintic, antispasmodic, the nut rind is anti-inflammatory.

Parts Used

J. regia
Leaves
In Europe, walnut leaves are a popular home remedy for both eczema and blepharitis in children. Recent research suggests antifungal properties, as well as an antiseptic action; the leaves are also used for intestinal worms and as a digestive tonic. Harvest throughout the growing season.

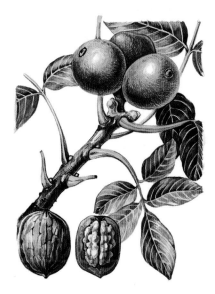

Outer nut rind & nuts
The fleshy green outer casing of the nut is rich in fruit acids and minerals. Traditionally infusions of walnut rind were used to darken the hair the infusion will also dye the skin dark brown so it needs careful handling. The nuts are now known to lower blood cholesterol levels and so help to reduce the risk of heart disease. Harvest in late summer.

Bach Flower Remedy
Recommended for times of change – as a "link-breaking, spell-breaking, bond-freeing remedy" to be taken at the menopause, puberty or when changing careers or moving house.

J. cinerea
Inner bark or quills
The quills and inner bark are one of the few potent laxatives that are safe to use in pregnancy.

Applications

J. regia
Leaves
Infusion: Use in standard doses for skin problems, eye inflammations. Also as a digestive tonic for poor appetite.
Wash: A standard infusion can be used as a wash for eczema or for wounds and grazes.
Eye bath: Use either a well-strained infusion or 5 drops of tincture in an eye bath of water for conjunctivitis and blepharitis.

Outer nut casing
Infusion: Used for chronic diarrhea or as a tonic in anemia.
Hair rinse: Use a standard infusion for hair loss.

Nut Oil
Oil: Take two teaspoons of unrefined walnut oil daily as a dietary supplement in cases of menstrual dysfunction or dry, flaky eczema.

J. cinerea
Inner bark
Decoction: Use standard doses as a stimulating laxative for constipation and sluggish digestion. Also used to stimulate the liver and as a cleansing remedy for skin diseases.
Tincture: As for the decoction: use up to 5 ml three times daily.

Juniperus communis
Juniper

Long associated with ritual cleansing, juniper was burned in temples as part of regular purification rites. Several medicinal recipes also survive in Egyptian papyri dated to 1550 BC. In central European folk medicine, the oil distilled from the berries was regarded as a cure-all for treating typhoid, cholera, dysentery, tapeworms, and other ills associated with unhygienic conditions and poverty.

Character: Pungent and slightly bitter-sweet, hot and dry.

Constituents: Volatile oil, flavonoids, sugars, glycosides, tannins, podophyllotoxin (an antitumor agent), vitamin C.

Actions: Urinary antiseptic, diuretic, carminative, digestive tonic, uterine stimulant, antirheumatic.

PARTS USED

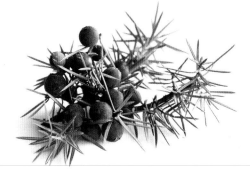

BERRIES
The ripe blue berries are mainly used for urinary infections and to clear acid wastes associated with arthritic and gouty conditions. They are also carminative, reducing flatulence and colicky pains, and the bitter taste helps to stimulate the digestion. Juniper also encourages uterine contractions and can be used before and during labor. Pick only after they have turned from green to purplish blue, a process that can take two years.

ESSENTIAL OIL
Made by steam distillation of the ripe berries, the oil is a popular external remedy for arthritic and muscle pains. Internally, the oil increases the filtration rate of the kidney and is effective against many types of bacteria.

OIL OF CADE
Made by dry distillation of the heartwood of various types of juniper tree and is also known as juniper tar oil. It contains phenol and has a mild disinfectant action. Applied externally it is a non-irritant and is mainly used for chronic skin conditions, such as eczema and psoriasis.

APPLICATIONS

Berries

Tincture: Use 2 ml three times daily for urinary infections (such as cystitis), or to stimulate the digestion. Can be used with herbs like celery seed, bogbean, or angelica for arthritic pains.

Infusion: Sip a weak infusion (15 g of berries to 500 ml water) for gastric upsets, stomach chills, or menstrual pains. The infusion can also be taken in the final weeks of pregnancy to aid parturition and sipped during the first stages of labor.

Essential oil

Massage oil: Use 10 drops of juniper oil in 5 ml of almond or vegetable oil as a massage for arthritic pain. Can also be combined with rosemary oil in an infused comfrey oil base.

Lotion: Use 5 drops of juniper oil to 50 ml of a rosewater/witch-hazel mixture for oily skins and acne.

Chest rub: Combine with thyme oil in a chest rub for stubborn coughs (up to 20 drops of essential oil in 20 ml of almond or vegetable oil).

Baths: Add 5 drops of juniper oil to bath-water for arthritic pains.

Cade oil

Hair rinse: Use 10 drops of oil in 1 pt of hot water (well-mixed) for psoriasis affecting the scalp. Leave for 15 minutes (longer if possible) and then rinse thoroughly.

Ointment: Add 10 drops of cade oil to 20 ml of melted ointment base. Allow to cool and use on chronic scaling eczema or psoriasis.

CAUTIONS:
- Do not take juniper oil internally without professional guidance.
- Avoid the herb in pregnancy although it may be taken during labor.
- Juniper may irritate the kidneys in long-term use so should not be taken for more than six weeks internally without a break. Do not use if there is already kidney damage.

Lavandula spp.
Lavender

One of most popular medicinal herbs since ancient times, lavender derives its name from the Latin *lavare,* to wash. In Arab medicine lavender is used as an expectorant and antispasmodic, while in European folk tradition it is regarded as a useful wound herb. Species used medicinally include *L. angustifolia* and *L. spica* as well as *L. stoechas* in southern Europe.

Character: Bitter tasting, dry, and mainly cooling.

Constituents: Volatile oil, tannins, coumarins, flavonoids, triterpenoids.

Actions: Relaxant, antispasmodic, circulatory stimulant, tonic for the nervous system, antibacterial, analgesic, carminative, cholagogue.

PARTS USED

L. angustifolia

FLOWERS

Less potent than the essential oil, the flowers are useful for nervous exhaustion, headaches, colic, and indigestion. Harvest towards the end of flowering when the petals have begun fade and dry in small bunches covered with paper bags to collect the florets as they fall.

ESSENTIAL OIL

One of the most popular aromatic oils, lavender oil can be used for muscular aches and pains, migraines, burns, asthma and bronchitis, digestive upsets, skin problems, to ease childbirth, soothe babies, or simply as a relaxing additive to the bath water at the end of the day. It is an essential component of any household first aid box.

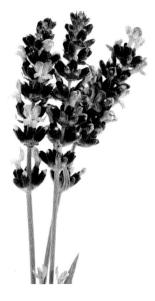

APPLICATIONS

Flowers

Infusion: Use a standard infusion as a relaxing tea for nervous exhaustion or tension headaches. Combines well with betony, chamomile, linden flowers, or vervain. Also for indigestion. A weak infusion (a quarter of normal strength) can be given by bottle to babies for colic, irritability, and nervous excitement. Drink lavender tea during labor.

Mouthwash: Use a standard infusion for halitosis.

Tincture: Use up to 5 ml twice a day for headaches, nervous tension and depression.

Essential oil

Massage: Use 10 drops in 10 ml of carrier oil for muscular pains – combines well with thyme and eucalyptus. Use neat for nervous tension or massaged into the temples and nape of neck for tension headaches or at the first hint of a migraine. The same oil can be applied for sunstroke or to help prevent sunburn (NB: It is not an effective sun-screen)

Chest rub: Use 20 drops of lavender oil and 5–10 drops of chamomile or yarrow oil in 5 ml of carrier oil for asthmatic and bronchitis spasm.

Baths: Add 10–20 drops of essential oil for a soothing and relaxing bath that can be helpful for insomnia. Add 2–5 drops to children's baths.

Creams: A few drops of lavender oil can be added to chamomile cream used for eczema.

Hair rinse: Dilute 5–10 drops in water as a hair rinse for lice or use a few drops of neat oil on a fine-toothed comb to run through the hair for nits. Lavender hair rinse may also help baldness.

Lotion: A few drops of oil in a little water can be used as a lotion for sunburn or minor scalds. use a stronger concentration of lavender oil for more severe burns.

Oil: Use the oil neat on insect bites and stings.

CAUTIONS:
- Avoid high doses during pregnancy.
- Do not take essential oils internally without professional advice.

Leonurus spp.
Motherwort

As the botanical name *L. cardiaca* suggests, motherwort has been an important heart herb since Roman times. The *Leonurus* part of the botanical name is from a Greek word meaning lion's tail, describing the shaggy shape of the leaves. Its common name also suggests a medicinal action for, in Gerard's words, ". . . them that are in hard travell with childe." Early herbals also recommend the plant for "wykked sperytis." Chinese herbalists use the related species *L. heterophyllus* mainly for menstrual problems.

Character: Pungent, bitter, drying, and cool.

Constituents: Alkaloids (inc. stachydrine), bitter glycosides, volatile oil, tannins, vitamin A.

Actions: Uterine stimulant, relaxant, cardiac tonic, carminative.

PARTS USED

L. cardiaca & L. heterophyllus
AERIAL PARTS/LEAVES
Useful as a tonic and for the heart, the aerial parts are ideal for palpitations associated with anxiety and nervous tension. Its alkaloids, stachydrine, and leonurine, also encourage and ease uterine contractions making it a valuable herb both for menstrual pains and during labor. It can also stimulate menstrual flow. In China leaves of *L. heterophyllus* are called *yi mu cao* and are used for eczema and sores. Harvest in summer.

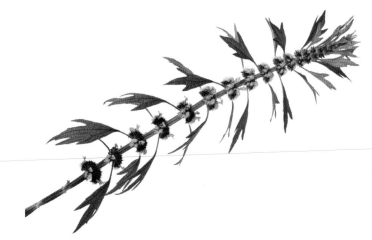

SEEDS

L. heterophyllus
In China, the seeds, *chong wei zi*, are used mainly for menstrual irregularities and as a circulatory stimulant. The Chinese consider that they act specifically on the liver and are therefore especially effective on the eyes to "brighten the vision."

APPLICATIONS

Aerial parts

L. cardiaca & L. heterophyllus
Infusion: As a tonic useful for menopausal syndrome, anxiety, and various heart weaknesses. Motherwort tea, flavored with cloves, can also be drunk during labor. Taken after childbirth motherwort tea helps restore the womb and reduce the risk of hemorrhaging.

Syrup: In an infusion it does not taste particularly pleasant, so traditionally syrups or conserves of motherwort have often been used instead for similar complaints.

Tincture: Used as the infusion or combined with other heart herbs like lily of the valley and hawthorn when a strengthening tonic is needed.

Douche: Use an infusion or diluted tincture for vaginal infections and discharges.

Seeds

L. heterophyllus
Decoction: Used for menstrual irregularities.

Eye bath: Use a weak decoction for conjunctivitis, sore or tired eyes.

CAUTIONS:
- Uterine stimulant: avoid in pregnancy although it can be used in labor.
- Seek professional advice for all heart conditions.

Ligusticum spp.
Alpine Lovage

Known as a fashionable cure-all and immune stimulant in North America, Colorado cough root or oshá (*L. porteri*) is also used for coughs and colds, digestive upsets, and menstrual problems. The herb originates in the Rocky Mountains, where it was once regarded as sacred by Native Americans who burned it to ward off evil influences. Several related species are also popular in China: *gao ben* (*L. sinense*) is used for pain relief, while *chuan xiong* (*L. wallichii*) is taken for menstrual and heart problems.

Character: Pungent, warm, dry.

Constituents: Essential oil, glycosides, ferulic acid, bitters.

Actions: *L. porterii*: carminative, diaphoretic, expectorant, stimulating.
L. sinense: antifungal, analgesic, antispasmodic.
L. wallichii antibacterial, hypotensive, sedative, uterine stimulant.

Parts Used

Root
L. porterii
Colorado cough root is a pungent warm herb that encourages sweating and is a good remedy for the chilling winds of the Rocky Mountains. It simulates the circulation and kidneys, improves digestion, and relieves spasmodic pains, toothache, and bronchitis. It is available in over-the-counter herbal products in North America and Europe.

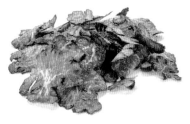

Root & Rhizome
L. sinense
Chinese folk tradition uses *gao ben* (*L. sinense*) or Chinese lovage for menstrual problems and as a strengthening remedy after childbirth, although its main medicinal uses are for chills and pain relief. It is taken for various types of headaches, migraines, joint pain, toothache, and arthritis, which can be associated with symptoms that develop in syndromes which the Chinese believe caused by external wind, cold, or damp.

Rhizome
L. wallichii
Chuan xiong, Sichuan lovage, has been used in China since the fourteenth century as an invigorating blood remedy for menstrual and heart problems and also for headaches. It is often combined with *dang gui*, *bai shao yao*, and *shu di huang* for menstrual irregularities, and anemia, and is included in several patent remedies for coronary heart disease.

Applications

Root

L. porterii
Maceration: Soak the root overnight and use in making syrups for coughs and colds or warm a cup of the maceration for menstrual pain, digestive upsets, and feverish colds.
Tincture: Use 20–30 drops per dose in a little water as the maceration. Combine with echinacea for colds and influenza.

Root & Rhizome

L. sinense
Decoction: Use for colds and chills associated with headaches and muscle pains; combine with fennel seed and *wu zhu yu* for abdominal cramps associated with cold.
Tincture: Use 10–20 drops per dose for headaches, stiff neck and toothache; combine with an equal amount of ginger or cinnamon. Use a cotton swab soaked in a little dilute tincture as a compress for toothache (apply to the adjacent gum).

Rhizome

L. wallichii
Decoction: Use with *shu di huang*, *dang gui*, and *bai shao yao* for anemia and poor circulation or with *chai hu* and *chi shao yao* for headaches associated with stagnant liver *qi*.
Pills: *Chuan xiong* is combined with other herbs in "*Ba Zhen Tang*," often made into tablets and marketed in the West as "Women's Precious Pills" used as a tonic for irregular menstruation and anemia.

Cautions
• Avoid sha and *chuan xiong* in pregnancy and heavy menstrual bleeding.
• *Gao ben* and *chuan xiong* should not be used in cases of *yin* deficiency or excess heat.

Linum spp.
Flax

As the source of linen fiber, flax (*L. usitatissimum*) has been cultivated since at least 5000 BC; today it is just as likely to be grown for its oil. The medicinal properties of the seeds (linseed) were known to the Greeks: Hippocrates recommended them for inflammations of the mucous membranes. In eighth-century France, Charlemagne passed laws requiring his subjects to eat the seeds in order to keep them healthy. In the Middle Ages, flax flowers were thought to provide protection against witchcraft. The related mountain flax (*L. catharticum*) was once popular as a strong purgative, but is less often used today.

Parts Used

L. usitatissimum
Ripe seeds
The ripe seeds can be used as a relaxing expectorant, a bulking laxative, and also extensively in poultices. The seeds are rich in mucilage so can be soothing for gastritis and sore throats. Linseed oil contains cis-linoleic and alpha-linolenic acids needed for the production of certain prostaglandins vital for many body functions. Harvest when ripe.

L. catharticum
Whole plant
Mountain or purging flax is a potent laxative and was often used as an alternative to senna. The whole plant was collected while flowering and used in infusions, often combined with carminatives like peppermint. The tea was also a traditional folk remedy for rheumatism and liver complaints, largely because its strong laxative action helps rid the body of toxins. Harvest while flowering.

Applications
L. usitatissimum
Ripe seeds

Poultice: Crushed seeds can be used for boils, abscesses and ulcers and also locally for pleurisy pain.

Oil: Linseed oil is an important source of essential fatty acids (cf. evening primrose oil) and can be usefully added to the diet in cases of eczema, menstrual disorders, rheumatoid arthritis, atherosclerosis, etc. Dose is typically 2 teaspoons of freshly pressed oil or 1–2 tablespoons of freshly crushed seeds daily.

Infusion: Used for coughs and sore throats – best flavored with honey and lemon juice.

Maceration: Linseed mucilage is made by soaking the seeds on water. The thick mucilage produced can be taken for inflammations of the mucous membranes such as gastritis, pharyngitis, etc.

Fresh seeds: For constipation eat 1–2 tablespoons of seeds followed by 1–2 glasses of water. The seeds swell in the bowel to produce a gentle, bulking laxative. The seeds can be mixed with muesli, porridge or honey and soft cheese and eaten at breakfast. Simultaneous high fluid intake is important.

L. catharticum
Whole plant

Infusion: Use the fresh herb for constipation, liver congestion, and rheumatic pain.

CAUTIONS:
- Linseed oil deteriorates rapidly and should be freshly prepared as required if possible.
- The seeds contain traces of prussic acid which is potentially toxic in large quantities, although no cases of prussic acid poisoning from linseed have ever been reported. Do not exceed the stated dose.

Lonicera spp.
Honeysuckle

Woodbine or English honeysuckle (*L. periclymenum*) was once widely used for asthma, urinary disorders, and in childbirth. Pliny recommended it to be taken in wine for spleen disorders, while almost 1600 years later Culpeper urged that honeysuckle conserve "should be kept in every gentlewoman's house" because it was such a valuable remedy. Today Chinese honeysuckle (*L. japonica* or *jin yin*) is more likely to be used medicinally. This was first listed in the *Tang Ben Cao* written in 659 AD and is one of the most important Chinese herbs for clearing heat and poisons from the body.

Character: Sweet and cold.

Constituents: Tannin, flavonoids, mucilage, sugars; salicylic acid reported in European spp.

Actions
L. japonica – antibacterial, hypotensive, anti-inflammatory, mild diuretic, antispasmodic;
L. periclymenum – diuretic, antispasmodic, expectorant, laxative, emetic.

PARTS USED

L. japonica
FLOWER BUDS
Known as *jin yin hua* in China, the flowers are widely used in feverish conditions, especially those attributed to "summer heat." They clear the toxins or "fire poisons" that in traditional Chinese theory cause conditions such as boils and dysentery. The Chinese warm the flower-buds slightly by stir-frying them to treat some types of diarrhea. Harvest in summer.

STEMS AND BRANCHES
Called both *jin yin teng* and *ren dong teng*, the stems and branches are generally used to remove heat from the channels by stimulating the circulation of *qi*. They are also used to treat feverish colds and dysentery and are recommended as a cooling remedy, in combination with other herbs, for the acute stages of rheumatoid arthritis.

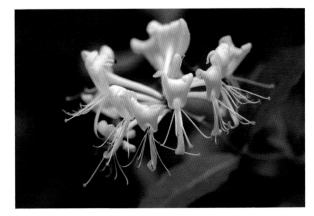

L. japonica

L. periclymenum
FLOWERS
Woodbine flowers were traditionally made into syrup taken as an expectorant for bad coughs and asthma. It was also used as a diuretic.

APPLICATIONS

L. japonica

Flower buds

Decoction: Use in the early stages of feverish colds characterized by headaches, thirst and sore throats. Use 10–15 g of flowers to 600 ml water or combine with *lian qiao*, *ban lang gen*, elderflowers, or peppermint. Add *huang lian* and *huang qin* for high fevers.

Tincture: Use standard doses for diarrhea or gastro-enteritis related to food poisoning.

Stems and branches

Decoction: Use 15–30 g to 600 ml of water in a similar way to the flowers and especially if the condition involves painful joints as in the aches associated with influenza or inflammatory diseases like rheumatoid arthritis when it should be used in combination with other herbs.

L. periclymenum

Flowers

Infusion: A standard infusion of the flowers can be used with other expectorant herbs for coughs and mild asthma.

Syrup: The standard infusion of the flowers preserved with sugar or honey (500 ml infusion to 500 g of sugar) can be used for coughs. Can be combined with other expectorant flowers like coltsfoot, mullein, mallow or marshmallow.

CAUTIONS:
• Honeysuckle berries are poisonous and should not be used.

Malus spp.
Apples

Despite the adage that "an apple a day keeps the doctor away," the apple's medicinal properties are often forgotten. Crab apples (*M. sylvestris*) were among the sacred herbs of the Anglo-Saxons, while fruits of *M. communis* have been cultivated since Roman times, with ripe apples used as laxatives and unripe ones used to counter diarrhea. In Galenical medicine, most apples were defined as cool and moist with juices and infusion prescribed for fevers or used in eye baths for conjunctivitis. Studies have shown that apples can reduce serum cholesterol levels.

Character: Cool and moist – ripe apples are generally sweet, unripe, and some cultivated varieties, sour.

Constituents: Sugars, fruit acids, pectin, vitamins A, B1, and C, minerals.

Actions: Tonic, digestive and liver stimulant, diuretic, antirheumatic, laxative, antiseptic.

PARTS USED

RAW FRUIT
Fresh apples are cleansing for the system, especially if eaten in the morning, while in the evening they have a more laxative action. They have also been traditionally used in poultices for skin inflammations. As a "cold" fruit too many apples can lead to digestive upsets and wind.

STEWED FRUIT
Traditionally used for diarrhea and dysentery, stewed apples can be especially helpful for babies and small children. They can also be soothing in gastric ulceration or ulcerative colitis.

PEEL
In France preparations made from apple peel have been used for rheumatism, gout, and urinary disorders as a diuretic.

BLOSSOM
Apple blossom has been used in the past as the basis for cough mixtures with a sedative rather than expectorant action.

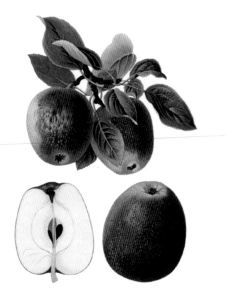

APPLICATIONS

Raw fruit

Infusion: Use an infusion of fresh, raw apple as a warming drink for both rheumatic pains and intestinal colic. The same tea can be used as a cooling remedy for feverish colds.
Juice: Use neat juice or juice mixed with olive oil as a household standby for cuts and grazes.
Fresh apples: Eat raw apples for constipation – effective where the cause is associated with overheated stomachs.

Use stewed apples for diarrhea, gastroenteritis, and intestinal infections. Apples are also a good source of minerals and vitamins in anemia and debility. Use sour apples as a diuretic in cystitis and other urinary infections.

Stewed fruit

Poultice: Use stewed apples for skin infections such as scabies.
Stewed apples: Use for diarrhea, gastroenteritis and intestinal infections.

Matricaria chamomilla
German chamomile

Called "ground apple" (*kamai melon*) by the Ancient Greeks because of its smell, chamomile was *maythen* to the Anglo-Saxons, one of the nine sacred herbs given to mankind by Woden. Two species of chamomile are used medicinally: the annual German chamomile (*Matricaria chamomilla*) and the perennial Roman chamomile (*Chamaemelum nobile*). They have virtually identical properties and applications, although the essential oil made from Roman chamomile is preferable. German chamomile is known as "*matricaria,*" referring to its role as a gynecological herb.

Character: Bitter, mainly warm, and moist.

Constituents: Volatile oil (inc. azulenes), flavonoids (inc. rutin), valerianic acid, coumarins, tannins, salicylates, cyanogenic glycosides.

Actions: Anti-inflammatory, antispasmodic, bitter, sedative, antiemetic.

PARTS USED

M. chamomilla or *Chamaemelum nobile*

FLOWERS
One flower of home-dried chamomile will often give more flavor that an entire tea bag of commercial offerings. Medieval herbalists developed double-flowered varieties to increase the yield of usable parts. Harvest throughout the summer and dry quickly so that the flowers retain their rich pungent scent for months.

Chamaemelum nobile

ESSENTIAL OIL
Distilled from fresh flowers of Roman chamomile since medieval times the oil is used for a very wide range of complaints including muscle pains, liver problems and menstrual disorders. True Roman chamomile oil is extremely expensive and is deep blue because of the azulenes – chemicals which are extremely anti-inflammatory, antispasmodic, and anti-allergenic – it contains. Because of the price colorless substitutes are common.

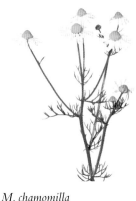

M. chamomilla

M. chamomilla or *Chamaemelum nobile*

ROOT
In homeopathic medicine chamomile extracts made from the root of either species are known as *Chamomilla* and are generally supplied in tablet form or as a mother tincture which is then further diluted before use. The remedy can be especially helpful for babies – for teething and colic – and it is also ideal for painful periods or during labor.

APPLICATIONS

M. chamomilla or *Chamaemelum nobile*

Flowers

Infusion: A standard infusion can be used for many digestive problems including irritable bowel syndrome, peptic ulcers, poor appetite, indigestion, liver stagnation, or menstrual problems. Drink a cup at night for insomnia or for anxiety and stress. Strong infusions can also help during the early stages of labor – combine with betony or rose petals.

Steam inhalation: Use 2 teaspoons of flowers to a basin of boiling water as an inhalant for catarrh, hay fever, to avert or reduce the severity of an asthmatic attack, or to ease bronchitis

Baths: Add 200–400 ml of strained chamomile infusion to baby's bath-water at night to encourage sleep.

Tincture: Standard doses (up to 5 ml three times per day) can be used for irritable bowel syndrome (combines well with hops, peppermint, or meadowsweet), insomnia, or nervous tension,

Mouthwash: Use an infusion or diluted tincture for gingivitis or other mouth inflammations.

Gargle: Use for sore throats – combine with sage, lady's mantle or purple coneflower.

Eye bath: Use 5–10 drops of tincture in an eye bath of warm water for conjunctivitis or tired, strained eyes.

Cream: Use in ointments and creams for insect bites, wounds, itching eczema, or anal/vulvar irritation.

Chamaemelum nobile

Essential oil

Inhalation: Put 2–3 drops in a saucer of warm water and leave by the bedside table at night in cases of asthma, whooping cough, bad nasal catarrh or other conditions which may make breathing difficult; 1–2 drops can similarly be put onto a handkerchief or pillow as a night-time inhalant.

Massage: For muscular aches and pains use 2–3 drops of oil to 5 ml of almond oil. Combine with thyme or rosemary.

Lotion: For eczema use 5 drops of chamomile oil to 50 ml of distilled witch hazel (or use equal amounts of rosewater and distilled witch hazel)

CAUTIONS:
* Do not use chamomile oil during pregnancy and also avoid excessive internal intake of chamomile herb (teas, etc.) during this time.
* Can cause contact dermatitis particularly if sunbathing on damp chamomile lawns.

Melaleuca alternifolia
Tea tree

Character: Warm, pungent.

Constituents: Terpinen-4-ol (up to 30%), ineol, pinene, cymene, terpinenes, other monoterpenes, and sesquiterpenes.

Actions: Antibacterial, antifungal, antiseptic, antiviral, diaphoretic, expectorant.

Tea tree was originally used by the Aborigines for colds, wounds, and general sickness, and by the Second World War it was included in field dressing kits used by Australian troops. The plant was first studied in Europe in the 1920s, when French researchers identified its impressive antibiotic properties. They found that the oil was a more effective antiseptic than phenol and five times more bactericidal than carbolic acid. Today, a thriving tea tree industry has developed, leading to a number of highly adulterated oils appearing on the market.

Parts Used

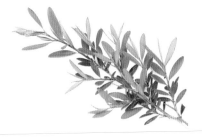

Dried Leaves
Leaves from the tea tree, so named by the botanist Joseph Banks as they made a pleasant-tasting infusion, were used by Australian Aborigines for treating colds, fevers, and vomiting: the sort of illnesses we know are often due to microorganisms.

Oil
True tea tree oil is one of the few that does not irritate mucous membranes and it can be used neat on the skin. However, adulterated products are all too common, so oils are best used diluted initially. The oil is antibacterial, antifungal, antiviral, and stimulates the immune system, so is suitable for a wide range of infectious conditions.

Cream
Tea tree cream is available commercially and is ideal in household first aid for minor cuts, grazes, and skin sores.

Applications

Oil

Pessaries: Add 2-3 drops of tea tree oil per teaspoon of melted cocoa butter for making pessaries for vaginal thrush. Alternatively, put 3-5 drops in a teaspoon of water and soak a little onto a tampon; insert and leave for no longer than four hours.

Lotion: Apply one drop of tea tree oil in 10 drops of almond oil to cold sores as soon as the prickling sensation that heralds the sore starts; it can often stop the sore developing completely. Use tea tree cream or 2-3 drops of oil in a teaspoon of water as a lotion to soothe the sores once they appear.

Oil: Use a drop of neat oil on warts 2-3 times daily. Dilute with an equal amount of almond oil if any irritation occurs. Neat oil can also be used to massage on gums in tooth abscesses.

Cream: Apply tea tree cream to athlete's foot, ringworm, and other infections. The cream can also be used for cuts, grazes, insect bites, and other skin infections. Alternatively combine equal amounts of tea tree oil and almond oil as a lotion.

Lotion: Add 5 ml of tea tree oil to 20 ml each of distilled witch hazel and rosewater and apply to acne pustules with cotton wool several times a day.

Hair rinse: Use 5 ml of oil in 250 ml of warm water as a final rinse to the hair after shampooing for nits and headlice. Alternatively, put several drops of oil on a fine-toothed comb and comb the hair thoroughly at night.

Leaves

Infusion: Use 10 g of leaves per 500 ml of water or half a teaspoon per cup for colds, glandular fever, cystitis, and urinary infections. The infusion is also a restorative nerve tonic in exhaustion and debility.

Gargle: Use 1 teaspoon of leaves per cup to make a gargle and mouthwash for throat infections and mouth ulcers.

Shampoo: Infuse a good handful of leaves in a 500 ml bottle of basic, soap-based shampoo for two weeks. Strain and then use the mix when washing children's hair to combat nits and head lice.

Melissa officinalis
Lemon balm

Balm and bees have been linked since ancient times. The name *Melissa* comes from the Greek for "honey bee," and lemon balm has similar healing and tonic properties to bee products such as honey and royal jelly. Gerard said that the herb "comforteth the hart and driveth away all melancholie and sadnesse," and it was a favorite in medieval "elixirs of youth" – praised as such by Paracelsus who made a preparation called *primum ens melissæ*. As late as the eighteenth century, lemon balm was still being recommended to "renew youth."

Character: Cold and dry with a sour, slightly bitter taste.

Constituents: Volatile oil (inc. citronellal), polyphenols, tannins, bitter principle, flavonoids, rosmarinic acid.

Actions: Sedative, antidepressant, digestive stimulant, peripheral vasodilator, diaphoretic, relaxing restorative for nervous system, antiviral (possibly due to polyphenols and tannins), antibacterial.

Parts Used

Aerial parts

Good for depression and tension, the aerial parts are also carminative so are ideal for anyone who suffers from digestive upsets when worried or anxious. As a cooling herb it is good in feverish colds while the fresh aerial parts make a refreshing and restorative lemon tea. Use both internally and externally to reduce the duration and discomfort of cold sore eruptions. Externally, the herb can be used on sores or painful swelling. Harvest just before flowering.

Essential oil

This concentrated essence of lemon balm has the same properties of the aerial parts but is far more potent: a few drops make an excellent restorative, antidepressant sedative. It has been shown to slow and calm the heart and is also a good carminative to settle the stomach and can be useful in colds, influenza and chest problems. Pure essential oil of lemon balm can be difficult to obtain commercially as it is often adulterated with lemon or lemon grass oils.

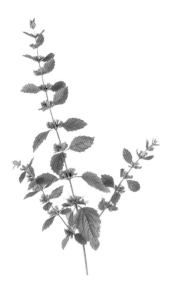

Applications

Aerial parts

Infusion: Make with fresh leaves, water which is off the boil and in a pot with a lid to avoid evaporating too much of the essential oil. Ideal for depression, nervous exhaustion, indigestion or nausea, and the early stages of colds and influenza.

Tincture: Best made from fresh leaves and with a rather stronger but similar action to the infusion. Small doses (5–10 drops) are usually more effective.

Ointment: Useful for sores and insect bites. The plant also contains citronellal which can help to repel insects.

Infused oil: Use as the ointment or as a gentle massage oil for tension or chest complaints. Make by the hot infusion method (less effective than essential oil-based extracts).

Compress: Use a pad soaked in the infusion for painful swellings such as gout.

Mouthwash: Use the infusion for mouth ulcers.

Essential oil

Massage oil: Use 5–10 drops of essential oil in 20 ml of almond or olive oil for depression, tension and as an antispasmodic for asthma and bronchitis.

Ointment: Use 5 ml of oil to 100 g of an ointment base for insect bites or as a preventative to deter pests.

Mentha spp.
Mint

There are thought to be around thirty different species of mint, but as they readily cross-pollinate and form hybrids, no one is entirely certain. Until the seventeenth century all mints were used in much the same way with little attempt to differentiate between varieties. Today, peppermint (*Mentha* x *piperita*) is preferred medicinally in the West, while the Chinese prefer field mint (*M. arvensis*), known as *bo he*. Garden mint is usually spearmint (*M. spicata*), which is not as strong as peppermint but can be used in similar ways and is good for children.

Character: Pungent and dry, generally cooling.

Constituents: Volatile oil (mainly menthol), tannins, flavonoids, tocopherols, choline, bitter principle.

Actions: Antispasmodic, digestive tonic, antiemetic, carminative, peripheral vasodilator, diaphoretic but also cooling internally, cholagogue, analgesic

Parts Used

M. x *piperita*
Aerial parts
Carminative and relaxing for the muscles of the digestive tract, peppermint also stimulates bile flow so is useful for indigestion, flatulence, colic, and similar conditions. Peppermint also reduces nausea and can be helpful for travel sickness. Its diaphoretic action is useful in fevers and influenza. Harvest just before flowering.

Essential oil
Peppermint oil contains large amounts of menthol. In fairly high doses it is analgesic and sedative while its cooling action is useful for feverish conditions or headaches and migraines linked to over-heating. It is antibacterial to combat many infections and used as an inhalant clears nasal congestion.

M. Arvensis
Aerial parts
The Chinese use *bo he* as a cooling remedy for head colds and influenza and also for some types of headaches, sore throats, and eye inflammations. As a liver stimulant it is also added to remedies linked with digestive disorders or liver energy (*qi*) stagnation.

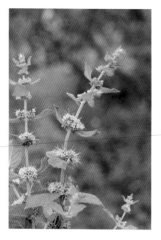

M. arvensis

Applications

Aerial parts

M. X piperita & M. arvensis
Infusion: Use water that is off the boil and in a pot with a lid to avoid evaporating too much of the essential oil. For nausea, travel sickness, indigestion, flatulence, and colic. In combinations for colds and catarrh. Can also ease migraines.

Steam inhalation: Use a few fresh leaves and boiling water for nasal congestion.

Compress: A pad soaked in the infusion can be used to cool inflamed joints or for rheumatism or neuralgia.

Tincture: Used in similar ways to the infusion. Small amounts often added to remedies as a digestive or liver stimulant.

Essential oil

M. X piperita
Wash: Use 20 drops of the oil in 100 ml of water for skin irritations, itching, burns and inflammations. Also as a mosquito repellent or for scabies and ringworm.

Massage oil: Use diluted in almond or vegetable oil as a massage for menstrual pains, or for milk congestion when breastfeeding. Combined with thyme and eucalyptus oils (up to a total of 25 drops of essential oil in 25 ml of carrier) it can be used as a chest rub during colds or influenza.

Inhalant: 2–3 drops of oil on a saucer of water left in the room at night can reduce nasal congestion during colds and influenza.

CAUTIONS:
- Avoid prolonged use of the essential oil as an inhalant.
- Peppermint should not be used for babies or young children.
- Peppermint can reduce milk flow and should be used with caution internally while breastfeeding.
- Spearmint (*M. spicata*) can be used as a gentle alternative to peppermint for children.

Morus spp.
Mulberry

In the sixteenth century, the berries, bark, leaves, and buds of the black mulberry (*M. nigra*) were all used medicinally: the berries for inflammations and to stop bleeding; the bark for toothache; the leaves for "the bitings of serpents"; and as an antidote to aconite. While mulberry has faded from the European *materia medica*, the white mulberry (*M. alba*) is still widely used in China as a remedy for coughs, colds, and high blood pressure, and as a *yin* tonic.

Character: Mainly sweet and cold; the leaves are also bitter and the branch is bitter and neutral.

Constituents: Flavonoids, coumarin, tannins, sugars; berries also contain vitamins A, B1, B2, C.

Actions
Root bark: Sedative, diuretic, expectorant, hypotensive;
Fruit: Tonic, astringent, laxative;
Leaf: Antibacterial, diaphoretic, expectorant;
Twigs: Antirheumatic, hypotensive, analgesic.

PARTS USED

M. alba & *M. nigra*

BERRIES
Known as *sang shen* in China, white mulberry fruits are used as a *yin* tonic to nourish the blood and vital essence and as a gentle laxative in constipation. In European tradition black mulberries are also regarded as a nourishing tonic. Harvest when ripe.

LEAVES
Called *sang ye* in China, white mulberry leaves are generally used for "wind heat evils" causing colds associated with fevers, headaches, and sore throats. They are also used for cooling heat in the liver meridian which can lead to sore eyes and irritability. In Europe, black mulberry leaves have been used to reduce blood sugar levels in diabetes. Harvest throughout the growing season.

ROOT BARK
White mulberry root bark, *sang bai pi*, is a good expectorant for coughs associated with thick, sticky yellow phlegm). In European tradition the root bark of the black mulberry was used to kill intestinal worms.

M. alba

TWIGS
Known as *sang zhi* these have been shown to be both analgesic and hypotensive although their traditional use is for rheumatic disorders. Branches grow upwards so in Chinese medicine they are considered more suitable for pain in the upper part of the body.

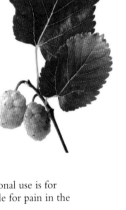

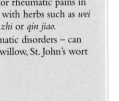

APPLICATIONS

M. alba & M. nigra

Berries

Tincture: Use as a tonic to nourish the blood and *yin* – combine with *wu wei zi* or *he shou wu* – or just eat the fresh fruits.

Gargle: Use the astringent juice from crushed fresh berries as a mouthwash or gargle for mouth ulcers and sore throats.

M. alba & M. nigra

Leaves

Infusion: Use a standard infusion for colds and chills – combines well with elderflowers and mint.

Chinese decoction: A typical remedy based on mulberry leaves for common cold will also include herbs such as *ju hua*, *lian qiao*, *jie geng*, peppermint and licorice.

Syrup: Combine a standard infusion with an equal quantity (weight to volume) of honey as a syrup for coughs and chronic lung weakness.

M. alba

Root bark

Decoction: Use for heat conditions affecting the lung or as a diuretic in cases of edema. For lung conditions mix with licorice, rice and *di gu pi*; for edema use with *fu ling*, *chen pi* and buchu.

Twigs

Decoction: Use a standard decoction for rheumatic pains in the upper part of the body – combined with herbs such as *wei ling xian*, Siberian ginseng, *fang feng*, *gui zhi* or *qin jiao*.

Tincture: Use standard doses for rheumatic disorders – can be combined with herbs such angelica, willow, St. John's wort or devil's claw.

CAUTIONS:

- Avoid excess fruits in diarrhea.
- Avoid leaves and bark if lungs are weak or cold; if in doubt seek professional advice.

Myristica fragrans
Nutmeg

First brought to Europe from the Banda Islands by Portuguese sailors around 1512, nutmeg rapidly gained the reputation of a cure-all and was widely eaten as a tonic. Its hallucinogenic properties were soon discovered with excessive nutmeg eaters becoming "deliriously inebriated." It was also taken, erroneously, to induce abortions and, equally erroneously, acclaimed as a cure for the plague. Known in China as *rou dou kou* it has been used there since the Tang Dynasty (c. 600 AD).

Character: Pungent and warm.

Constituents: Volatile oil (inc. borneol, eugeneol).

Actions: Carminative, digestive stimulant, antispasmodic, antiemetic, appetite stimulant, anti-inflammatory.

Parts Used

Kernel

Mainly used today is as a digestive remedy for nausea, vomiting, and indigestion, nutmeg is also taken for diarrhea, especially if related to food poisoning. In trials it has been successfully used for Crohn's disease. The Chinese take *rou dou kou* to warm the stomach and regulate *qi* flow. As in the West, it is also used for diarrhea, especially the "cock crow" variety, which occurs on rising and can be related to *qi* weakness.

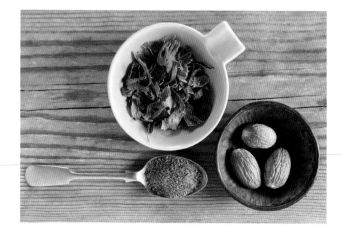

Essential oil of nutmeg

Externally, the oil is used for rheumatic pain and, like clove oil, it can also be used as an emergency treatment to dull toothache. In France it is given in drop doss in honey for digestive upsets or used for bad breath.

Mace

Mace is the outer fleshy aril of the nutmeg fruit and is mainly used as a culinary herb. Oil of mace has similar properties to nutmeg oil and was also used in the past to flavor medicines. In folk medicine mace is made into an ointment used for rheumatism.

Applications

Nutmeg

Powder: Use 1–2 x 200 mg capsules three times daily for nausea, indigestion, gastric upsets, and chronic diarrhea.

Decoction: Decoct 5 g with ginger (2 g), licorice (2 g), *wu wei zi* (5 g), *wu zhu yu* (5 g), and *bu gu zi* (10 g) in 600 ml of water (three doses) and use for early morning diarrhea or chronic colitis.

Nutmeg Oil

Massage oil: Dilute (5%) in vegetable oil and use for muscular pains associated with rheumatism or over-exertion. Can also be combined with essential oils of thyme or rosemary. To prepare for childbirth, massage the abdomen daily in the three weeks before the baby is due with a mixture of 5 drops of nutmeg oil and 5 drops of sage oil in 25 ml of vegetable oil.

Neat oil: Use 1–2 drops on a cotton swab applied to the gum around an aching tooth until dental treatment can be obtained. Use 3–5 drops on a sugar lump or teaspoon of honey for nausea, gastro-enteritis, chronic diarrhea and indigestion.

CAUTIONS:
- Large dose (7.5 g or more in a single dose) is hallucinogenic and can lead to convulsions and palpitations.

Nardostachys grandiflora
Spikenard

Highly valued since Biblical times, spikenard was the substance used to anoint Jesus at the Last Supper, and was regarded as a rejuvenating tonic by the Moghul emperors. Known as *jatamansi* in India, it shares the sedative properties of its relative valerian, although it also has a more spiritual dimension – believed in Ayurvedic medicine to promote awareness and strengthen the mind. It is listed by CITES as endangered, and trade in the wild plant is permitted only under licence.

Character: Sweet, bitter, astringent.

Constituents: Volatile oil including borneol acetates.

Actions: Antifungal, antibacterial, relaxing nervine, carminative, laxative, anti-pasmodic, diuretic.

Parts Used

Root and Rhizome
In India, *jatamansi* is used for a wide range of acute and chronic disorders including dysentery, consumption, bronchitis, smallpox, and menstrual and digestive upsets. It is used in Ayurveda to balance the humours (*doshas*) and promote spiritual awareness as a rejuvenating tonic. It is also an effective cardiac tonic and respiratory stimulant.

Oil
The oil is strongly antimicrobial and has sedative actions. It can be used in massage treatments for stress and nervous tension as well as added to external remedies for athlete's foot and other skin infections.

Aerial Parts
The aerial parts can be collected from garden-grown specimens and used in infusions as a gentle sedative and antibacterial for infections and fevers.

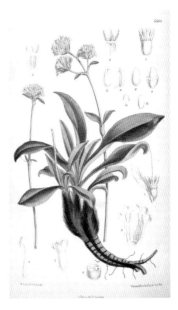

Applications

Root

Decoction: Simmer 1 teaspoon of dried root in a cup of milk as a restoring tonic for tension and nervous upsets. Use the standard decoction to strengthen and stimulate the digestive system in poor appetite, constipation, and sluggish digestion. Add a pinch of powdered cinnamon to each cup or combine with an equal amount of gotu kola infusion to enhance the action.

Syrup: Use the decoction as the base for a syrup and take 1-2 teaspoons for chesty coughs and bronchitis.

Maceration: The root can be macerated (as with valerian) as an alternative to the decoction and used as a calming sedative and tonic.

Tincture: Use as an alternative to valerian as a calming sedative or combine with gotu kola as a digestive and energy. Take up to 40 drops per dose.

Oil

Lotion: Add 1-2 drops of oil to 1 teaspoon of almond oil as a lotion for athlete's foot and ringworm.

Aerial Parts

Infusion: Drink a cup as a calming and soothing tea after a stressful day.

Wash: Use the infusion to bathe cuts, grazes, and fungal skin infections, such as athlete's foot.

Nelumbo nucifera
Lotus

The lotus, or *padma*, is revered as India's most sacred plant: its unfolding petals symbolizing the growth of spiritual awareness. In the East, the plant holds much the same place as the rose in Western Europe – a potent symbol of love and compassion. The lotus is sacred to Lakshmi, the goddess of prosperity, and it is believed to bring both material and spiritual wealth. It has been used medicinally since ancient Egyptian times and almost all parts are used in China for a wide range of ailments.

Character: Most parts are cooling or neutral, sweet, and astringent; flower stems are warm, bitter and astringent. Leaves are also bitter.

Constituents: *Rhizome nodes*: asparagine, tannin, vitamin C; *Seeds*: carbohydrates (inc. raffinose), calcium, phosphorus, iron, proteins; *Plumule/radicle*: flavonoids, alkaloids, glucosides; *Stamens*: flavonoids, alkaloids, glucosides; *Penduncle*: proteins, carbohydrates, carotene, riboflavin, ascorbic acid; *Leaves*: alkaloids, flavonoids, oxalic acid, citric acid, malic acid, tannin.

Actions: Aphrodisiac, astringent, stops bleeding, tonic, nervine.

PARTS USED

RHIZOME & RHIZOME NODE/*ou jie*
The root and rhizome are used in India as a rejuvenating tonic specifically for problems affecting the root *chakra* (including diarrhea, uterine disorders and hemorrhoids). In China, the nodes of the rhizome (*ou jie*) are used to stop bleeding.

PENDUCLE/RECEPTACLE (flower stalk with receptacle)/*lian fang*
The flower stalk (*lian fang*) is used in Chinese medicine to disperse congealed blood and stop internal bleeding from gastric ulcers, abnormally heavy periods, blood in the stool, or post-partum haemorrhage.

STAMENS/*lian xu*
The stamens (*lian xu*) are believed in Chinese medicine to act on the heart and kidney.

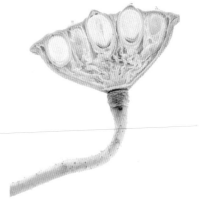

SEED/*lian zi*
In China, the seeds (*lian zi*) are used as a tonic for the spleen and stomach to combat diarrhea and stimulate the appetite. They are a kidney tonic and act as a calming sedative for insomnia and palpitations. In India the seeds are taken in powder format with rice as a tonic for the heart and reproductive organs. They are believed to help the heart *chakra* and to encourage devotion, aspiration and concentration, as well as improve speech and help reduce stammering.

SEED PLUMULE & RADICLE/*lian zi xin*
The plumules and radicles (*lian zi xin*) from the seeds are specifically used to "sedate the fire of the heart."

LEAVES/*he ye* & LEAF STEM/*lian geng*
The leaves (*he ye*) and leaf stems (*lian geng*) are mainly used in Chinese medicine as a cooling remedy for fevers associated with "summer heat." They are given as a spleen tonic for weaknesses associated diarrhea and upsets following summer fevers.

APPLICATIONS

Leaves and Leaf stem

Infusion: Take a cup three times daily for summer colds and fevers.
Wash: Use as a wash to bathe the forehead and body in fevers.

Seed

Powder/capsules: Take 1–2 x 200 mg capsules or half a teaspoon of powder stirred into water as a tonic for heart and kidneys. In India, the same mix is used to strengthen the heart *chakra* and encourage devotion, aspiration, and concentration, as well as improve speech and help reduce stammering.
Decoction: Combine with *dang shen* and goldenseal for insomnia, palpitations, irritability, and urinary dysfunction associated with kidney and heart energy weakness.

Rhizome node

Tincture: Soak a swab in the tincture and use as a plug for nosebleeds.
Decoction: Combine with *sheng di huang* and elecampane for bronchitis and congestive coughs with blood streaked phlegm; seek professional help if symptoms continue for more than 24 hours.
Juice: Use 10 ml the fresh juice for blood in the urine or heavy periods, three times daily.

Penduncle/receptacle/flower stalk

Infusion: Combine with motherwort for heavy menstrual bleeding and irregularity; with shepherd's purse for cystitis with blood in the urine.
Tincture: Use as the infusion.

CAUTIONS:
• Avoid in constipation.

Ocimum basilicum
Basil

From its native India, sweet basil (*O. basilicum*) was introduced into Europe in ancient times. Views and traditions associated with the herb have been mixed. Some cultures associate it with hatred and misfortunes, while others regarded it as a love token. Dioscorides said that it should never be taken internally, while Pliny advised smelling it in vinegar for fainting fits. In Ayurvedic medicine, holy basil (*O. sanctum*) is known as *tulsi* and the juice is an important tonic.

Character: Sweet, pungent and slightly bitter, very warm and dry.

Constituents: Volatile oil (inc. estragol), tannins, basil camphor.

Actions: Antidepressant, antiseptic, stimulates the adrenal cortex, antiemetic, tonic, carminative, febrifuge, expectorant.

PARTS USED

LEAVES
Good for rubbing on insect bites, the leaves can also be taken as a warming and uplifting tonic for nervous exhaustion or any cold condition. Harvest before and during flowering.

OIL
The essential oil, extracted from the aerial parts, is a light greenish-yellow color, and in aromatherapy is often combined with hyssop, bergamot, or geranium oils as a stimulating massage for depression.

O. sanctum
JUICE
In Ayurvedic medicine the juice is an important tonic and is also recommended for snakebites, chills, coughs, and skin problems, or used as ear drops for earache.

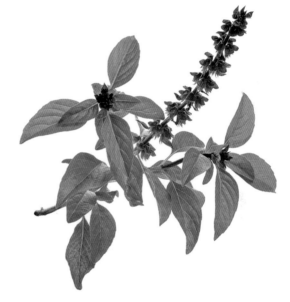

APPLICATIONS

Essential oil
Baths: Use 5–10 drops in a bath for nervous exhaustion, mental fatigue, melancholy, or fear.
Chest rub: Use 5 drops in 10 ml or almond oil as a rub for asthma or bronchitis. Can be combined with thyme or hyssop oils.
Massage oil: Use the diluted oil for nervous weakness; can also be applied to prevent insect bites.

Leaves
Fresh herb: Rub leaves on insect bites to reduce itching and inflammation.
Tincture: This is almost as potent as the essential oil and can be combined with wood betony and skullcap in nervous conditions or with elecampane and hyssop for coughs and bronchitis.
Steam inhalant: Pour boiling water on basil leaves as an inhalant for head colds. Alternatively add 2–3 drops of the essential oil to a basin of very hot water and inhale.
Infusion: Combine with motherwort and drink a standard infusion immediately after childbirth to prevent a retained placenta.
Juice: Mix with a decoction of cinnamon and cloves for chills; combine 50:50 with honey as a syrup for coughs or use the same honey/basil juice mixture externally for ringworm and itching skin.

CAUTIONS:
• Basil oil should not be used in pregnancy.

Paeonia spp.
Peony

Although now regarded in the West as no more than a decorative garden flower, the peony has a long tradition as a medicinal herb, and used in the past to treat nervous conditions including epilepsy. Today, the root is highly valued in Chinese medicine, where two species are used: both the red- and white-flowered *P. lactiflora* and *P. suffruticosa*, the tree peony. The name reputedly derives from Paeos, a physician during the Trojan Wars.

PARTS USED

ROOT

P. lactiflora (red)
Known as *chi shao yao*, the root of the red peony is used to cool the blood, move stagnating blood and relieve pain. It was successfully used in combination with other Chinese herbs in a project at Great Ormond Street Hospital in London to treat childhood eczema.

P. lactiflora (white)
White peony has a much more specific action on the liver than red peony, soothing liver energy and improving function. Called *bao shao yao* in Chinese medicine, it is seen as nourishing the blood rather than cooling and is regarded as more yin in character that chi shao yao. It is considered one of the great women's tonics of Chinese medicine and is often used for menstrual disorders.

P. suffruticosa
ROOT BARK
In China, the root bark of the tree peony is known as *mu dan pi*. Like *chi shao yao* this is considered to cool the blood and is also used in the eczema project at Great Ormond Street Hospital. It is also a good antibacterial used for boils and abscesses.

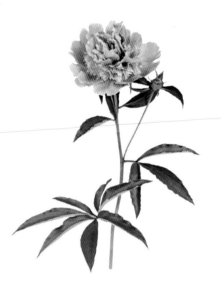

APPLICATIONS

Root

P. lactiflora (red)
Decoction: Used, mainly in combination with other herbs, for any condition involving over-heated blood including certain types of eczema, skin inflammations, nose bleeds, and inflammations and pain associated with injuries. The usual dose is around 10–15 g of *chi shao yao* per dose (i.e. a decoction containing up to 45 g of herb in 600 ml water)
P. lactiflora (white)
Decoction: Used for liver-associated problems including menstrual disorders. One of the classic Chinese formulas is the "Four Things Decoction," which includes *shu di huang* (10 g), *dang gui* (10 g), *chuan xiong* (5 g), and *bai shao yao* (10 g) in 600 ml water and is used for anemia and irregular periods.

As a regular tonic, ideal for women and reputed to beautify the skin, decoct 20 g of *bai shao yao* and 5 g of licorice root for 15 minutes with 500 ml of water and drink two wineglass doses daily.

Root bark

P. suffruticosa
Decoction: Used in combination with other herbs for feverish conditions involving nosebleeds and is also added to remedies for some types of eczema. It is often combined with *shu di huang*, *shan zhu yu*, *fu ling*, *ze xie*, and *shan yao* for liver disharmonies. The usual amount used is around 10 g of *mu dan pi* per dose (i.e. 30 g to 600 ml of water).

CAUTIONS:
• Avoid during pregnancy.

Panax spp.
Ginseng

Used in China for more than 5,000 years, ginseng (*P. ginseng*) was known to Arab physicians of the ninth century. Marco Polo wrote of this highly prized wonder drug, and when a delegation from the King of Siam visited Louis XIV at Versailles, they presented him with a root of "gintz-aen." From then on ginseng was widely used by wealthy Europeans for exhaustion and debility. By the eighteenth century it was also popular in America, especially when a very similar plant (*P. quinquifolius*) was found to be indigenous.

Character: Sweet and slightly bitter. *P. ginseng* and *P. notoginseng* are warm, *P. quinquifolius* is cool.

Constituents: Steroidal glycosides, saponins, volatile oil, vitamin D, acetyleneic compounds, sterols.

Actions: Tonic, stimulant, reduces blood sugar and cholesterol levels, immunostimulant.

PARTS USED

ROOT

P. ginseng

Root: Korean or Chinese ginseng, *ren shen*, is one of the most highly prized and expensive herbs. It is a *yang* tonic replenishing *qi* especially of spleen and lung. It also strengthens the immune system and reduces fatigue. Modern research has identified steroidal components similar to the human sex hormones in the root.

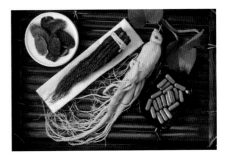

P. quinquifolius

American ginseng, *xi yang shen*, is a *yin* tonic, taken in China for fevers or where exhaustion is due to chronic, wasting disease such as tuberculosis. It can be helpful for coughs related to lung weakness.

P. notoginseng

Known as *san qi* or *tienchi* in China, this is used as an analgesic and to stop both internal and external bleeding. It is also added to treatments for coronary heart disease and angina. *San qi* was used extensively by the Vietcong during the Vietnam war to increase recovery rates from gun wounds.

APPLICATIONS

Root

P. ginseng

Powder: Use in capsules or tablets in 1–4 g doses as a general tonic. It is often best to take ginseng for one month as the seasons change in the autumn to strengthen the body for winter. If taking ginseng regularly have a break of at least 2–3 weeks every two months.

Tincture: Use standard doses for diarrhea related to weak digestive function: combine with specific digestive remedies. Combine with walnut and a little ginger for asthma and chronic coughs. Can be used as a general tonic for fatigue and extreme weakness as with the powder.

Decoction: Use 3–10 g in 500 ml water. Featured in many traditional formulas, for example in a Taoist "longevity" mixture using ginseng with *he shou wu*, *wu wei zi*, and *gou qi zi*.

P. quinquifolius

Powder: Use in capsules or tablets in 1–2 g doses for yin deficiency (e.g. may be suitable for women at the menopause) or for chronic lung weakness.

Tincture: Use standard doses as a tonic or combine with herbs like elecampane and mulberry bark for chronic cough and weak lungs or TB.

Decoction: Use 3–6 g in 500 ml of water as a yin tonic or for lung weakness.

P. notoginseng

Powder: Use in capsules or tablets in 1–2 g doses for wounds, internal bleeding, traumatic injuries or pain. Combine with slippery elm for the pain of gastric ulceration or with hawthorn berry for blood stagnation.

Tincture: Use standard doses for painful injuries. Combine with shepherd's purse or mugwort for uterine bleeding. Combine with cornsilk, couchgrass or buchu for severe urinary tract inflammations with blood in the urine. Can be combined with herbs such as hawthorn or linden flowers in coronary heart disease.

Decoction: Use 2–6 g in 600 ml water for wounds, bleeding or coronary heart disease

CAUTIONS:
- *P. notoginseng* should be avoided in pregnancy.
- Although *P. ginseng* is generally safe side effects have been reported, high doses or prolonged use should be avoided in pregnancy and hypertension.
- It is best to avoid other stimulants, such as tea, coffee, or Coca Cola, when taking *P. ginseng*.

Passiflora incarnata
Passion flower

Passion flower takes its name from the religious symbolism of its flowers: the three stigmas to represent the nails of the Crucifixion, the five anthers for Christ's five wounds, a finely cut corona for the Crown of Thorns, and the ten sepals representing the Apostles present at the Cross. The herb originates in North America, where it is known as maypop. It was first sent to Europe as a gift for Pope Paul V in 1605. By the nineteenth century it was established as a remedy for epilepsy and later as a cure for insomnia.

Character: Cooling, bitter.

Constituents: Flavonoids (including rutin), cyanogenic glycosides, alkaloids, sapanarin.

Actions: Analgesic, antispasmodic, bitter, cooling, hypotensive, sedative, heart tonic, relaxes blood vessels.

PARTS USED

AERIAL PARTS (Dried leaves and flowers)

The Houmas in Louisiana traditionally used passion flower as a blood tonic while the Maya Indians used the crushed plant as a poultice for swellings and as a decoction for ringworm. Today, it is mostly used as a sedative, painkiller, to reduce blood pressure, and in homeopathy as a remedy for nervous insomnia. Although a potent remedy, it is gentle enough for children and can be used for hyperactivity and restlessness. It can ease tremors in the elderly, including those associated with Parkinson's disease, and it can also be helpful in relieving the vertigo and dizziness of Ménière's disease, which affects the inner ear. Tablets are readily available over the counter for insomnia and nervous tension.

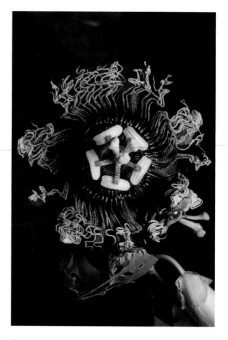

APPLICATIONS

Aerial parts

Tablets: Take 1–2 tablets at night (or as directed on the pack) for insomnia; the tablets can be used for nervous tension during the day although excess can cause drowsiness.

Tincture: Combine with equal amounts of valerian and hops for insomnia and nervous tension; take 50 drops three times daily in a little water. The same can be used for high blood pressure associated with nervous stress. Use up to 4 ml three times daily for tremors and vertigo or to ease the pain associated with shingles and toothache.

Powder/capsules: Take 1–2 x 200 mg capsules or half a teaspoon of powder night and morning for anxiety, tension, and nervous headaches.

Infusion: Take a cup for menstrual pain, tension headaches, and to help calm underlying tension in conditions like irritable bowel syndrome and irregular heartbeats. Dilute a standard infusion with an equal amount of water and give half a cup for hyperactivity in children. Combine with an equal amount of raspberry leaf for menstrual pain.

CAUTIONS:
- Use only low doses in pregnancy.
- May cause drowsiness.

Phyllostachys nigra
Bamboo

Bamboo is an important Asian cash crop used for just about everything from musical instruments to drainpipes and scaffolding. Extracts of bamboo are used in both Chinese and Ayurvedic medicine mainly as a cooling lung remedy for coughs and congestion and as a rejuvenating tonic after chronic illness. Bamboo extracts can be rich in silica leading some Western suppliers to promote the herb as helpful for bone and joint disorders and to prevent bone loss after the menopause.

Character: Sweet, cold.

Constituents: Cellulose, sugars, triterpenes.

Actions: Antispasmodic, antimicrobial, demulcent, expectorant, tonic, stops bleeding.

Parts Used

Sap
Like the shavings, the sap (*zhu li*) is used in Chinese medicine to clear heat and phlegm. It is ideal for coughs with thick yellow sputum and is often combined with ginger to reduce its very cold nature.

Shavings
Bamboo shavings (*zhu ru*) are usually supplied by Chinese herbalists in balls looking rather like raffia. They are used as a cooling remedy for the blood and to clear dampness and phlegm and to clear heat from the stomach, which in Chinese terms may include such symptoms as bad breath, nausea, and vomiting. In Ayurveda both shavings and sap are combined as *vamsha rochana* or bamboo manna and are regarded as strongly anti-*pitta* to stop bleeding and clear fevers. *Vamsha rochana* is also nourishing and a rejuvenative tonic for the lungs to speed recovery from chronic illnesses and debility.

Leaf
The leaves (zhu ye) are mainly used in Chinese medicine as a cooling remedy for fevers, nausea and nosebleeds. They are also used in combination with other cooling herbs in the classic decoction *Zhu Ye Shi Gao Tang* taken for heat in the stomach associated with nausea, poor appetite, sunstroke, and thirst.

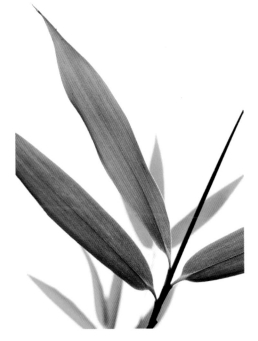

Applications

Sap

Juice: The sap is generally used singly as a juice for congestive coughs; it can be combined with an equal amount of ginger juice to warm the mixture. Take in teaspoon doses.

Shavings

Decoction: Combine with an equal amount of elecampane as a tonic following flu or use with a pinch of ginger for congestive coughs. The decoction is often made with milk in Ayurvedic medicine.

Tincture: Take 20–40 drops to soothe the nervous systems.
Powder: Use 250 mg to 1 g (up to a teaspoon) per dose as a lung tonic after flu or other debilitating disorders.

Leaf

Infusion: Take a cup for feverish colds and nausea. Soak a swab in the infusion and use to plug nosebleeds; the infusion taken internally will also help.

CAUTIONS:
• Avoid in diarrhea and coughs associated with cold.

Phytolacca americana
Pokeroot

Called *pocon* by Native Americans, pokeroot was mainly used either as an emetic or externally for skin diseases. The Delaware Indians took it as a heart stimulant while in Virginia it was regarded as a strong purgative. Even today in the Appalachians, backwoodsmen chew the seeds for arthritis, all the more remarkable because the fresh plant is extremely toxic. It arrived in Europe in the nineteenth century and is used as an important lymphatic cleanser.

Character: Pungent, drying, and slightly cold.

Constituents: Saponins, tannin, alkaloids, bitter principle, sugars.

Actions: Antirheumatic, stimulant, anti-catarrhal, purgative, emetic, antiparasitic, anti-inflammatory, immune stimulant, lymphatic stimulant, mild analgesic.

PARTS USED

DRIED ROOT
Used today as a lymphatic cleanser, particularly suitable for glandular fever and tonsillitis, the dried root can also be helpful for mastitis and is added to rheumatic remedies. Externally the herb is used occasionally for skin infections such as scabies and ringworm and can be applied in poultices for ulcers and piles.

BERRIES
Generally described as "milder" in action to the root, the fresh and dried berries are toxic, so the Appalachian practice of chewing them is not recommended. In the past they were used externally for skin complaints and in poultices for rheumatism. The juice was once used externally for ulcers and tumors but is not particularly effective.

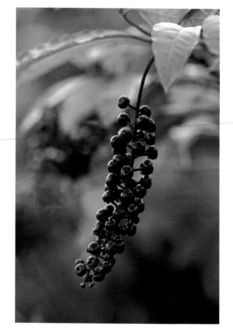

APPLICATIONS

Root

Powder: Can be taken in small doses of 50–250 mg for lymphatic disorders including mastitis, tonsillitis, etc. or for rheumatism. Use a little of the powder as a dust for skin fungal infections, dry eczema, psoriasis or scabies.

Tincture: Use a maximum dose of 1 ml or 20 drops for acute lymphatic congestion and infection including conditions like mastitis, tonsillitis, scrofula, and in glandular fever. Combine with wild indigo, purple coneflower, or cleavers. Can also be added to herbal remedies for rheumatism and rheumatoid arthritis.

Poultice: Use poultices of the dried root or berries on inflamed joints.

Lotion: Use the diluted tincture or powder dispersed in water as a lotion for lymphatic swellings.

CAUTIONS:
- All parts of the fresh plant are toxic and can cause vomiting. Fatalities have been reported in small children who have eaten the berries and care should be taken if growing it in domestic gardens.
- In large doses the dried root is an extremely violent emetic and purgative. Do not exceed stated doses.
- Both fresh and dried berries are toxic.
- Avoid in pregnancy as it can cause fetal abnormalities.

Piper spp.
Pepper

Many forms of pepper are used medicinally, notably black pepper (*P. nigrum*), a common seasoning, and long pepper (*P. longum*), which is known in India as *pippali* and in China as *bi ba*. These peppers originate in the East Indies, but have been imported into Europe since ancient times. Pliny cites numerous uses for pepper, with dill and cabbage, for example, as a cough remedy, while Hildegard of Bingen recommends it with hart's tongue fern (*Scolopendrium vulgare*) and cinnamon as a remedy for strengthening the liver and cleansing the lungs.

Character: Pungent, hot.

Constituents: Alkaloids (including piperine), camphene, beta–bisabolene and other terpenes, proteins, minerals.

Actions: Antiseptic, antibacterial, carminative, digestive and circulatory stimulant; topically rubefacient.

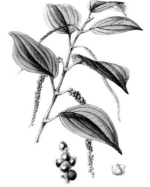

PARTS USED

FRUIT
P. nigrum
Black pepper is an effective warming stimulant for the digestive tract. It was traditionally used in cooking to counter cold, damp vegetables, such as beans, with their tendency to cause flatulence and stomach chills. In China, the herb is known as *hu jiao* and is used as a warming remedy for stomach chills.

ESSENTIAL OIL
P. nigrum
Black pepper oil, made by steam distillation, is used in aromatherapy massage for coughs, chills, digestive upsets aches and pains. It can be irritant in large quantities so needs to be used in moderation.

FRUIT
P. longum
Pippali is used in Ayurveda for strengthening *pitta* and controlling the *vata* and *kapha* humors. It is used in cold conditions affecting the digestive and respiratory systems. It is also regarded as aphrodisiac, strengthening reproductive organs, and is a rejuvenating tonic for the lungs and *kapha*. In China, *bi ba* is also used for abdominal chills and discomfort. It is believed to reverse the upward flow of *qi* to combat nausea and acid regurgitation and is also used as a painkiller for headache, toothache, and sinus pains. A combination of long and black pepper with dry ginger is known in Ayurveda as *trikatu*, or the three spices, and is the main remedy for stimulating *agni*, the digestive fire, to clear *ama* (toxic wastes).

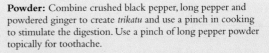

APPLICATIONS

Fruit

P. nigrum
Decoction: Simmer 10 peppercorns and a slice of galangal per cup for nausea, vomiting, diarrhea and abdominal bloating associated with cold and chills.

P. longum
Infusion: Use as a tonic in chronic respiratory problems; in Ayurveda a milk decoction rather than infusion is often used – simmer three pods in a cup of milk and take each morning.
Decoction: Simmer three pods with a slice of galangal and take a cup for stomach chills and diarrhea. Use with a slice of ginger, a small piece of *dang shen*, and a pinch of cinnamon powder for chronic diarrhea associated with cold.

Powder: Combine crushed black pepper, long pepper and powdered ginger to create *trikatu* and use a pinch in cooking to stimulate the digestion. Use a pinch of long pepper powder topically for toothache.

Essential oil

P. nigrum
Massage rub: Use 10 drops of oil in 20 ml of infused cayenne oil (see p. 39) for rheumatic aches and pains associated with cold. Use 1 drop in 5 ml of infused St. John's wort oil for neuralgia and sprains.
Cream: Add 10 drops of oil to 20 g of arnica cream for chilblains (on unbroken skin only).

Piper methysticum
Kava kava

Character: Pungent, bitter, warm.

Constituents: Resin containing kava lactones, glycosides, piperidine alkaloids (including pipermethysticine).

Actions: Analgesic, antispasmodic, antiseptic, sedative, diuretic, tonic, urinary antiseptic, encourages sleep.

Great ritual significance is attributed to kava kava in the South Sea Islands; it is offered in ceremonies to honor guests, used in religious rites, and recommended for an impressive list of ailments. Traditional ritual drinks were made from the macerated root as a calming potion to increase mental awareness, while the leaves, juice, and stumps are all used medicinally. The plant smells slightly of lilac with a pungent taste. It has become heavily commercialized and is regarded rather as a cure-all in North America.

PARTS USED

ROOT

The root is most commonly used. It was traditionally chewed to a pulp, mainly by young girls, which fermented the root with saliva before it was infused in cold water, strained, and served in half coconut shells. Nowadays mechanical grinding is more common and regarded as more hygienic. The root extract is given for urogenital infections, menstrual syndromes, headaches, general debility, colds and chills, chest pains, or as a tonic. Kava is traditionally taken before the evening meal, as a full stomach can reduce the appreciation of its psychoactive properties. The root is usually harvested after three or four years, although some may be grown for up to twenty years before cropping.

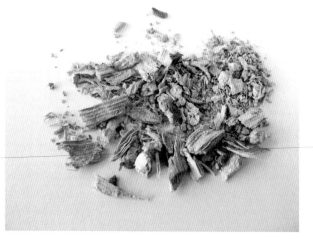

STUMP

In many parts of Polynesia the underground stump of the plant is prepared by chewing and soaking. It is preferred for rheumatic pains, digestive upsets, obesity, asthma, chest infections, and as a poultice for skin diseases. The stump can be up to 60 cm long, while the creeping roots attached to it can reach 3 metres.

LEAVES

The leaves are burned in parts of the South Seas as a general fumigant for infectious diseases, and they were also inserted into the vagina to cause abortion.

APPLICATIONS

Root

Tincture: Use drops doses on the tongue to relieve pain.

Infusion: Drink a cup as a calming sedative, to relieve tension and insomnia. It will also relieve the pain of rheumatic complaints and urinary tract infections. Regular cups will also help in debility and convalescence. High doses of the infusion can induce euphoria although excess will lead to stupor and drowsiness.

Capsules and tablets: Available commercially, use for pains, stress and tension headaches, or to increase resistance to infections.

Mouthwash: Use the infusion as a mouthwash and gargle for toothache and gum disorders.

Wash: Use the infusion as an antiseptic to bathe cuts and grazes.

Stump

Poultice: Use the crushed and soaked root or stump as a poultice for skin infections and suppurating sore.

Juice: Take 5–10 ml per dose for chronic respiratory disorders.

CAUTIONS:

- Kava kava should not be taken in pregnancy or for longer than one month without a break.

- Kava acts as an appetite suppressant and is always followed by a small meal, as overeating after taking the herb can lead to nausea.

Plantago spp.
Plantain

Called waybread by the Anglo-Saxons, common plantain (*P. major*) and was one of the nine sacred herbs given to mankind by Woden. t was considered an important healing herb; Pliny even suggests that if several pieces of flesh are put in a pot with plantain then the herb will join them back together again. Common plantain is still used as a healing astringent to stop both external and internal bleeding while ribwort plantain (*P. lanceolata*) is more often used for catarrhal conditions. The seeds of related species, *P. ovata* and *P. psyllium*, are used as laxatives.

Character: Slightly sweet, salty and bitter, cool and mainly drying.

Constituents
Leaves: Mucilage, glycosides, tannins, minerals;
Seeds: Mucilage, oils, protein, starch.

Actions
Leaves: relaxing expectorant, tonifying to mucous membranes, anti-catarrhal, antispasmodic, topically healing;
Seeds: demulcent, laxative.

PARTS USED

LEAVES
P. major & P. lanceolata
These can both be used to soothe urinary tract infections and irritations and to ease dry coughs. Ribwort leaves are anti-catarrhal and useful in allergic rhinitis, while common plantain leaves tend to be more suitable for gastric inflammations. Both are topically healing for sores and wounds. Harvest throughout the year.

SEEDS
P. psyllium & P. ovata
Both black *P. psyllium* seeds are known as flea seeds while the pink *P. ovata* seeds are ispaghula are used as bulking laxatives for sluggish or irritable bowels. Rich in mucilage their demulcent action is useful for topical wound healing, infections or boils. Harvest when ripe.

P. asiatica
Chinese plantain seed are called *che qian zi* while the aerial parts of the plant are known as *che qian cao*. Both are used much as our ribwort and common plantain herbs as soothing anti-inflammatories, expectorants and for urinary irritations. Like common plantain, *che qian cao* is also diuretic and used for urinary tract infections.

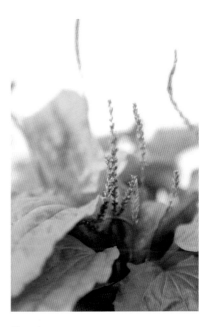

P. major

APPLICATIONS

Leaves
P. major & P. lanceolata
Juice: Pressed from fresh leaves for inflamed mucous membranes in, for example, cystitis, diarrhea, lung infections (e.g. whooping cough). Use 10 ml three times daily.
Infusion: Second best to the juice but suitable for similar conditions.
Tincture (*P. lanceolata*): Make from fresh leaves if possible. Good for catarrhal conditions or where a more astringent effect is needed.
Syrup: Combine honey with the juice or infusion to make a cough syrup useful if the throat is sore or inflamed.
Poultice: Use fresh leaves for slow-healing wounds or chronic ulcers. Apply fresh leaves (*P. major*) to insect stings.

Wash: Use the juice or infusion for inflammations, sores, or wounds.
Ointment (*P. major*): For wounds, burns, and hemorrhoids.
Gargle: Use the infusion or diluted juice for sore throats, mouth or gum inflammations.
P. asiatica
Juice: Pressed from the fresh leaves and used as a diuretic.
Decoction: Unusually in Chinese medicine, *che qian cao* is often used as a simple for lung and urinary infections rather than in complex formulas with other herbs.

Seeds
P. psyllium & P. ovata
Infusion: Pour a cup of boiling water onto a teaspoon of seeds. Allow to cool and then drink the mucilage and seeds as a bulking laxative for constipation. Best taken at night.

Primula spp.
Cowslip and primrose

Cowslips (*P. vera*) take their name from the Anglo-Saxon *cu-sloppe*, a reminder or the days when they bloomed in meadows among the dairy herds. Given their current rarity, primroses (*P. vulgaris*) are now regarded as a good second-best, and the two herbs are used almost interchangeably. The roots, and to a lesser extent the leaves, are rich in saponins, irritant chemicals that have expectorant properties, making them a favorite for chesty coughs. They also contain salicylates so can be helpful for arthritic conditions.

Character: Sweet, dry, and slightly warm.

Constituents: Saponins, glycosides, salicylates, volatile oil, flavonoids.

Actions
Root: Stimulating expectorant, antispasmodic, anti-inflammatory, astringent.
Flowers: Sedative nervine.

Parts Used

Root
Once a popular European standby for arthritis, today, the root is mainly used as an expectorant for stubborn coughs, as in chronic bronchitis. It helps to stimulate and warm the lungs and can be very effective where there is a lot of sticky, white sputum suggesting a "cold" condition. Harvest the roots of established plants in autumn.

Flowers
These contain neither saponins nor salicylates so have markedly different properties from the roots. The petals are very sedating and calming – ideal for over-excited states or what Gerard described as the "frenzies." They also have a diaphoretic and astringent action and can be used for feverish colds with headache and nasal congestion. Harvest in spring.

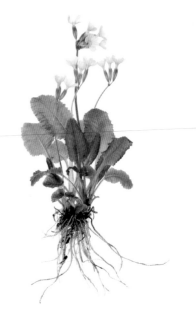

Applications

Root

Decoction: Use a standard dose for stubborn coughs to clear phlegm – especially suitable for chronic bronchitis. The decoction can also be used for arthritic and rheumatism.
Tincture: Use as the decoction – up to 5 ml three times a day.
Compress: A compress soaked in the decoction can be applied to painful arthritic joints.

Flowers

Tincture: Take 5–10 drops for insomnia, anxiety or over-excitement.

Infusion: A standard infusion can be sipped for headaches and feverish chills.
Compress: For facial or trigeminal neuralgia.
Ointment: Traditionally used for sunburn and skin blemishes.
Essential oil: Can be used in ointments and massage oils or 5–10 drops in bath-water at night for insomnia.

Cautions
- High in salicylates so should be avoided by those with sensitivity to aspirin.
- Uterine stimulant so high doses should be avoided in pregnancy.
- Should be avoided by patients on warfarin therapy.

Prunella vulgaris
Self-heal

A highly regarded European wound herb, self-heal is widely used to stop bleeding from "inward and outward wounds." In the past, the flower spikes were considered to resemble to throat and under the doctrine of signatures theory whereby plants cured those parts of the body that they most resembled, so it was used for inflammations of the mouth and throat. In Chinese medicine the flower spikes are known as *xia ku cao*, which translates as "summer dry herb."

Character: Slightly bitter and pungent, cold and drying.

Constituents: Flavonoids (inc. rutin), vitamins A, B, C, K, fatty acids, volatile oil, bitter principle.

Actions
Leaves/aerial parts: Antibacterial, hypotensive, diuretic, astringent, wound herb.
Flower spikes: Liver stimulant. hypotensive, antibacterial, antipyretic.

PARTS USED

AERIAL PARTS
Western herbalists use the leaves and young shoots gathered before flowering to stop bleeding and are applied fresh in poultices as emergency first aid on clean cuts. Culpeper recommended them for "green" (i.e. fresh) wounds, suggesting that they would be ideal to "close the lips of them" in the days before stitches. Harvest before flowering.

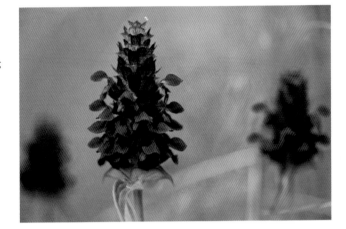

FLOWER SPIKES
In China, *xia ku cao* is regarded as being very specific for the liver and gallbladder: cooling in over-heated conditions and soothing the eyes, which the Chinese traditionally associate with the liver. The Western expression, "gung-ho" is derived from the Chinese for "liver fire" (*gan hao*) and self-heal is ideal for cooling this over-exuberance.

APPLICATIONS

Aerial parts

Tincture: Best made from the fresh plant. Can be used for all sorts of bleeding – including heavy periods, blood in the urine, etc.

Infusion: Use as the tincture, allowing the brew to cool. Can also be helpful as an astringent and bitter herb in diarrhea. the infusion also makes a useful Spring tonic.

Mouthwash: Use a weak infusion or dilute tincture for bleeding gums and mouth inflammations.

Gargle: Use a weak infusion or dilute tincture for sore throats.

Eye bath: Use a very weak, well strained infusion in an eye bath for hot, tired eyes or conjunctivitis.

Poultice: Use the fresh leaves on clean wounds.

Ointment: Can be used for bleeding piles.

Flower spikes

Decoction: Used to clear heat from the liver which may be associated with irritability and anger, over-excitability, high blood pressure, headaches, hyperactivity in children or eye problems. Often combined with *ju hua* (Chinese chrysanthemum flowers).

Prunus spp.
Plum Family

Character: *P. armeniaca*, bitter, slightly warm, toxic; *P. japonica*, pungent, sweet, bitter, neutral; *P. mume*, sour, warm; *P. persica*, sweet, bitter, neutral; *P. serotine*, pungent, astringent, warm, toxic.

Constituents: Amygdalin (cyanogenic glycosides), amygdalase, prunase, salicylates, plant sterols, vitamin C, fruit acids, sugars.

Actions: Most species show antitussive, astringent, antibacterial, analgesic, diuretic, and anti-inflammatory activity.

Many members of the plum family are used in herbal medicine, including wild apricot (*P. armeniaca*), Chinese plums and bush cherries (*P. mume and P. japonica*), peaches (*P. persica*), and wild cherry (*P. serotina*). Seeds, stalks, fruits, bark, and flowers have all been used medicinally, although most of the therapeutic activity is due to cyanogenic glycosides. These chemicals break down in the body to form tiny amounts of cyanide-like compounds, which act as a stimulant for the digestive, respiratory, and nervous systems.

PARTS USED

SEEDS
P. japonica, P. persica, and P. armeniaca
Seeds of Chinese bush cherries (*yu li ren*) are a mild laxative and diuretic used for constipation and fluid retention and will help to reduce blood pressure. Peach seeds (*taoren*) are used to invigorate the blood and circulation, as a mild laxative, and a cough remedy. They are included in many formulas for menstrual problems and constipation due to old age or debility. Wild apricot seeds (*xingren*) are mainly used for respiratory problems such as asthma and bronchitis.

FRUIT
P. armeniaca
Wild apricots are rich in iron and are used in the West in tonic mixtures for anemia and debility.

UNRIPE FRUIT
P. mume
The unripe fruits are used as an expectorant for chronic coughs, for diarrhea and to relieve the symptoms of diabetes. It is also an effective anthelmintic for hookworms.

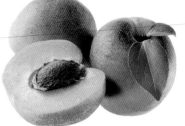

P. armeniaca

BARK
P. serotina
The bark of the North American wild cherry is one of the most widely used cough remedies in Anglo-American herbalism. The tree was popular with many Native American peoples who used the bark to relieve labor pains, diarrhea, eye inflammations, skin sores, and as a pain-killing poultice after amputations. The fruit, leaves, and root bark were also important for treating diarrhea, colds, and stomach upsets, although these parts are rarely used today.

APPLICATIONS

Seeds

P. armeniaca
Tincture: Use 10 drops in 1 teaspoon of mulberry leaf tincture for dry coughs associated with feverish colds.
Decoction: Combine with dang gui for constipation associated with debility and dryness.
P. persica
Tincture: Use with dang gui to stimulate blood and circulation.
Decoction: Use with rhubarb root, liquorice, cinnamon twigs (guizhi) and dang gui for menstrual problems associated with blood stagnation.
P. japonica
Decoction: Use as a gentle laxative for mild constipation.

Fruit

P. armeniaca
Tonic: Simmer 250 g of apricots in 500 ml of water for 8-12 hours or leave in a slow cooker overnight. Remove the stones and blend the mixture in a food processor. Add 500 ml of red wine and 100 ml of dang guitincture and mix well. Take 10 ml twice a day for iron-deficient anaemia.

Unripe Fruit

P. mume
Syrup: Simmer the fruits with water and add sugar to make a syrup for coughs and lung weakness.
Decoction: Use for chronic diarrhea and colitis.

Bark

P. serotina
Tincture: Use 40-80 drops per dose to ease irritant hacking coughs and whooping cough. Combine with mullein or hyssop. Avoid for productive coughs as wild cherry bark acts as a cough suppressant rather than expectorant.
Decoction: Use ½ teaspoon of dried bark per cup and take in ½ cup doses, up to three times daily. Combine with elecampane or liquorice.
Syrup: Use the decoction as a base for syrups.

CAUTIONS
- All *Prunus* spp., especially the seeds, are potentially toxic in high doses because of the cyanogenic glycosides. Use in moderation.
- High doses may also cause drowsiness.
- Do not take wild cherry bark for productive coughs as it acts as a cough suppressant and not an expectorant.

Pueraria lobata
Kudzu

Introduced into the U.S. from Japan in the 1870s as a food, fodder, and fiber crop, by 1945 some 500,000 acres in the Southeast were infested with the vine. Today the plant is described as a "vegetative plague" throughout many of the Southern states and is the subject of a strenuous eradication program. Despite its bad press, kudzu is an important Chinese remedy for fevers, headaches, and heart disease, and it is also effective at combating alcohol addiction.

Character: Sweet, pungent, cool.

Constituents: Isoflavonoids, beta-sitosterol, arachidinic acid, daidzein (estrogenic), genistein, starch.

Actions: Circulatory stimulant, diaphoretic, mild hypotensive, febrifuge, reduces blood sugar.

PARTS USED

ROOT
The root is known as *ge gen* in China and is mainly used for treating "superficial syndromes" associated with colds and chills. It is believed to combat both "wind-cold" and "wind-heat" problems, which are typified by aches and pains, fever, and headaches, as in a severe cold or flu. It is also used for measles and to reduce high blood pressure. In folk tradition, *ge gen* is taken to reduce the effects of alcohol and sober up drunkards. Studies have demonstrated that it will also help to discourage alcohol addiction. It has also been used to treat angina pectoris and sudden deafness.

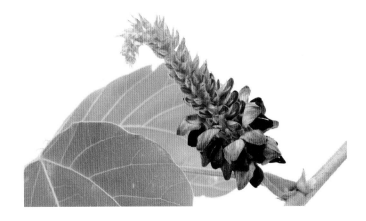

FLOWERS
The flowers (*ge hua*) are used in folk tradition to combat alcoholic poisoning and alcoholism. They are taken for hangovers, and symptoms of nausea and vomiting associated with excess alcohol consumption.

STEMS OR LEAVES
The stems (*ge man*) are used for treating boils and sore throats while a poultice of the leaves (*ge ye*) is a folk remedy used to stop bleeding from knife wounds.

APPLICATIONS

Root

Tincture: Use with half as much each of *huang qin*, licorice and goldenseal for diarrhea associated with food poisoning. Take 5 ml of the mix per dose.

Decoction: Use with cinnamon twigs, ginger and licorice for "wind-cold' syndromes associated with common colds, feverish chills, stiffness in the neck and headaches.

Tincture: Use 10–20 drops in hot water to combat the symptoms of alcohol poisoning.

Juice: Used to reduce severe drunkenness – traditionally enough juice to fill 12 liqueur glasses is needed for the drunkard to regain consciousness.

Tablets/capsules: Used to stimulate and normalize blood flow through the coronary artery in angina pectoris (30–120 mg daily divided into two doses). Tablets containing the equivalent of 5 g of crude root (take two, three times daily) have been successfully used in trials for headaches and sudden deafness associated with spasms of the internal auditory artery.

Powder: Take ½ teaspoon of powder in water for high blood pressure associated with stiff neck and pain.

Flower

Infusion: Drink a cup for nausea and vomiting associated with hangovers.

Rheum palmatum
Rhubarb

Originating from Northwest China and Tibet, rhubarb has been used in medicine for more than 2,000 years. Its use gradually spread through India reaching Europe via Asia Minor, hence its common name of Turkey rhubarb. The plant was a favorite with early Persian and Arabian physicians and was adopted in Europe at the Renaissance. The variety grown for cooking in pies is usually *R. rhabarbarum*, an eighteenth-century cultivar.

Character: Bitter, cold and dry.

Constituents: Anthroquinones, tannins, calcium oxalate, resins, minerals.

Actions: Laxative, digestive remedy, astringent.

PARTS USED

ROOT

This is known as *da huang* in China, which translates literally as "big yellow," an accurate description of the color of rhubarb tinctures and decoctions. It is used in very similar ways in both East and West as a purgative and liver cleanser. Rhubarb root is intrinsically cold, and the Chinese use it to clear pathogenic heat from the stomach and liver in such cases as acute jaundice and appendicitis. It is also added to remedies used to clear heat from the blood and is believed to move stagnant blood. Harvest in winter after the aerial parts have died down.

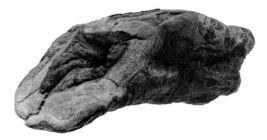

APPLICATIONS

Root

Tincture: The action of rhubarb root varies considerably depending on the dose. Low doses (5–10 drops) are astringent and can be used in diarrhea. A slightly higher dose (1 ml) acts as a good liver stimulant and gentle laxative while very high doses (up to 2.5 ml) have a strong cooling and purgative effect. Use increasing doses of carminatives such as fennel or mint with higher doses of rhubarb to prevent griping pains.

Decoction: A weak decoction (up to 0.5 g of root per dose) can be used for diarrhea while a strong decoction (3 g of root per dose) is effective for chronic constipation or period cramps associated with delayed menstruation.

Wash: Rhubarb root is also antibacterial and astringent and a strong decoction can be used on boils and suppurating skin diseases.

CAUTIONS
- Avoid in pregnancy.
- Contains oxalates – best avoided in arthritic conditions and gout.
- Do not use the leaves which are toxic and can cause fatal oxalate poisoning.

Rosa spp.
Rose

There is a saying that roses are good for "the skin and the soul," and they have a long tradition of medicinal use in all cultures for an enormous variety of ailments. In Roman times the wild or "dog" rose (*R. canina*) was recommended for the bites of rabid dogs. Roses continued as an official medicine well into the 1930s, when tincture of apothecary's rose (*R. gallica* var. *officinalis*) was still prescribed for sore throats. Today roses are still highly prized: the oil is expensive and is one of the most important oils in aromatherapy. The plant was originally held sacred to Venus, but by the Middle Ages it had become symbolically associated with the Virgin Mary.

Character: Sweet, astringent, and generally either neutral or slightly cooling.

Constituents: Volatile oil, vitamins C, B, E and K, tannins. Rose oil contains some 300 chemical constituents of which only around 100 have as yet been identified.

Actions: Antidepressant, antispasmodic, aphrodisiac, astringent, sedative, digestive stimulant, choleretic, cleansing, expectorant, antibacterial, antiviral, antiseptic.

PARTS USED

FRUITS

R. x *laevigata*
In China, the hips from this rose are known as *jin ying zi* and are mainly used as a kidney *qi* tonic prescribed for urinary dysfunction. Like other rose remedies, these are also astringent and are recommended for chronic diarrhea. Harvest when ripe in winter.

R. canina
Valued as an important source of vitamin C during and after the Second World War, rosehips from the dog rose are still used in commercial teas, syrups, and fruit drinks. The leaves were once used as a substitute for tea. Harvest when ripe in winter.

FLOWERS

R. rugosa
The hardy Japanese rose is popular in European gardens, but the Chinese use the flower-buds (*mei gui hua*) as a *qi* stimulant and blood tonic, to relieve stagnant liver energies. They are used for digestive irregularities or with motherwort for heavy periods. Harvest before the flowers are fully open.

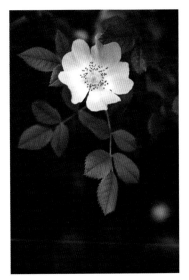

R. canina

ESSENTIAL OIL

R. x *damascena*
Unlike modern hybrid roses the damask rose blooms for only a couple of weeks when the petals are collected and steam distilled to produce true Bulgarian rose oil used in around 96% of all women's perfumes. Medicinally it is an important nervine used for depression and anxiety and can be helpful for those who lack love in their lives. It can be added to many skin remedies or used for digestive problems. Recent research also suggests that the oil has anti-HIV activity.
Rosewater: This is a by-product of the steam distillation of rose oil and is a good skin remedy.

R. centifolia
The cabbage rose is used to produce French rose oil which differs significantly in its chemical composition from the damask rose oil. It contains considerably more phenyl ethanol, for example, which has a narcotic action and could account for the reputation of French rose oil as an aphrodisiac.

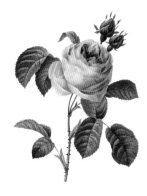

R. centifolia

PETALS

R. gallica var. officinalis
Red rose petals were listed in the official British
Pharmacopoeia until the 1930s when they were widely
as mild astringents and to flavor other medicines.

R. indica
Roses are known as *shatapatra* in Ayurvedic
medicine and are cooling and a good tonic for the
mind. The "temperature" of rose preparations can
be varied in Eastern tradition by leaving them in
moonlight to cool the mixture or in sunshine to
produce a more heating brew.

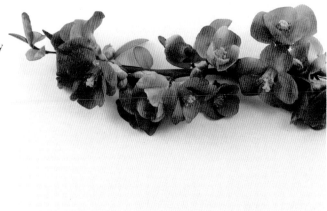

R. rugosa

APPLICATIONS

Essential oil

R. x damascene & R. centifolia
Baths: Add two drops of rose oil to bath-water for depression,
sorrows or insomnia. Massage oil: Use up to 10% rose oil in
a carrier oil to relieve stress and exhaustion or for a sluggish
digestion.
Cream: Add a few drops of rose oil to creams for dry
or inflamed skin conditions. Lotion: Use rosewater with
10% lady's mantle tincture for vaginal itching. The same
combination can be made into a cream using a standard base.
Use 50:50 rosewater and distilled witch-hazel as a cooling,
moisturising lotion for skin prone to spots or acne.

Petals

R. gallica var. officinalis
Tincture: Use up to 3 ml, three times a day for diarrhea or
sluggish digestion. Can be combined with other herbs for
irregular menstruation or heavy periods (such as lady's mantle.
white deadnettle, or shepherd's purse).
Gargle: Use a standard infusion as a gargle for sore throats,
could also be combined with sage.

Flower buds

R. rugosa
Decoction: Use with motherwort for heavy menstrual
bleeding (mild cases). Combine with *bai shao* and *xiang fu* for
liver qi dysfunction.

Fruits

R. canina
Syrup: Used to flavor other medicines and added to cough
mixtures or as a source of vitamin C.
Tincture: Use a standard tincture as an astringent for
diarrhea, to relieve colicky pains, or as a component in cough
remedies.

R. laevigata
Decoction: Use with *dang shen, bai zhu,* and *shan yao* for
chronic diarrhea associated with stomach weakness. Also used
with other herbs for kidney weakness.

CAUTIONS:

- Because of the high price of rose oils adulteration is commonplace and only the best quality, genuine oils should be used medicinally.

- Rose oil is non-toxic and can be taken internally – but seek professional advice first if you are new to herbs.

- Use only the rose species listed here and not garden hybrids.

Rosmarinus officinalis
Rosemary

A favorite herb both medicinally and as a symbol for remembrance, rosemary is a Mediterranean shrub that gradually spread north and was reputedly first grown in England by Philippa of Hainault, wife of Edward III in the fourteenth century. The plant is an excellent tonic and stimulant for the nervous system and has always been regarded as uplifting and energzing. Gerard said that it "comforteth the harte and maketh it merrie."

Character: Warming and dry with a pungent, slightly bitter taste.

Constituents: Volatile oil (inc. borneol), bitter principle, tannin.

Actions: *Leaves/aerial parts*: astringent, digestive remedy, nervine, carminative, antiseptic, diuretic, diaphoretic, antidepressant, circulatory stimulant, antispasmodic, restorative tonic for nervous system; cholagogue, cardiac tonic.
Essential oil: topically – rubefacient, analgesic, antirheumatic.

PARTS USED

LEAVES/AERIAL PARTS
Ideal in exhaustion, debility, and depression, the aerial parts invigorate the circulation, stimulate the digestion and are good in any "cold" conditions including chills and rheumatism. They are useful for headaches that are eased by warm towels rather than ice packs. It is evergreen and can be gathered fresh throughout the year although avoid cutting in frosty conditions.

ESSENTIAL OIL
This makes a good stimulating rub for arthritic conditions and has also traditionally been used for hair problems – to stimulate growth in premature baldness and restore the color to gray hair. Extracts are a common ingredient in commercial shampoos.

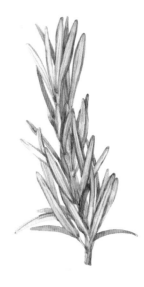

APPLICATIONS

Leaves and aerial parts

Infusion: For colds and flu or for rheumatic pains use a standard infusion and drink while hot. Also as a general stimulating drink for fatigue or headaches. Also has a gentle carminative action for indigestion.

Hair rinse: Use an infusion as the final rinse for dandruff.

Compress: A pad soaked in hot rosemary infusion can be used for sprains. Alternate 2–3 minutes of the hot compress with 2–3 minutes applying an ice pack to the injury.

Tincture: Use whenever a stimulant tonic is needed (up to 5 ml three times a day). Combines well with oats, skullcap, or vervain in depression.

Essential oil

Massage rub: For arthritis and rheumatism dilute 1 ml of rosemary oil in 25 ml of sunflower or almond oil and massage a little into aching joints and muscles. The same oil can be massaged into the scalp to stimulate hair growth or used on the temples for headaches.

Baths: Use 10 drops of oil in the bath for aching limbs or as a stimulant in nervous exhaustion.

Rubus idaeus
Raspberry

The raspberry plant was a favorite household remedy with raspberry vinegars used for sore throats or to "cut the phlegm" in coughs; the leaves were used in infusions for diarrhea or as poultices for piles; and raspberry syrup was used to prevent a build up of tartar on teeth. Gerard considered the fruit "of a temperate heat" and so it was easier on the stomach than strawberries which could cause excess phlegm and chilling. Today raspberry leaf tea is still taken to prepare for childbirth.

Character: Dry and astringent with a generally cooling nature.

Constituents: *Leaves*: fragarine (uterine tonic), tannins, polypeptides; *Fruit*: vitamins A, B, C and E, sugars, minerals, volatile oil.

Actions: Astringent, partus preparator, stimulant, digestive remedy, tonic, diuretic, laxative.

PARTS USED

LEAVES

Used for period cramps and discomfort, the leaves, taken during late pregnancy, also help to prepare the womb for childbirth. They are also astringent so are useful for diarrhea, wounds, sore throats, and mouth ulcers. They have also been used as a cleansing diuretic, included in rheumatic remedies, and in France they are regarded as a tonic for the prostate. Harvest in summer before and during fruiting.

BERRIES

Traditionally recommended for indigestion and rheumatism, the berries are rich in vitamins and minerals and highly nutritious. The juice has been used in folk medicine as a cooling remedy in for fevers, childhood illnesses, and cystitis. Harvest when ripe in summer or autumn.

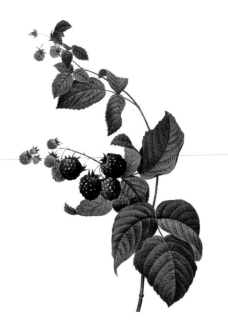

APPLICATIONS

Leaves

Infusion: To ease childbirth, take one cup daily of the standard infusion in the last six to eight weeks of pregnancy and drink plenty of the warm tea during labor. The infusion can also be used for mild diarrhea.

Mouthwash: Use a standard infusion for mouth ulcers or as a gargle for sore throats.

Wash: The infusion can be used for bathing wounds or regularly on varicose ulcers and sores. In eye baths it can ease conjunctivitis and other eye inflammations.

Tincture: This is more astringent than the infusion and is useful, diluted, on wounds or inflammations or used as a mouthwash for ulcers or gum inflammations.

Berries

Vinegar: Steep 500 g fruit in 1 liter of wine or cider vinegar for two weeks to produce a thick red liquid that can be added to cough mixtures as an expectorant or used in gargles for sore throats. It tastes quite pleasant and can help disguise the flavor of other herbal expectorants.

CAUTIONS:

• Avoid raspberry leaf tea in early pregnancy as it can stimulate the uterus.

Salix alba
Willow

In traditional herbal medicine, white willow was classified as a cool, moist plant and was widely used for fevers and other "hot" conditions. It was one of the first herbs to be scientifically investigated, and in the nineteenth century a French chemist, Leroux, extracted the active constituent and named it salicine. By 1852 this same chemical was being produced synthetically, and by 1899 a less irritant and unpleasant tasting variant of this substance (acetylsalicylic acid) was manufactured and marketed as aspirin; the first of the modern generation of plant-derived drugs.

Character: Cool and dry with a slightly bitter taste.

Constituents: Salicin, tannins, flavonoids, glycosides.

Actions: Antirheumatic, anti-inflammatory, antipyretic, anti-hydrotic, analgesic, antiseptic, astringent, bitter digestive tonic.

PARTS USED

BARK
In modern herbal medicine only the bark is used. It is prescribed for many inflammatory conditions, including rheumatism and arthritis. It was popular in fever management and can relieve neuralgia, headaches and pains in general. As a gentle bitter it also acts as a mild digestive stimulant and is used for gastro-enteritis and diarrhea related to heat and inflammation. Harvest in autumn or winter, taking only a little from each tree.

LEAVES
In the past, the leaves were a popular home remedy used much as the bark is today. Willow leaf tea was used in fevers or colicky pains and the infusion was also used as a rinse for dandruff.

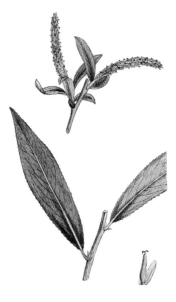

APPLICATIONS

Bark
Fluid extract: Stronger than a standard tincture and it is generally used for rheumatic conditions in standard doses. It can also be used for headaches and neuralgia.

Tincture: Use up to 15 ml doses for fevers. Combine with other suitable herbs – such as boneset, elder, or bitters.

Powder: The powdered root can be used in doses of up to 10 g for fevers and headaches. Take mixed with a teaspoon of honey.

Decoction: Use standard doses for feverish chills, headaches or as part of arthritic treatments.

Leaves
Infusion: Use a standard infusion after meals for digestive problems.

CAUTIONS:
- Avoid in aspirin allergy.

Salvia officinalis
Sage

Traditionally associated with longevity, sage has a reputation for restoring failing memory in the elderly. Like other herbs associated with memory it was also planted on graves. It is said that when the British started importing tea from China, the Chinese so valued the herb that they would exchange two cases of tea for one of dried English sage leaves. Green sage (*S. officinalis*) is often mixed with Greek sage (*S. fruticosa*), although the two have very similar properties. Purple sage (*S. officinalis* Purpurescens Group) is preferred by some herbalists instead.

PARTS USED

LEAVES
S. officinalis & S. officinalis Purpurescens Group
Sage has a special affinity with the mouth and throat, making it ideal as a gargle and mouthwash. Its antiseptic property is attributed to thujone found in the essential oil, which is highly antibacterial. It is also a good bitter digestive stimulant and its drying property, coupled with the estrogenic action, make it a useful herb both for menopausal problems and at weaning. Sage is strongly antioxidant to reduce symptoms of ageing; extracts have been used to relieve Alzheimer's and senile dementia. Harvest throughout the summer and autumn.

ROOT
S. miltiorrhiza
In China, the root, known as *dan shen*, is primarily regarded as "moving blood" and is used wherever there is stagnation or stasis, as in some types of menstrual pain and heart conditions. It is also considered sedative and cooling to reduce heat, particularly in the heart and liver, conditions that the Chinese associate with symptoms such as insomnia, palpitations, and irritability.

Character: Pungent, bitter, slightly cold, and drying.

Constituents
Leaves (*S. officinalis*): volatile oil (includes thujone, linalool, and borneol); bitter, tannins, triterpenoids, flavonoids, estrogenic substances, resin, saponins;
Root (*S. miltiorrhiza*): ketones, vitamin E.

Actions
S. officinalis Leaves: Carminative, antispasmodic, astringent and healing to mucosa, antiseptic, peripheral vasodilator, suppresses perspiration, reduces salivation and lactation, uterine stimulant, systemically antibiotic, hypoglycemic, cholagogue.
Essential oil: Antiseptic, antispasmodic, astringent, hypertensive, stimulant, emmenagogue, antioxidant.
S. miltiorrhiza: Circulatory stimulant used to move blood, sedative, clears pathogenic heat.

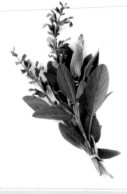

APPLICATIONS

Leaves

S. officinalis & S. officinalis Purpurescens Group
Infusion: Use 20 g to 50 ml water as a general tonic. Also as a liver stimulant and to improve digestive function and circulation in debilitated conditions. Can also be used to reduce lactation at weaning and for night sweats and other menopause symptoms.
Gargle/mouthwash: Use a weak infusion as a gargle for sore throats, tonsillitis, quinsy, or as mouthwash for mouth ulcers, gingivitis, and similar problems.
Tincture: Used in menopausal remedies for night sweats and as a digestive stimulant. Also used to reduce salivation in Parkinsonism, giving symptomatic relief.
Cream: Popular in France to treat minor skin sores, grazes, and insect bites.
Hair rinse: For dandruff or to restore the color to gray hair.

Root
S. miltiorrhiza
Decoction: For menstrual pain caused by stagnation; also used in Chinese medicine for angina pectoris and coronary heart disease

CAUTIONS:
- Do not take therapeutic doses of sage leaf in pregnancy.
- *Dan shen* should only be used where the condition is caused by blood stasis. Seek professional help for all heart disorders.
- *S. officinalis* contains thujone which can trigger fits in epileptics who should avoid large amounts of the herb. *S. fruticosa* contains significantly less thujone so should be used in preference.

Sambucus nigra
Elder

A wealth of folklore is associated with the elder, which is often described as a "complete medical chest" because of its numerous therapeutic and prophylactic qualities. Classed as "hot and dry" by Galen, the herb was used for cold, damp conditions such as catarrh, excessive mucous or water retention. In the seventeenth century, it was a favorite for "clearing phlegm," both as an expectorant for coughs and as a diuretic and violent purgative. Elderflower water was a favorite in the eighteenth century for whitening the skin and removing freckles.

PARTS USED

FLOWERS
These are anti-catarrhal and encourage sweating so are ideal for feverish colds and influenza. They are also helpful for hay fever, taken as a prophylactic early in the year to strengthen the upper respiratory tract before the pollen count rises. Topically, they are anti-inflammatory, used in skin creams and for chilblains. Harvest in early summer.

BARK
Warming in character, the bark is an effective liver stimulant taken in the past for stubborn constipation, fluid retention, gout and arthritic conditions. Harvest the inner layer of bark in autumn from young trees.

LEAVES
The leaves were once popular in green elder ointment, known officially as *unguentum sambuci viride*, used for bruises, sprains, wounds and hemorrhoids. Harvest in summer after flowering.

BERRIES
The berries were once an important source of vitamin A and C. In the days before imported winter fruits, elderberry wines and syrups were a useful prophylactic against seasonal colds. Harvest in autumn when ripe.

Character: Mainly bitter and drying – flowers and berries also cool and slightly sweet; bark is hot.

Constituents: Volatile oil, flavonoids, mucilage, tannins, vitamins A & C, cyanogenic glycoside, viburnic acid, alkaloid.

Actions: *Flowers:* expectorant, anti-catarrhal, circulatory stimulant, diaphoretic, diuretic; locally – anti-inflammatory.
Berries: diaphoretic, diuretic, laxative.
Bark: internally – strong purgative, emetic (in large doses), diuretic; externally – softening.
Leaves: externally – softening, wound-healing; internally – purgative, expectorant, diuretic, diaphoretic.
Root: violent emetic and purgative (not used nowadays).

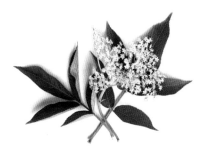

APPLICATIONS

Flowers

Infusion: Drink hot for feverish and catarrhal conditions involving the lungs or upper respiratory tract (including hay fever); can be combined with yarrow, boneset, and peppermint in equal proportions.
Gargle: Use a standard infusion as a mouthwash and gargle for mouth ulcers, sore throats, tonsillitis.
Eye bath: Use a cold, well-strained infusion for inflamed or sore eyes.
Tincture: Use a standard infusion for colds and flu or take from February to April to help reduce hay fever symptoms.

Bark

Decoction: Use 10 g to 800 ml water for stubborn constipation or as a general digestive cleanser, also for chronic gout and arthritis.

Leaves

Ointments: For bruises, sprains, wounds, chilblains or hemorrhoids.

Berries

Syrup: As a prophylactic for winter colds or in combination with expectorants (e.g. thyme) for coughs.
Tincture: Can be useful in combination with other herbs for rheumatic conditions.

CAUTIONS:
- The bark should be avoided in pregnancy and standard doses should not be exceeded.
- The root can be a violent purgative and emetic and should not be used.
- For home use, the leaves should only be used externally, but the berries and flowers are safe in long-term use.
- The plant should be avoided if further drying or fluid depletion would worsen the condition.

Scrophularia spp.
Figwort

In both Eastern and Western traditions, figwort (*S. nodosa*) is a very cleansing herb: it was known as the scrofula plant – hence its botanical name – and used to treat abscesses, purulent wounds and the "king's evil" or scrofula (tuberculosis of the lymph nodes). Culpeper called the herb "throatwort" because of its use in treating this disease. The Chinese use a related species (*S. ningpoensis*) known as *xuan shen*, as a prime remedies for "fire poisons," the same sort of purulent conditions associated with it in the West.

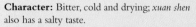

Character: Bitter, cold and drying; *xuan shen* also has a salty taste.

Constituents: *S. nodosa*: Saponins, cardioactive glycosides, alkaloids, flavonoids, bitters; *S. ningpoensis*: Saponins, phytosterol, essential fatty acids, asparagine.

Actions: *Aerial parts* (*S. nodosa*): diuretic, laxative, heart stimulant, circulatory stimulant, anti-inflammatory, diuretic, laxative; *Root* (*S. ningpoensis*): tonic, antipyretic, anti-inflammatory, antibacterial, heart tonic, hypotensive, sedative.

PARTS USED

AERIAL PARTS
S. nodosa
Best known for treating skin problems, the aerial parts are used for cleansing. For example, in rheumatic disorders and gout; when there is stagnation in the lymphatic system; or for a sluggish digestion with constipation. Harvest in summer after flowering.

ROOT
S. ningpoensis
Also used as a cleansing plant, but it has a more relaxing action on the heart than *S. nodosa*, reducing blood pressure and with a slight sedating effect. It also replenishes *jing* or "vital essence" – one of the fundamental substances which traditional Chinese medicine believes underlies all life.

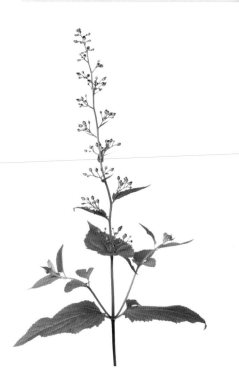

APPLICATIONS

Aerial parts
S. nodosa
Infusion: Use whenever there is a build-up of toxins to cleanse – in rheumatic conditions, lymphatic disorders, or for skin conditions like eczema and psoriasis.
Tincture: In combination with other digestive herbs for constipation and sluggishness or with herbs like yellow dock, bitter sweet, or burdock in skin conditions.
Wash: Use the infusion for eczema, skin inflammations, fungal infections, etc.

Compress: Use a pad soaked in the infusion for painful swellings, wounds, ulcers, etc.

Root
S. ningpoensis
Decoction: For deep-seated abscesses and lymphatic swellings. Also for throat problems – swollen glands, tonsillitis, etc. As *yin* tonic it is used with salt.

CAUTIONS:
• Figwort is a heart stimulant; avoid in cases of abnormally raised heartbeat.

Scutellaria spp.
Skullcap

A comparative newcomer to the European *materia medica*, Virginian skullcap was used by Native Americans for rabies and to promote menstruation. It is characterized by its dish shaped seed-pods and flowers grow on only one side of the stem, hence its botanical name *S. lateriflora*. Today it is considered as one of the best herbal nervines – sedative, tonic, and antispasmodic. The Chinese plant, *S. baicalensis* (*huang qin*), is very different and mainly used for the stomach and lung problems.

Character: Bitter, cold, and drying.

Constituents
Aerial parts (*S. lateriflora*): Flavonoids, tannins, bitter, volatile oil, minerals;
Root (*S. baicalensis*): Flavonoids, sitosterols.

Actions
S. lateriflora: Relaxing and restorative nervine, antispasmodic;
S. baicalensis: Antibacterial, antipyretic, diuretic, antispasmodic, cholagogue.

USED

AERIAL PARTS
S. lateriflora
Calming for many nervous conditions, such as tension, excitability, insomnia, and depression, the herb also has a tonic effect on the central nervous system making it ideal in nervous exhaustion. It can also be helpful in premenstrual tension and has been used for epilepsy. Harvest late in the flowering period when some of the characteristic skullcap-shaped seed pods have formed.

ROOTS
S. baicalensis
In China *huang qin* is mainly used to clear heat from the respiratory and digestive systems and is used in diarrhea, jaundice, gastro-enteritis, or bronchitis, for example. It can also be useful in urinary tract infections and for skin infections. It is believed to contain high levels of melatonin which help combat insomnia and chronic headaches. Korean research suggests it may reduce the risk of gum and tooth disease.

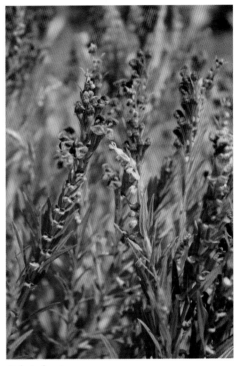

S. baicalensis

APPLICATIONS

Aerial parts
S. lateriflora
Infusion: Use the fresh herb if possible as a calming tea in nervous exhaustion, excitability, over-anxiety, etc. The tea can also be helpful for PMT or taken – combined with wild lettuce or passionflower – at night for insomnia.
Tincture: Best made from the fresh herb and a very potent calming nervine. Take 5 ml as a simple or combine with lemon balm (1 ml) for any nervous stresses or depression.

Root
S. baicalensis
Decoction: Usually in combination with other cold, bitter herbs to purge heat from the system in gastric, chest, and urinary infections. Also combined with other herbs to reduce high blood pressure.

Senna alexandrina
Senna

For centuries, senna leaves and pods have been used as a potent laxative. In China, the leaves are known as *fan xie ye*, while in Sanskrit the plant is called *rajavriksha*, meaning "king of trees." When using senna in herbal remedies, it is best to start with low doses of the pods, which are milder than the strongly purgative leaves, and move on to the leaves if need be. Today the herb is commonly found in many over-the-counter remedies.

Character: Bitter, sweet, cold.

Constituents: Sennosides (rhein-dianthrone diglucosides), monoanthraquinone glycosides, dianthrone diglycosides, aglycones, flavonoids.

Actions: Stimulating laxative, cooling, antibacterial, anthelmintic.

Parts Used

Leaves
Generally, the leaves are used in infusions, powders, or tablets. They irritate the digestive tract and encourages peristalsis so long-term, habitual use can weaken the digestive system. Senna should be avoided if there is inflammation in the gut, as in Crohn's disease or ulcerative colitis. Senna produces a soft stool so it is used where there are problems with bleeding piles or anal fissures. The Chinese use dried senna leaf as a cooling remedy to clear heat from the digestive system, which can lead to abdominal bloating and discomfort, as well as a purgative for habitual constipation. In India, senna is also used to clear *pitta* and as a cooling and cleansing remedy for skin inflammations, obesity, and hypertension associated with that humor.

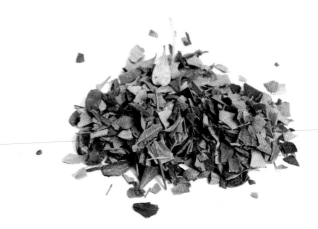

Pods
Senna pods are rather milder than the leaves and are generally preferred by Western practitioners. Pods are often classified as "Alexandrian senna" (*Cassia senna*) or "Tinnevelly senna" (*Cassia angustifolia*) although botanists now regard these as the same species renamed *S. alexandrina*.

Applications

Pods
Infusion: The usual recommendation is 15–30 mg per dose, which generally means 3–6 pods. Leave the pods in a cup of warm water overnight and drink first thing in the morning. Add a slice of fresh ginger root or a teaspoon of fennel seeds to the maceration to help combat any griping pains which may be caused by increase in peristalsis.

Tablets/powders: Many commercial preparations are available: the usual dose is 1–2 teaspoons of granules or 2–4 tablets, taken in the morning.

Leaves
Tincture: 10–30 drops per dose; taken in the morning with a little water.

Infusion: Use ½ teaspoon of dried leaf with 1 teaspoon of fennel seeds per cup of boiling water for severe constipation. Do not continue for more than seven days and ensure a break of at least two weeks before repeating the treatment.

CAUTIONS:
- Do not take senna in pregnancy, while breastfeeding or in cases if inflammatory bowel disease.

Silybum marianum
Milk thistle

Milk thistle, or Mary thistle, takes its name from its traditional use in stimulating milk flow in nursing mothers. The plant is another example of the medieval doctrine of signatures with its white-streaked leaves said to symbolise splashes of milk. Milk thistle was once cultivated as a vegetable with the flower heads eaten like globe artichokes, the young leaves as spinach, and the root as salsify. Today it is regarded as one of our most important liver tonics and restoratives.

Character: Bitter, astringent, warm.

Constituents: Flavo-lignans (including silymarin), bitters.

Actions: Bitter tonic, stimulates bile flow, antidepressant, antioxidant, antiviral, stimulates milk flow.

PARTS USED

SEEDS

The seeds are rich in silymarin, which research studies since the 1970s have identified as being highly protective for the liver, helping to combat damage from pollutants and toxins. Extracts of silymarin have been used to treat liver cirrhosis and hepatitis, while taking milk thistle seeds is an effective way to prevent damaging the liver in alcohol abuse. The seeds can also help reduce high cholesterol levels and soothe inflammations of the gallbladder. Studies have also shown that milk thistle is a more powerful antioxidant than vitamin E so can help prevent damage to tissues caused by free radicals.

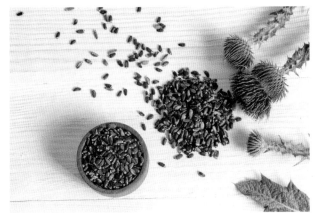

LEAVES

The leaves were traditionally used for stimulating milk flow and to ease menstrual problems. They can also be used in infusions to help stimulate the digestion. Harvest before flowering.

FLOWER HEADS

Like globe artichokes, milk thistle flower heads, eaten before the flowers open, make as a bitter-tasting vegetable that will also stimulate the liver and digestive system.

APPLICATIONS

Seeds

Tincture: Take 20–50 drops on a little water for liver and gallbladder problems or to stimulate the digestion. Take up to 5 ml daily in water as a preventative if there is a history of gall stones or liver disease: combine with an equal amount of dandelion root tincture. Instead of water, you can also add the tincture to a cup of peppermint infusion as a digestive tonic.

Capsules: Use 1–2 x 200 mg capsules to combat symptoms of a hangover or before drinking alcohol to reduce the risk of liver damage. Regular capsules can help combat the liver damage caused by drug and alcohol abuse.

Powder: Use topically to dust varicose ulcers.

Infusion: Drink a cup for any liver and gallbladder weakness: combines well with vervain. Use with lady's mantle and St. John's wort for premenstrual syndrome.

Leaves/Flower Heads

Infusion: Drink a cup to stimulate milk production when breastfeeding. Also helps to stimulate digestive function.

Solanum lycopersicum
Tomato

Spanish conquistadors introduced tomatoes into Europe from Peru in the fifteenth century. The first tomatoes to arrive were yellow in color, hence the Italian name *pomodoro*, or "golden apples." By the time the fruit arrived in Britain in the sixteenth century, via France, this had been corrupted to *pommes d'amours*, giving the old English name "love apples." The fruits were originally thought to be highly poisonous, as tomatoes are a member of the Solanaceae family and the flowers are similar to those of its relative, deadly nightshade (*Atropa belladonna*).

Character: Cold, sour, sweet.

Constituents: Vitamins A, B1, B2, B6 C, E, folic acid, malic acid, citric acid, bioflavonoids (including rutin), calcium, magnesium, phosphorous.

Actions: Antiscorbutic, antimicrobial, diuretic, mild laxative, digestive stimulant, reduces acidity in the blood.

PARTS USED

FRESH FRUIT
The fruit of the tomato is rich in nutrients: 100g provides the necessary daily intake of vitamins A, B1, C, and folic acid. It also contains rutin, so it can help to strengthen the capillaries. Research in the U.S. suggests that men who eat at least 10 servings of tomatoes a week have a 45% reduction in the risk of prostate cancer. This is probably due to the presence of lycopene, a type of carotene, which may be antitumor. Lycopene is also believed to reduce the risk of heart disease – one study suggests by as much as 50%.

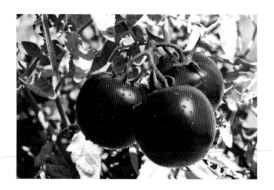

JUICE
Drinking tomato juice before a meal makes a good aperitif to stimulate the digestion, particularly the pancreas. It is an ideal tonic in debility and convalescence and makes an effective lotion for acne. A pilot study suggests a daily glass is as effective as vitamin D or calcium in preventing osteoporosis in postmenopausal women.

LEAVES
Hanging bunches of tomato leaves above the bed is at traditional way to deter mosquitoes and gnats at night.

APPLICATIONS

Juice

Plain Juice: Drink three glasses of juice each day as a restorative tonic during debility and convalescence. Drink a glass before meals to stimulate the digestion.

Lotion: Mix 100 ml of tomato juice with 50 ml of vodka or other strong alcohol and shake well. Use as a lotion to help prevent acne.

Poultice: Use chopped fresh tomatoes as a face pack to clear acne pustules. Leave for half an hour and then rinse with clean water.

Leaves

Fresh: Rub crushed leaves on insect bites to relieve itching and discomfort.

Fruit

Cooked fruit: Cooking tomatoes make the lycopene easier to absorb. Use tomatoes daily in sauces, casseroles, and stews as a preventative for prostate cancer and heart disease.

Fresh fruit: Eat fresh tomatoes to ease arthritis, rheumatism, and gout: the plant is oxalate free and will clear uric acid and toxins from the system.

Stachys officinalis
Wood betony

Wood betony was the most important herb in the Anglo-Saxon repertoire, wood betony had around thirty uses listed in the *Leech Book of Bald*. As well as internal and external applications, it was possibly the most popular amulet herb, used well into the Middle Ages to ward off evil or ill humors. Gerard, in 1597, gives a very long list of applications, adding that "it maketh a man to pisse well." Today, wood betony is neglected by many herbalists; it is, however, very well worth rediscovering.

Character: Cool, drying and with a bitter-sweet taste.

Constituents: Alkaloids (inc. stachydrine and trigonelline), tannins, saponins.

Action: Sedative, bitter digestive remedy, nervine, circulatory tonic particularly for cerebral circulation, astringent.

Parts Used

Aerial parts
Mainly used for headaches and nervous disorders, the herb is also a good digestive remedy – stimulating and cleansing for the system – with a mild diuretic action. It can be used as a pain killer and wound herb and may be helpful for catarrh and coughs. Harvest in summer while flowering.

Root
Although not commonly used nowadays, betony root is regarded as more bitter and specific for the liver with a gentle laxative action. Harvest in early autumn.

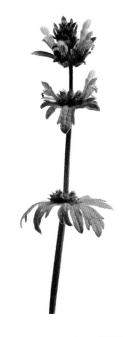

Applications

Aerial parts

Infusion: Use in low doses (1 teaspoon per cup) as a general relaxing and tonic herb for everyday drinking. In therapeutic doses it can be used for menstrual pain, migraines, and other headaches, nervous tension, as a digestive stimulant and cleanser. Combine with elderflower or yarrow and drink hot at the onset of colds or flu. The hot infusion can also be drunk during difficult or painful labor.

Tincture: Use as the infusion. Especially helpful for nervous headaches when it combines well with lavender. For catarrhal conditions use with ground ivy or coltsfoot. Also useful as a cleansing herb in toxic and arthritic conditions.

Poultice: For wounds and bruises.

Tonic wine: Macerate 50 g of betony with 25 g each of vervain and hyssop in 750 ml of white wine for two weeks. Use for nervous headaches and tension in liqueur glass doses.

Mouthwash: Use an infusion for mouth ulcers and gum inflammations. Also as a gargle for sore throats.

Wash: Use an infusion for leg ulcers and infected wounds.

CAUTIONS:
- Uterine stimulant; avoid high doses during pregnancy but drink betony tea during labor.

Stellaria spp.
Chickweed

Character: Sweet, moist, and cool.

Constituents: Mucilage, saponins, silica, minerals, vitamins A, B and C, fatty acids.

Action: Astringent, antirheumatic, wound herb, demulcent.

As the name suggests, chickweed is a favorite with small birds and in Gerard's day chickweed (*S. media*) was given as a tonic to caged linnets. It is probably one of the most common weeds, growing in virtually all corners of the world. Instead of rooting it out, it is worth remembering that chickweed was once gathered as a vegetable. It was also used to heal wounds and in poultices for drawing boils. can should be sweated without water like spinach and served with butter or used as a salad herb. In China, the root of close relative *S. dichotoma*, or *yin chai hu*, is used.

PARTS USED

AERIAL PARTS
S. media
Made into creams, the aerial parts are used today for eczema and skin irritations. In mainland Europe, the plant is generally taken internally as a cleansing diuretic and tonic used for rheumatic pains and debilitated conditions. Harvest throughout the growing season.

ROOT
S. dichotoma
In China *yin chai hu* is used as a cooling herb in fevers and also to stop nose bleeds, heavy menstrual bleeding, and similar bleeding disorders. It is also given as a tonic for malnourished children reflecting its European use as an emergency free food in poor country districts.

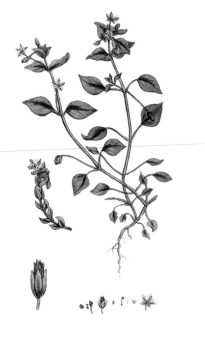

APPLICATIONS

Aerial parts

S. media
Infusion: Use the fresh herb, if possible, to produce a tonic, cleansing mixture for tiredness and debility. Also helpful for urinary tract inflammations such as cystitis.
Poultice: Use the fresh plant for boils and abscesses; also for rheumatic pain.
Tincture: Can be added to remedies for rheumatism.
Compress: Use the hot decoction or soak a hot pad in the tincture for rheumatic pains.

Cream: Used for eczema – especially if it is itching.
Infused oil: Use the cold infusion method for fresh herb or the hot method for dried, either can be used as an alternative to creams for irritant skin rashes or add 1 tablespoon to the bath-water for eczema sufferers.

Root

S. dichotoma
Decoction: Use for hot fevers related to weakness in chronic illness.

Symphytum officinale
Comfrey

A country name for comfrey is knitbone, a reminder of its traditional use in healing fractures. The herb contains allantoin, which encourages bone, cartilage, and muscle cells to grow: the chemical is absorbed through the skin and speeds up healing. Poultices of the leaves were once regularly spread on broken limbs. The botanical name is derived from the Greek *sympho*, meaning to unite, and in the past comfrey baths were popular before marriage in the belief that they would repair the hymen and restore "virginity" before the wedding night.

Character: Cool and moist with a sweet taste.

Constituents: Mucilage, steroidal saponins, allantoin (mainly flowering tops), tannin, pyrrolizidine alkaloids (mainly root), inulin, vitamin B12, protein.

Actions: Cell proliferator, astringent, demulcent, wound herb, expectorant.

PARTS USED

AERIAL PARTS
Rich in allantoin, the flowering tops and leaves are mainly used externally in ointments and infused oils for sprains, arthritic joints, and other injuries. Internally the plant is equally healing and is used for ulceration in the digestive tract. Harvest in summer.

ROOT
This has similar properties to the leaves but is more mucilaginous. It should only be used externally because of the high pyrrolizidine alkaloid content. Harvest in spring or autumn when the allantoin levels are highest.

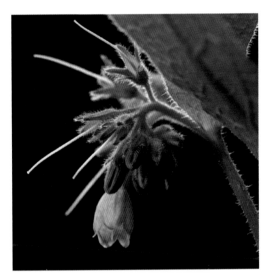

APPLICATIONS

Aerial parts
Tincture: Use a standard dose internally for gastric ulceration, oesophagitis, hiatus hernia and ulcerative colitis. Treatment should not be continued beyond 6–8 weeks because of the potential risk of liver damage due to pyrrolizidine alkaloids.
Infused oil: Make by the hot infusion method and use as a massage for arthritic joints, sprains, bruises, and other traumatic injuries. Can also be used for inflamed bunions.
Compress: Soak a pad in the diluted tincture for bruises, sprains and other painful injuries
Cream: For any bone, cartilage, or muscle damage. For osteoarthritis apply cream twice daily for at least two months.
Syrup: Sweeten 500 ml of the infusion with 500 g of honey for dry coughs or stubborn, thick, phlegm.
Poultice: Use the puréed leaves on minor breaks that would not normally be set in plaster – such as broken toes, ribs, or hairline cracks in larger bones.

Root
Poultice: Make a paste of powdered root with a little water and use on varicose ulcers and other stubborn wounds. The same paste can be used on bleeding hemorrhoids.

CAUTIONS:
- Only take internally under professional guidance; the plant contains pyrrolizidine alkaloids which have been linked by some researchers to liver cancer in rats whose diets were composed of 33% comfrey leaf. Do not take the root internally.
- Do not use on dirty wounds as rapid healing may lead to trapped dirt.
- Use is restricted in Australia, New Zealand, Canada, and Germany.

Tanacetum parthenium
Feverfew

Character: Bitter, warm, and drying.

Constituents: Sesquiterpene lactones, parthenolides, volatile oil, pyrethrin, tannins.

Actions: Anti-inflammatory, vasodilator, relaxant, digestive stimulant, emmenagogue, anthelmintic.

In the 1980s, feverfew was hailed as a "cure" and prophylactic for migraine thanks to the parthenolides it contains, but although there is a tradition of using the plant for headaches this was largely in external applications as the herb's bitterness was regarded as potentially damaging if taken internally. Frying the herb first was said to make it more palatable for internal medicinal use. The name feverfew is a corruption of featherfew, a description of its fine petals.

PARTS USED

AERIAL PARTS

In the past, feverfew was primarily known as a woman's herb for womb disorders or delayed menstruation. It was mainly used externally in poultices or "squatting inhalations" (where the woman crouches over a bowl of the steaming decoction, absorbing the herb into the vagina). Today it is mainly used for migraines and, as an anti-inflammatory, is also recommended by some for rheumatoid arthritis. Harvest in summer before flowering.

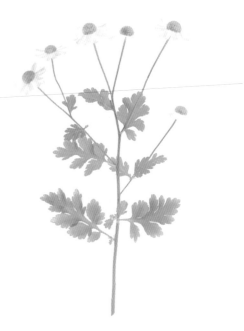

APPLICATIONS

Aerial parts

Fresh herb: Eat one leaf daily as a prophylactic against migraines.

Tincture: Use 5–10 drops at 30 minute intervals at the onset of migraines. It is best for "cold" type migraines involving vasoconstriction and eased by applying a hot towel to the head. For the acute stages of rheumatoid arthritis add up to 2 ml of tincture, three times a day to other herbal remedies.

Poultice: Use the hot herb fried in a little oil as an abdominal poultice for colicky pains.

Infusion: Drink a weak infusion (15 g to 500 ml of water) after childbirth to encourage cleansing and tonifying of the womb; also for menstrual pain associated with sluggish flow and congestion.

CAUTIONS:
- Mouth ulcers are a common side-effect of eating fresh leaves.
- The herb has a salicylate-like anti-prostaglandin action and it should be avoided by patients on warfarin, heparin and other blood-thinning drugs as it can affect blood clotting rates.

Taraxacum officinale
Dandelion

A comparative newcomer to the medicinal repertoire, dandelion was not mentioned in Chinese herbals until the seventh century, while in Europe, it first appears in the *Ortus Sanitatis* of 1485. The name dandelion was apparently invented by a fifteenth century surgeon who compared the shape of the leaves to a lion's tooth or *dens leonis*. In the West, we use the leaves and root separately, but the Chinese prefer just the aerial parts of various Asiatic species of dandelion, including *T. mongolicum*.

Character: Cold with a bitter and sweet taste.

Constituents: *Leaves*: bitter glycosides, carotenoids, terpenoids, choline, potassium salts, iron and other minerals, vitamins A, B, C, D. *Root*: bitter glycosides, tannins, triterpenes, sterols, volatile oil, choline, asparagine, inulin.

Actions: *Leaves*: diuretic, hepatic and digestive tonic. *Root*: liver tonic, cholagogue, diuretic, laxative, antirheumatic.

Parts Used

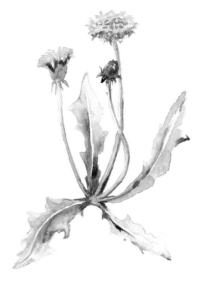

Leaves
T. officinale

An effective diuretic, the leaves are rich in potassium, which is lost from the body by frequent urination, so using them both encourages urination and maintains potassium levels. Like the root, the leaves are also an effective liver and digestive tonic. Harvest throughout the growing season.

Root
T. officinale

A favorite liver stimulant with many modern herbalists, the root is used as a gentle cleansing tonic for a wide range of problems including gallstones and jaundice. Harvest the long tap root in spring.

Sap
T. officinale

The white sap from dandelion stems and root can be used as a topical remedy for warts.

Whole plant
T. mongolicum

Called *pu gong ying*, the Chinese use this Asian species much as in the West, as a diuretic and liver stimulant. It is also considered to clear heat and toxins from the blood so is used for boils and abscesses. Harvest in summer before the flowers are fully open.

Applications

Leaves

T. officinale

Juice: Either the juice or fluid extract should be used when a diuretic action is needed. Up to 20 ml three times daily can be used.

Infusion: This is less effective than the juice but can be used as a cleansing herb in toxic conditions. The freshly dried leaves should be used.

Fresh herb: The leaves can be added to spring salads as a cleansing remedy.

Tincture: This is often added to remedies for failing heart and ensures adequate potassium intake.

Root

T. officinale

Tincture: Fresh root should be used as a liver stimulant in hepatic disorders and for toxic conditions such as gout, eczema, or acne.

Decoction: Used as the tincture, but is less effective as a diuretic than the leaf.

Aerial parts

T. mongolicum

Decoction: Use 10–30 g to 300 ml of water per dose for urinary tract infections, boils, and similar "hot" infections.

Terminalia spp.
Myrobalan

Character: Astringent, sour/sweet/bitter, warm.
Constituents: Tannins, triterpenoid saponins, flavonoids, phytosterols.
Actions
T. belerica / T. chebula: Astringent, rejuventative tonic, expectorant, laxative, anthelmintic, antiseptic.
T. arjuna: Cardioprotective, liver protective, mild diuretic.

Several species of the *Terminalia* genus of trees are used in Ayurvedic medicine among them *T. belerica* (*bibhitaki* or beleric myrobalan), *T. arjuna* (*indradrum* or *arjuna*) and *T. chebula* (*haritaki* or chebulic myrobalan). They are all important rejuvenating and tonic herbs that are now starting to be investigated by modern researchers. *Haritaki* is also used in Chinese medicine, where it is known as *he ti* and is used for persistent coughs and dysentery; in Tibet it is regarded as "the king of medicines."

PARTS USED

FRUIT
T. belerica
Bibhitaki is mainly used in Ayurveda as a *kapha* tonic, helping to strengthen the lungs, voice and vision. The unripe fruit is an effective laxative for cleansing the system and is used as an anthelmintic to expel intestinal parasites. The ripe fruit is preferred for indigestion and diarrhea. *Bibhitaki* is often combined with *haritaki* in the classic "three fruits" or *triphala* remedy.

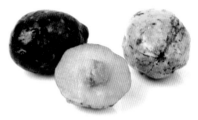

BARK
T. arjuna
Arjuna has been used for treating heart problems for at least 3,000 years. Modern studies have had mixed results but most have confirmed a degree of efficacy and the plant is known to reduce cholesterol levels, improve the supply of nutrients to the heart muscles, and reduce the risk of attacks among patients suffering from angina pectoris.

FRUIT
T. chebula
Haritaki is one of the most important Ayurvedic tonic herbs. It is the main ingredient in *triphala* – with *amalaki* (*Emblica officinalis*) and *bibhitaki* – a widely used laxative and antiseptic tonic for the digestive system. *Haritaki* is believed to strengthen the brain and nerves and increase spiritual awareness. Like *bibhitaki* it is used for both diarrhea and constipation and is said to promote vision, voice, and longevity. As an astringent, it is also used for vaginal discharges and excessive menstrual bleeding.

APPLICATIONS

Fruit

T. belerica
Poultice: Use crushed fruits spread on gauze as a poultice for sore eyes: put the gauze onto closed eyelids and relax for 10–15 minutes.
Powder: Mix 1 teaspoon of powder with 1 teaspoon of honey for sore throats and vocal problems.
Gargle: Use an infusion of the dried fruits or a juice extract of fresh fruit as a gargle for sore throats.

Bark

T. arjuna
Tincture: Take 40 drops to 5 ml daily, in three doses to help protect against heart disorders or to combat angina pectoris and irregular heartbeat.
Decoction: Take half a cup three times daily to help improve heart energies and performance.

Fruit

T. chebula
Decoction: Use 1 teaspoon of dried fruit per cup of decoction as a strengthening tonic for respiratory and digestive systems.
Wash: Use the infusion or decoction as a wash for ulcerated skin sores and infections. The same wash can also be used as a douche for vaginal discharges and infections.
Eye bath: Use a well-strained weak decoction as an eye bath for inflammations like conjunctivitis.
Syrup: Use the decoction and honey to make a syrup for persistent, rasping coughs or hoarseness.
Mouthwash: Use the strained decoction or ½ teaspoon of powder in water as a mouthwash for mouth ulcers and bleeding gums; the powder was traditionally used to whiten teeth and prevent decay and gum diseases.

CAUTIONS:
- Avoid all *Terminalia* spp. in pregnancy and severe exhaustion or excess heat syndromes.

Thymus spp.
Thyme

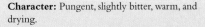
Character: Pungent, slightly bitter, warm, and drying.

Constituents: Volatile oil (inc. thymol), bitter, tannins, saponins, triterpenes, flavonoids.

Actions: Antiseptic expectorant, antispasmodic, astringent, antimicrobial, diuretic, antitussive, antibiotic, wound herb, topically rubifacient.

Common or garden thyme (*T. vulgaris*) is the cultivated form of wild thyme, *T. serpyllum,* which is known as "mother of thyme," possibly because of its traditional use for menstrual disorders. Wild thyme derives its botanical name from its creeping or serpent-like growth pattern and Pliny recommends it as an antidote for serpent bites and "the poison of marine creatures" as well as for headaches. The Romans also burned the plant in the belief that the fumes would also repel scorpions and "all such creatures."

PARTS USED

AERIAL PARTS

T. vulgaris

Mainly used as an expectorant and antiseptic, thyme is ideal for deep seated chest infections characterized by thick yellow sputum, as in chronic bronchitis, asthma, or whooping cough. Like many culinary herbs, thyme is also a digestive remedy and has been shown to inhibit *Heliobactor pylorii,* associated with gastric ulcers. Harvest before and during flowering discarding any woody stems.

T. serpyllum

Similar in action to common thyme, but slightly more stimulating and antispasmodic; the aerial parts are also used for menstrual pain. Harvest before and during flowering.

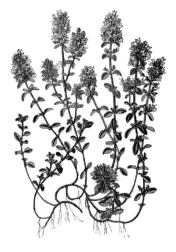

ESSENTIAL OIL

T. vulgaris

Extremely antibacterial, antifungal, and stimulating for the immune system, thyme oil is good for respiratory and digestive problems. Recent studies suggest that when used with evening primrose and fish oils it can help improve concentration skills in hyperactive and dyslexic children.

APPLICATIONS

Aerial parts

T. vulgaris & T. serpyllum

Infusion: Combine with chamomile as a general purpose everyday tonic tea (1 teaspoon of the mixed dried herbs per cup of boiling water). In therapeutic doses use for chest infections, stomach chills or irritable bowel syndrome.

Tincture: Use for diarrhea associated with stomach chills or combine with other expectorant herbs for chest infections.

Gargle: Use the infusion or diluted tincture for sore throats.

Compress: Use a hot pad soaked in tincture for both lung complaints and muscle pain.

Mouthwash: For gum disease.

Syrup: Use the infusion preserved with honey or sugar for coughs and lung infections. Combines well with licorice and white horehound.

Essential oil

Oil: Diluted thyme oil (10 drops in 20 ml of water) can be used for insect bites and infected wounds.

Bath: Add 5 drops to baths for debility and arthritic conditions. Combines well with rosemary.

Chest rub: Use 10 drops in 20 ml of almond or vegetable oil for bronchitis and chest infections. Can be combined with anise, hyssop, or eucalyptus oils.

Massage oil: Use 10 drops each of thyme and lavender oils in 25 ml of almond or vegetable oil for rheumatic pains or strained muscles.

CAUTIONS:

- Often repeated recommendations to avoid thyme and thyme oil in pregnancy are not based on secure clinical evidence and some argue that the herb is actually quite safe to use then.

- The essential oil should not be used internally without professional guidance.

- Thyme oil can irritate the mucous membranes and must always be used well-diluted.

Trifolium pratense
Red clover

Although red clover has been grown as a fodder crop for cattle for at least 500 years, it also has a long history as a medicinal herb. Gerard called it, meadow trefoil and "three-leaved grasse," and its familiar three-lobed leaves were associated with the Trinity by medieval Christians who carried a bunch to help identify witches and sorcerers. The Romans used strawberry-leaved clover (*T. fragiferum*), a Mediterranean plant, which Pliny recommended taking in wine for urinary stones, while the root was used for dropsy.

Character: Slightly sweet and cool.

Constituents: Phenolic glycosides, flavonoids, salicylates, coumarins, cyanogenic glycosides, mineral acids.

Actions: Alterative, antispasmodic, diuretic, possible estrogenic activity.

Parts Used

Flowers
Mainly used as a cleansing herb for skin complaints, especially in childhood. The flowers are also useful for coughs, possibly because of the cyanogenic glycosides, and have been widely used for bronchitis and whooping coughs. In the 1930s they because popular as an anti-cancer remedy and may still be used for breast, ovarian, and lymphatic cancers. As a gentle, anti-inflammatory, and cleansing wound herb it can be useful for persistent sores, eye inflammations, and insect bites. Harvest during flowering.

Applications

Flowers

Tincture: Use a standard dose internally eczema and psoriasis. Combines well with heartsease for childhood eczema.
Syrup: Use a standard syrup for stubborn, dry coughs and especially for whooping cough: combine with marshmallow, hyssop, or mullein.
Fresh: Use the crushed flowers directly on insect bites and stings.

Eye bath: Use diluted tincture or a well-strained infusion for conjunctivitis.
Compress: Use a hot pad soaked in diluted tincture for arthritic pains and gout.
Ointment: Use fresh flowers and simmer with water in a slow cooker for 48 hours. Strain, evaporate the residue to semi-dryness and combine with a standard ointment base for lymphatic swellings.
Douche: Use a standard infusion for vaginal itching.

Trigonella foenum-graecum
Fenugreek

Highly regarded by Hippocrates, fenugreek is one of our oldest medicinal herbs: seeds were found in the tomb of Tutankhamun and it was used in Ancient Egypt to ease childbirth and to increase milk flow. Today, it is still taken by Egyptian women for menstrual pain and as *hilba* tea is a popular standby to ease abdominal cramps for tourists afflicted by gastric upsets. In China, the herb, called *hu lu ba*, is also used for abdominal pain. Western research has highlighted its hypoglycemic properties.

Character: Very warming with a pungent, bitter taste.

Constituents: Steroidal saponins, alkaloids (inc. trigonelline), mucilage, bitter, protein, vitamins A, B, C, minerals.

Actions
Seeds: Anti-inflammatory, digestive tonic, galactagogue, locally demulcent, uterine stimulant, hypoglycemic.
Whole herb: Antispasmodic.

PARTS USED

SEEDS
Warming for the kidneys and reproductive organs, it is used in China to treat male impotence. The herb can be used for menstrual pains and for menopausal problems related to kidney weakness. Traditionally it was used as an aphrodisiac since the steroidal saponins it contains mimic the body's sex hormones. It is a bitter digestive remedy also used to regulate glucose metabolism in diabetes. Externally demulcent and anti-inflammatory, it can be used on skin inflammations and boils. Harvest the seeds when ripe.

AERIAL PARTS
Taken in the Middle East and Balkans as a folk remedy for abdominal cramps associated with menstrual pains, gastroenteritis, and diarrhea. The herb is also used to ease labor pains during childbirth. The young sprouted shoots may be used.

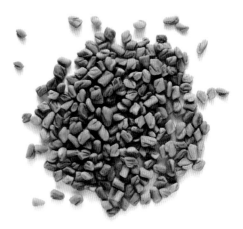

APPLICATIONS

Seeds
Decoction: A standard decoction can be used as a warming drink for menstrual pains, stomach upsets, and to increase milk flow in nursing mothers. It has a bitter taste, which can be disguised with a little fennel or aniseed.

Tincture: Used for reproductive disorders and conditions involving kidney qi weakness. May be combined with other hypoglycemic herbs in diabetic treatments.

Capsules: Two or three taken after meals can help control glucose metabolism in late-onset diabetes and to lower cholesterol levels in those at risk from heart disease.

Poultice: The powdered herb can be made into a paste and used for boils and cellulitis.

Aerial parts
Infusion: The dried plant is available in parts of the Middle East and Balkans and a standard infusion is used for abdominal cramps, labor, and menstrual pains.

CAUTIONS:
- Insulin dependent diabetics should seek professional advice before using fenugreek as a hypoglycemic.
- A uterine stimulant, so avoid in pregnancy although it may be taken during labor.

Tussilago farfara
Coltsfoot

Smoking coltsfoot for coughs and asthma was recommended by Dioscorides. Its botanical name means "cough dispeller" and even now herbal cigarettes often contain the plant. The flowers appear in late winter and only when they have died down do the leaves come – hence the plant's old name *filius ante patrem* (the son before the father). In China only the flowers, known as *kuan dong hua*, are used.

Character: Warm, with a pungent, slightly sweet taste.

Constituents: Mucilage, tannins, pyrrolizidine alkaloids, inulin, zinc, bitter principle, sterols, flavonoids (inc. rutin), potassium, calcium.

Actions: Relaxing expectorant, anti-catarrhal, demulcent.
Topically: Tissue healer and demulcent.

PARTS USED

FLOWERS
The expectorant, anti-catarrhal and antispasmodic action makes these ideal for a wide range of chest problems including bronchitis, whooping cough, asthma, and stubborn, irritating coughs. Chinese medicine considers them specific for chronic coughs with profuse phlegm and to force rising lung *qi* to descend. Harvest in late winter when they appear.

LEAVES
Used to treat for coughs, as with the flowers. The leaves are also rich in zinc, which is very healing and can be applied, fresh, to a variety of skin sores and chronic wounds. Harvest in summer.

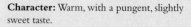

APPLICATIONS

Flowers

Decoction: Use for irritable coughs and catarrh. Also for coughs associated with the common cold or flu.

Syrup: Add 500 g of honey or sugar to 500 ml of infusion and heat gently to form a syrup. Use in 5 ml doses for coughs. The syrup is more moistening for dry, stubborn coughs.

Tincture: Used for chronic or persistent coughs. Combines well with thyme and elecampane.

Leaves

Poultice: Use the fresh leaf for ulcers, sores, and other slowly healing wounds.

Cigarettes: The dried leaf can be rolled in cigarette paper and smoked for asthma and bronchitis. Can be combined with dried thyme and eyebright leaf.

Decoction: As for flowers.

Tincture: As for flowers.

CAUTIONS:
- Contains pyrrolizidine alkaloids which are believed to cause liver damage. However, Swedish research suggests that in coltsfoot these are destroyed in making a decoction and the quantity is too minute to be harmful.

Urtica dioica
Stinging nettle

Tradition has it that Caesar's troops introduced the Roman nettle (*U. pilulifera*) into Britain because they expected the climate to be so cold that they would need to whip themselves with nettles to keep warm. "Urtication", or beating with nettles, is a standard folk remedy for arthritis and rheumatism still sometimes recommended today. Perennial stinging nettles (*U. dioica*) are still used medicinally and make good cleansing spring tonics and a nourishing vegetable if gathered when the leaves are young.

Character: Cool and dry with an astringent, slightly bitter taste.

Constituents: Histamine, formic acid, acetylcholine, serotonin, glucoquinones, many minerals (inc. silica), vitamins A, B & C, tannins.

Actions: Astringent, diuretic, tonic, nutritive, hemostatic, circulatory stimulant, galactagogue, hypoglycemic, antiscorbutic.

PARTS USED

AERIAL PARTS
Nettles "rob the soil," making them rich in vitamins and minerals, including iron, so a good tonic for anemia. The high vitamin C content also ensures that the iron is properly absorbed. They help clear uric acid from the system so are good for gout and arthritis, while the astringency makes them valuable in stopping bleeding. Nettles "sting" because of histamine and formic acid in the hairs, which trigger an allergic response. Harvest (with care) while flowering.

ROOT
Traditionally used as a conditioner for falling hair and dandruff. Recent research has confirmed that it is also effective in controlling benign prostate enlargement.

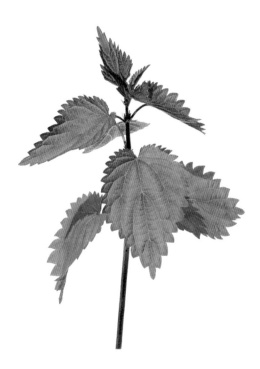

APPLICATIONS

Aerial parts

Juice: The juice from the whole fresh plant makes a good tonic for debilitated conditions and anemia. It can also be used for nettle stings. The fresh juice is also diuretic and is used for cardiac insufficiency with edema.

Infusion: Use the young fresh shoots to make a spring tonic. A standard infusion can be used to stimulate the circulation and cleanse the system in arthritis, rheumatism, gout, and eczema. Also to increase milk flow in nursing mothers.

Tincture: Used in combinations with relevant herbs for arthritic disorders, skin problems or heavy uterine bleeding.

Wash: For burns, insect bites, wounds.

Compress: A pad soaked in the tincture can be applied to painful arthritic joints and used for gout, neuralgia, sprains, tendonitis, and sciatica.

Ointment: For hemorrhoids (piles).

Powder: The powdered leaves can be inhaled as snuff for nosebleeds.

Root

Hair rinse: A decoction can be used for dandruff, falling hair, and as a general conditioner.

Decoction: Use with saw palmetto for benign prostate enlargement.

Vaccinium myrtillus & V. vitis-idaea
Bilberry & cowberry

Once highly regarded medicinal herbs, bilberry and cowberry plants are near relatives of bearberry (*Arctostaphylos uva-ursi*), an important urinary antiseptic, and their leaves have been used in very similar ways in folk medicine. Elizabethan apothecaries made a syrup of the berries with honey, called rob, which was used as a remedy for diarrhea. In recent trials the juice of another near relative, cranberry (*V. oxycoccos*) has proved effective in treating cystitis.

Character: Sour, astringent, cold, and drying.

Constituents: Tannins, sugars, fruit acids, glucoquinone, glycosides. Some species (not bilberries) contain arbutin.

Action: Astringent, hypoglycemic, tonic, antiseptic, antiemetic. Some species also diuretic.

PARTS USED

FRUIT
V. myrtillus
Bilberries are mainly used for diarrhea; they contain a pigment believed to kill or inhibit the growth of bacteria cells, so are especially useful in dysentery. Large quantities of fresh fruit, however, have a laxative effect. Harvest in late summer and autumn.

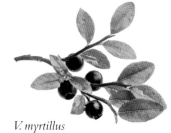

V. myrtillus

LEAVES
V. myrtillus
Bilberry leaves are hypoglycemic so reduce blood sugar levels in late-onset diabetes. Modern research suggests that they increase insulin production in some way. Harvest before the berries ripen.

V. vitis-idaea
These contain up to 7% arbutin, which is an effective urinary antiseptic, and are used for conditions such as cystitis. Like bilberry leaves, they also appear to stimulate insulin production and can be used for late-onset diabetes. Harvest in summer.

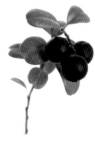

V. vitis-idaea

APPLICATIONS

Fruit

V. myrtillus
Juice: The unsweetened juice is most effective for diarrhea – use 10 ml doses. The diluted juice can also be used as a mouthwash for ulcers and inflammations. Diluted with witch hazel, it makes a cooling lotion for sunburn and other skin inflammations.
Powder: This is useful for babies and infants, mix 150 mg per 1 kg bodyweight into the baby's feed: best used heated or slightly cooked.
Fresh raw berries: Eat a large bowl of the whole fresh berries with sugar and milk or cream for constipation.
Decoction: Use one glass of a standard decoction daily for chronic diarrhea.

Leaves

V. myrtillus
Infusion: Use in standard doses as an adjunct to dietary controls in late-onset, non-insulin dependent diabetes mellitus. Combines well with goat's rue and may be flavored with peppermint in long-term use.
Mouthwash: Use a standard infusion as a mouthwash or gargle for ulcers and throat inflammations.

V. vitis-idaea
Infusion: Use a strong infusion (40 g to 500 ml of water) in standard doses for cystitis and other urinary tract infections. The leaves can also be used instead of bilberry leaves with goat's rue and peppermint in diabetic therapy.

CAUTIONS:
• Insulin dependent diabetics should not use hypoglycemic teas without professional guidance.

Valeriana officinalis
Valerian

Sometimes described as nature's tranquilizer, valerian calms the nerves without the side effects of comparable orthodox drugs. It has a distinctive, rather unpleasant smell and was aptly called *phu* by Galen. In recent years, it has been well-researched, and chemicals called valepotriates, which develop in valerian extracts, have been identified. These seem to have a depressant effect on the nervous system, while the fresh plant is more sedating.

Character: Pungent, slightly bitter, cool, and dry.

Constituents: Volatile oil (inc. isovalerianic acid, borneol), valepotriates, alkaloids, iridoids.

Actions: Tranquilizer, antispasmodic, expectorant, diuretic, hypotensive, carminative, mild anodyne.

PARTS USED

ROOTS
Good for all types of nervous tension, especially anxiety and insomnia, the roots are also strengthening for the heart and can sometimes be help to reduce high blood pressure. Valerian is a healing herb for wounds and ulcers and can be effective, topically, for muscle cramps. It is an expectorant, and coupled with its sedating action, can help tickling, nervous coughs. Harvest in autumn.

LEAVES
Although no longer used, these were once recommended as a poultice for headaches and an infusion was recommended for mouth ulcers and sore gums.

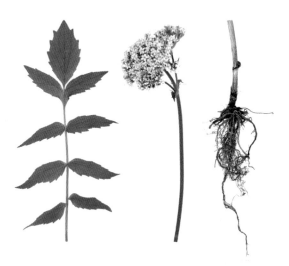

APPLICATIONS

Roots
Maceration: Soak two teaspoons of the chopped, preferably, fresh root for 8–10 hours in a cup of cold water. Used as a sedating brew for anxiety and insomnia. Add 2–3 drops of peppermint water to disguise the flavor.
Tincture: Dosage can vary considerably with individuals – up to 5 ml may be required but in some people this can cause headaches so start with low doses. Use as a sedative or for insomnia. The tincture can be combined with licorice and other expectorants for coughs.
Wash: Use the infusion or maceration for chronic ulcers, wounds or for drawing splinters.

Compress: A pad soaked in the tincture can ease muscle cramps.

CAUTIONS:
* Easily confused with the popular garden plant red "American" valerian (*Centranthus ruber*).
* Do not use for more than two or three weeks without a break as continual use or high doses may lead to headaches and palpitations.
* Enhances the action of sleep-inducing drugs so avoid if taking this type of medication.

Verbascum thapsus
Mullein

The tall stems of mullein covered in fine down were once burned as tapers in funeral processions. Dioscorides used it for scorpion stings, eye diseases, tooth-ache, tonsillitis, and coughs. It was also traditionally used in wasting diseases such as tuberculosis. An infused oil made from the flowers was a household standby in many parts of Europe for ailments as diverse as piles, frost bite, and ear infections.

Character: Slightly sweet, cool, and moist.

Constituents: Mucilage, saponins, volatile oil, bitter, flavonoids, glycosides (inc. aucubin).

Action: Expectorant, demulcent, mild diuretic, sedative, wound herb, astringent, anti-inflammatory.

PARTS USED

FLOWERS
A relaxing expectorant for dry, chronic, hard coughs such as in whooping cough, tuberculosis, asthma, and bronchitis. The flowers are also effective for throat inflammations including tracheitis, laryngitis and tonsillitis and they can be helpful for relieving hay fever symptoms. The infused oil can be used to soothe inflammations and wounds as well as in its traditional role for earache. Harvest flowers individually when in bloom.

LEAVES
Used for respiratory disorders, the leaves were once made into herbal "tobacco" and smoked for asthma and tuberculosis. The plant is also generally antiseptic and loaves and fruits were traditionally wrapped in the large leaves to help preserve them. Harvest before flowering in the second year. In commercial supply the flowers and leaves are not often separated and in such mixes the leaves predominate.

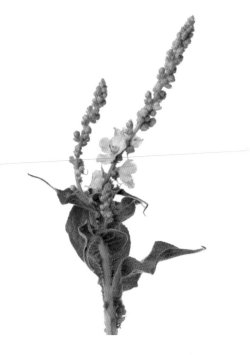

APPLICATIONS

Flowers

Syrup: Use a standard syrup in 5–10 ml doses for chronic, hard coughs. Combine with elecampane or hyssop if desired.

Gargle: Use a standard infusion of the flowers as a gargle for tracheitis, tonsillitis, or laryngitis.

Tincture: Use up to 20 ml daily for all sorts of chronic, dry chest conditions. Also for throat inflammations. Combine with eyebright for hay fever.

Infused oil: Make the oil using the cold infusion technique and use drops for the pain of ear infections. The same oil can be used as a salve on wounds, hemorrhoids, eczema, swollen glands, or in conditions like blepharitis.

Leaf

Infusion: Use a strong infusion of dried herb (50 g to 500 ml water) for chronic coughs and throat inflammations. This also has a diaphoretic effect so can be useful for feverish chills with hard coughs.

Tincture: Use standard doses for chronic respiratory disorders – combine with elecampane, white horehound, mulberry bark, or hyssop.

Cigarettes: Crushed dried leaves can be rolled in cigarette papers and smoked for asthma and bronchitis; alternatively, they can be smoked in a pipe. Can be combined with coltsfoot leaf.

CAUTIONS:
* Do not use as eardrops if the ear drum is perforated.

Verbena officinalis
Vervain

Vervain was one of the Druids' most sacred herbs, vervain was called it *hiera botane* (sacred plant) by the Romans who used it to purify homes and spread it on Jove's temple. Its association with magic and ritual persisted well into the seventeenth century, and Gerard warns against using it for "witchcraft and sorceries." The herb was traditionally used for dropsy, and cardioactive glycosides have now been identified in the plant to support this use.

Character: Pungent, bitter, and cool.

Constituents: Volatile oil (inc. citral), glycosides, bitter, tannins.

Actions: Relaxant tonic, galactagogue, diaphoretic, nervine, sedative, antispasmodic, hepatic restorative, laxative, uterine stimulant, bile stimulant.

Parts Used

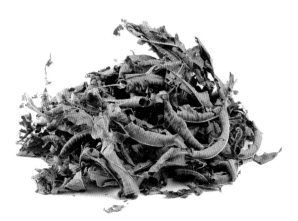

Aerial parts
An effective nerve tonic, liver stimulant, urinary cleanser, and fever remedy, vervain also encourages milk flow and can be taken during labor to stimulate contractions. It has a number of topical uses for sores, wounds and gum disorders. In China, the plant is known as *ma bian cao* and is used mainly as fever herb for malaria and flu. Traditional Chinese medicine holds that it stimulates the circulation, and the herb is used for scanty and painful menstruation as well as for urinary disorders. Traditionally harvested in July and August when the dog star can be seen in the heavens.

Bach flower remedy
Vervain is one of Dr. Bach's original twelve remedies. It is used for mental stress and overexertion with related insomnia and inability to relax.

APPLICATION

Aerial parts

Tincture: For nervous exhaustion and depression – combines well with oats; as a liver stimulant for sluggish digestion, toxic conditions, or jaundice; and with other urinary herbs for stones and conditions related to excess uric acid, such as gout.

Infusion: Can be sipped during labor or to simulate milk flow in nursing mothers. Also for insomnia and nervous tension or to encourage sweating and stimulate the immune system in feverish conditions.

Mouthwash: Use the infusion for mouth ulcers and soft, spongy gums.

Ointment: Use on eczema, wounds, and running sores. Also for painful neuralgia.

Poultices: Use on insect bites, sprains, and bruises.

CAUTIONS:
- Uterine stimulant; avoid in pregnancy.
- May cause vomiting in excessive doses.

Viburnum spp.
Guelder Rose & Black Haw

An alternative name for guelder rose (*V. opulus*) is cramp bark which neatly sums up its main medicinal action as a muscle relaxant. The plant was known in the fourteenth century as Chaucer suggests eating the berries. It was also used by Native Americans for mumps and other swellings. A close relative, black haw (*V. prunifolium*) is an important American variety known for its significant relaxing action on the womb was soon recognised. Black haw was a favorite with the Eclectics of nineteenth century America.

Character: Astringent and bitter, cool, and dry.

Constituents: Bitter (viburnin), valerianic acid, tannins, saponins. V. prunifolium also contains scopoletin (a coumarin) which is a uterine relaxant.

Action: Antispasmodic, sedative, astringent, muscle relaxant, cardiac tonic, uterine relaxant, sedative. anti-inflammatory.

PARTS USED

ROOT BARK
V. prunifolium

A potent relaxant for both smooth and skeletal muscle, black haw has a very specific action on the womb and is one of the best remedies for menstrual pains. It can be helpful for pain after childbirth and is also used in remedies for post-partum haemorrhage as well as in cases of heavy menstrual bleeding associated with menopausal syndrome. It is used to treat vaginal discharges, morning sickness, and threatened miscarriage. It may also be a component of high blood pressure remedies and is used for cramping pains. Harvest in the autumn.

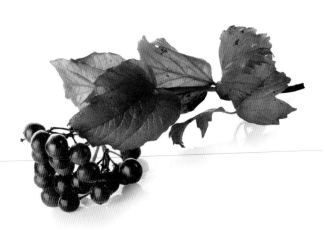

BARK
V. opulus

Guelder rose bark is used to relax both smooth and skeletal muscle. It also has a sedating action on the nervous system and is useful when physical and emotional tensions combine: sufferers typically suffer from tense raised shoulders or tight breathing. It helps to relax the cardiovascular system in high blood pressure, lowering the diastolic reading, and also soothe the gut in irritable bowel syndrome and constipation associated with tension. Used externally, it can quickly ease muscle cramps. Strip bark from stems in spring before flowering.

APPLICATIONS

Root bark
V. prunifolium

Tincture: Use as a simple for menstrual pain either in 20–30 drop doses taken frequently or as a single 20 ml dose taken at the first hint of muscle cramps. Both approaches are effective but one or other may be more effective for a particular individual. Take a similar approach for post-partum pain. Use in standard doses for other menstrual irregularities and menopausal syndrome. Can also be added to hypertensive remedies.

Decoction: Less effective than the tincture. Drink a cup of string decoction for menstrual pains.

Bark
V. opulus

Tincture: Use in standard doses as a relaxant for nervous or muscular tension. Useful for colicky conditions of the intestines, gallbladder, or urinary system. Combine with skullcap or valerian for nervous tension. Add to digestive remedies for irritable bowel or with butternut or rhubarb root for constipation associated with tense personalities who do not "let go." May be helpful with chamomile for asthmatic spasms and with cinnamon twigs for vasospasm associated with poor peripheral circulation.

Cream: Mix the tincture with a standard base (such as emulsifying ointment) to make a cream and apply for muscle cramps, as in the legs, or for shoulder tension. Add 10 drops of lobelia tincture per 50 ml of cream if required.

Viola spp.
Sweet violet & heartsease

Sweet violet (*V. odorata*) and heartsease (wild pansy, *V. tricolor*) have been used medicinally since ancient times. Homer related that the Athenians used violets to "moderate anger," while Pliny recommended wearing a violet garland on the head to dispel wine fumes and prevent headaches and dizziness. Heartsease takes its name from its early use in love potions it was also once used for heart disorders. The Chinese use a related species (*V. yedoensis*) in very similar ways.

Character: Moist, pungent, cold, and slightly bitter.
Constituents: Saponins, salicylates, alkaloids, flavonoids (inc. rutin), volatile oil.
Actions
V. odorata: anti-inflammatory, stimulating expectorant, diuretic, antitumor remedy.
V. tricolor: expectorant, anti-inflammatory, diuretic, antirheumatic, laxative, stabilizes capillary membranes.
V. yedoensis: antimicrobial, anti-inflammatory.

PARTS USED

AERIAL PARTS
V. tricolor
Used for a wide range of skin disorders (from diaper rash to varicose ulcers) while the saponin content also makes it a good expectorant for coughs. The herb also acts on the blood vessels, tonifying and strengthening them thanks to the flavonoids it contains. Harvest while flowering.

V. odorata
Mainly used for coughs, bronchitis and catarrh although like heartsease they also have a role in treating skin disorders. In the 1930s they were widely used in treating breast and lung cancer. Harvest in spring.

FLOWERS
V. odorata
Once popularly made into a syrup used for insomnia, epilepsy, pleurisy, jaundice, sore throats, sore eyes, and headaches. Today the flowers are more likely to be crystallized for cake decorations.

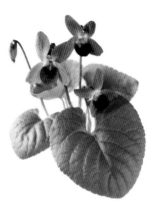

Viola odorata

WHOLE PLANT
V. yedoensis
Called *zi hua di ding* in China, the plant is mainly used for infectious skin conditions including boils and erysipelas as well as for snake bites. It is also used for breast abscesses and lymphatic inflammations.

APPLICATIONS

Aerial parts

V. tricolor
Infusion: Use a standard infusion as a cleansing remedy toxic conditions and as a gentle stimulant for the circulation and immune system; useful in such conditions as for rheumatic disorders, chronic skin problems, and chronic infections.
Wash: Use the standard, well-strained infusion, for conditions such as diaper rash, cradle cap, weeping sores, varicose ulcers, and oozing insect bites.
Powdered herb: This can be used as a paste on skin sores and ulcers.
Tincture: Add to remedies for capillary fragility, urinary disorders, digestive upsets, and lung problems. Useful for complex syndromes affecting many body systems.
Cream: Make a standard cream for skin rashes and irritant eczema.

V. odorata
Infusion: Use a standard infusion for catarrh and chesty coughs.

Mouthwash: Use a standard infusion for mouth and throat infections.
Syrup: Sweeten a standard infusion with honey or sugar (500 ml infusion to 500 g honey) for coughs. Can combine with coltsfoot flowers.
Tincture: Use 10–15 ml of a standard tincture three times day after surgery for cancer of the breast, lungs or digestive tract. Can be used in standard doses with other expectorant herbs for bronchitis and coughs.

Whole plant

V. yedoensis
Decoction: The herb is used in combinations for skin diseases and abscesses. Often combined with *chi shao yao, fang feng, mu dan pi, sheng di huang*, and similar cooling, cleansing herbs in eczema treatments.

CAUTIONS:
*   High doses of saponin-containing herbs can lead to nausea and vomiting.

Withania somnifera
Ashwagandha or Winter Cherry

Ashwagandha, the Sanskrit name for winter cherry, translates as "that which has the smell of a horse," as the plant was believed to endow any who took it with the strength, vitality, and sexual energy of a horse. Also called "Indian ginseng," it is one of Ayurveda's most important tonic herbs. It is less expensive than Korean ginseng, can be just as effective, and is becoming more readily available in the West. In extensive studies, it has proved an invigorating tonic for the elderly and shown significant antitumor activity in laboratory tests.

Character: Bitter, astringent, sweet, hot.

Constituents: Alkaloids (including anaferine and isopelietierine), steroidal lactones (including withanolides, and withaferins), saponins, iron.

Actions: Tonic, nervine, sedative, anti-inflammatory, antitumor.

Parts Used

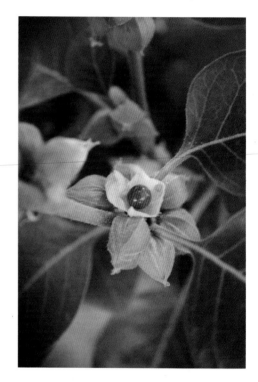

Root
The root is used as a tonic to encourage healthy growth in children and combat emaciation caused by famine. It is important for the elderly increasing vigor and energy and, in one clinical trial, improved sexual performance in more than 70% of the men over age fifty involved. Studies have also shown that it can help increase body weight, slow the development of lung cancers in laboratory animals, and apparently encourage tumor regression in some cases. Studies also suggest *ashwagandha* can nourish the blood, improving hemoglobin levels in anemia. The plant shows strong anti-inflammatory activity similar in action to human steroidal hormones.

Leaves
The leaves are traditionally used as a calming, sleep-inducing remedy in exhaustion and fevers.

Applications

Root

Powder/capsules: Use 250 mg to 1 g per dose as a restorative tonic in overwork, exhaustion, sleep problems, and debility caused by chronic disease. Up to 5 g per day can be used in warm milk sweetened with a little sugar. Regular use can also help in degenerative disorders such as arthritis.

Decoction: Drink a cup for weakness in pregnancy or use ½ cup to encourage healthy growth in children or to help strengthen weak and emaciated children. The root is also decocted in milk to enhance its tonic effects or can be combined with half as much long pepper to similarly increase its potency.

Wash: Use the decoction externally as a wash for wounds, sores, and skin inflammations.

Tonic wine: Use the tonic wine or tincture as the basis for an iron tonic in anemia, which will also encourage hemoglobin production.

Leaves

Infusion: Used as a calming narcotic for those suffering from debilitating fevers and stress. Drink a cup at night.

Powder: Studies suggest the leaves may help act as a preventative for cancer: take ½ teaspoon in a little water each day.

Zingiber officinalis
Ginger

Originally from tropical Asia, ginger has been used as both culinary and medicinal herb in the West for at least 2,000 years. It was introduced into the Americas by the Spaniards and is now cultivated extensively in the West Indies. As a hot, dry herb it was traditionally used for to warm the stomach and dispel chills. In the eighteenth century, ginger was added to many remedies to modify their action and reduce the irritant effects on the stomach. The herb is also used in this way in China to reduce the toxicity of some herbs.

Character: Pungent, hot, and dry.

Constituents: Volatile oil (inc. borneol, citral), phenols, alkaloid, mucilage.

Actions: Circulatory stimulant, peripheral vasodilator, diaphoretic, expectorant, antiemetic, antispasmodic, carminative, antiseptic. *Topically:* rubefacient.

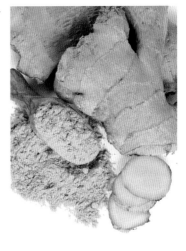

Parts Used

Fresh root
In China, the fresh root is known as *sheng jiang* and is mainly used as a diaphoretic and expectorant for colds and chills and is also roasted with hot ashes and used for diarrhea or as a styptic. As well as using the root for chills, Western herbalists regard the plant as an effective circulatory stimulant.

Dried root
Called *gan jiang* in China, the dried root is used to warm and stimulate the stomach and lung in such conditions as diarrhea related to digestive weakness or chronic bronchitis. The herb is an effective restorative and is often added to classic Chinese tonic formulas. In the West, dried ginger is similarly used as a warming remedy for the stomach and for both travel sickness and sickness in pregnancy. It has a stimulant, warming effect on the womb and can be helpful for menstrual cramps and other irregularities.

Ginger peel
Peeled root skin (*jiang pi*) is considered as cold in China and is used for edema and abdominal bloating in China.

Essential oil
Used in both East and West for at least 400 years, the oil is recommended in China for malaria and coughs characterized by copious phlegm. In France it is prescribed in drop doses on sugar lumps for both flatulence and fevers and taken before meals as an appetite stimulant. The oil can be added to massage rubs for rheumatic pains and bone injuries.

Applications

Fresh root

Decoction: Use 1–2 slices of root to a mug of water, simmer for 10 minutes and drink for chills and catarrhal colds. A pinch of cinnamon can be added to the mixture.

Tincture: Use 2–10 drops of a 1 in 5 tincture per dose as a warming circulatory stimulant where poor circulation may be contributing to chilblains, very cold feet and hands, etc. Also for flatulence, indigestion and nausea.

Dried root

Capsules: Take 1–2 200 mg capsules before travelling for seasickness, travel sickness, etc. Up to 1 g doses can be used for morning sickness in pregnancy.

Decoction: Used in many Chinese tonic formulas in combination with herbs such as ginseng, *bai zhu*, or specially prepared monkshood as a restorative for *yang* or spleen energies. Also combined with herbs such as *ban xia*, *huang lian*, and *huang qin* for abdominal fullness, nausea, and excess phlegm.

Essential oil

Massage rub: Add 5–10 drops of essential oil to 25 ml of almond oil as a rub for rheumatism or lumbago. Combine with juniper or eucalyptus oil.

Essential oil: Use 1–2 drops on a sugar lump or in a half a teaspoon of honey for flatulence, menstrual cramps, nausea, or stomach upsets.

CAUTIONS:
- Avoid excessive amount of ginger if the stomach is already hot and over-stimulated as in peptic ulceration.
- Use with respect in early pregnancy although it can be safely taken for morning sickness in the doses described.

Ayurvedic Herbs

Out of India

The Ayurvedic healing tradition in India dates back to the *Rigveda*, written between 3500 and 1800 B.C. Later theories have also influenced the therapeutic uses of the many thousands of medicinal herbs used in the subcontinent. The *Siddha* system, which attains spiritual perfection through meditation, for example, started around 2000 B.C. among the Dravidian people of Southern India and was believed to originate directly from the Hindu deity Shiva and his wife, Parvati. Later Arab traders brought the Unani-Tibb tradition (based on ancient Greek theories), which was a favorite with the Moghul emperors from the fourteenth century. Many plants are common to all three systems, but there can often be subtle differences, which can make interpretation of Indian plant therapeutics more complex. India's many different languages also mean that the same plant can be known by a dozen different names.

Around 75% of India's population still depend on traditional medicines, which significantly outsell conventional drugs. Many products are complex, and adulteration is all too common; for example, "*ashtavarga*" used as a fertility tonic, should be made of eight herbs, most of them from the lily family, but analysis has shown at least 42 different plants in samples. Many prepared remedies also contain heavy metals and gemstones and are often regarded suspiciously by Western medicines regulators.

Santalum album – *chandana*, sandalwood

Traditionally, sandalwood (*chandana*) is used to cool and calm the body and mind, awaken the intelligence, and open the third eye to increase devotion and meditation. Aromatherapists combine it with rose, neroli, or benzoin oils as a calming, sedative, and antidepressant massage. The wood is used in decoctions for fevers and inflammations and as a circulatory and digestive stimulant. It is known as *tan xiang* in China and is believed to normalize energy flows to the stomach and spleen, to stimulate the digestion and relieve pain.

Parts used: Inner heartwood, volatile oil.

Key uses: Sandalwood is strongly antiseptic and antibacterial and can be used as a wash or made into a paste for external sores. The oil is used in massage for urinary problems, including cystitis, and digestive upsets with abdominal discomfort. It can be added to warm compresses for dry skin, itching, and irritation, and also added to rosewater as a lotion for acne. A few drops to the brow *chakra* (third eye) can improve concentration and cool the body in fevers and thirst.

Cautions: Do not take the essential oil internally.

Cinnamomum camphora – camphor, *karpura*

In Ayurvedic medicine camphor (*karpura*) is used to open the senses, clear the mind, and help mediation. In India, a pinch of powdered camphor is taken as snuff for nasal congestion and headaches and in infusion for a range of respiratory problems and emotional upsets. It is not used internally in the West since it is known to contain safrole, which is carcinogenic. Instead it is used in medicated oils traditionally used for chest rubs and muscular aches and pains.

Parts used: Crystalized distilled oil.

Key uses: In the West, camphorated oils are used externally for coughs, influenza, bronchitis and breathing difficulties. In aromatherapy, it is used to stimulate heart and respiration and to raise low blood pressure. It can also help balance the nervous system – stimulating in depression and calming in hysteria. A compress soaked in weak camphor infusion can relieve backache, and it is used in lotions for cold sores and chilblains. Camphorated oil can be made by dissolving 25 g of camphor crystals in 500 ml of sesame oil.

Cautions: Do not take camphor internally and use only pure raw camphor, not synthetic substitutes.

Commiphora mukul – **guggul/guggula**

A close relative of myrrh, *guggul* (*guggula*) is purifying and rejuvenating and forms the basis of a series of Ayurvedic remedies known as *gugguls*. Traditionally it was used as a remedy for arthritis and applied externally in plasters for aches and pains. Like myrrh it is also added to gargles and mouthwashes for sore throats and mouth ulcers. Research suggests that *guggul* will also reduce high blood cholesterol levels – studies suggested by ancient Sanskrit texts which recommended the herb for treating obesity and lipid disorders.

Parts used: Oleo-gum-resin.

Key uses: In India *guggul* is combined with herbs such as *gokshura* (*Tribulis terrestris*) and the *trikatu* combination for urinary problems or with *triphala* and *pippali* for ulcers and arthritic conditions. The herb is also anti-inflammatory, stimulates white blood cell production, reduces blood clotting, and helps protect heart tissue in degenerative diseases. In the West, extracts are starting to be used to reduce cholesterol.

Cautions: Avoid in pregnancy and breastfeeding.

Picrorrhiza kurroa – **katuka**

Katuka is an important bitter digestive remedy used in India to stimulate the digestion, improve appetite, and treat jaundice, diarrhea, and constipation. Modern research has confirmed that it acts to protect the liver from a variety of toxins and in some studies has proved more effective than silymarin from milk thistle. It is the main ingredient in *arogyavardhini* – a complex remedy used for liver disorders and is also included in *ayush-64* – another patent remedy used as an antimalarial.

Parts used: Root.

Key uses: Katuka is used by Western practitioners to stimulate the immune system in acute and chronic infections and in cases of weakened immunity. It has also been used for combating autoimmune disorders such as rheumatoid arthritis and vitiligo. As a bile stimulant, it help to cleanse the gallbladder. It also shows significant antioxidant activity. Typical dosage is 500–2000 mg daily.

Cautions: High doses may cause diarrhea, abdominal griping, and flatulence. It is extremely bitter, which some patients find totally unpalatable, and cases of allergic skin reaction have been reported.

Curcuma longa – **turmeric**

Turmeric (*haridra* in Sanskrit, *haldi* in Hindi and *jiang huang* in China) is a familiar Indian spice used in flavoring and coloring curries and sauces. Traditionally, it is used in Ayurveda as a digestive, circulatory, and respiratory stimulant, cleansing for the *chakras* and purifying the body. In folk medicine it is used for scabies, poor eyesight, to encourage milk flow in breastfeeding, and for rheumatic pains. The flowers are used in parts of India for sore throats and indigestion. Modern research has shown turmeric to be anti-inflammatory and antioxidant, to reduce cholesterol levels, stimulate bile production, and possibly act as a cancer preventative.

Parts used: Rhizome.

Key uses: Taken as a digestive stimulant and to combat infections as in gastroenteritis and food poisoning. Externally it was used with honey for sprains and bruises or taken as a milk decoction to cleanse and improve the skin. It is now also being used as an anti-inflammatory for arthritic conditions, to help thin the blood and lower cholesterol levels in cardiovascular disease. Typical dose is 250–1000 mg daily.

Cautions: Turmeric can cause skin rashes in sensitive individuals and may increase sensitivity to sunlight.

Tinospora cordifolia – **guduchi**

Guduchi powder is used in India as a popular remedy for liver problems, malaria, urinary disorders, and as a tonic during convalescence. It is taken in ghee (clarified butter) twice a day as a bitter tonic. The root is used for diarrhea and dysentery, the stem in infusions as an anti-inflammatory and antispasmodic in urinary diseases and fevers, while the fruits are regarded as a liver tonic and the leaves are cooling for fevers.

Parts used: Root, stem, fruit, leaf, whole plant.

Key uses: Used mainly as a bitter digestive tonic for liver congestion, and jaundice; it is also cooling in fevers and headaches and as a poultice for fractures. Typical dose is 1-2 g, twice a day.

BUSH HERBS

REMEDIES DOWN UNDER

For the Australian Aborigines, any illness that did not have an obvious cause, such as traumatic injuries or battle wounds, was likely to be "sung" – the result of a curse in the form of a ritual drawing placed on a tree. Recovery was only certain if the offending image was found and destroyed. In New Zealand, the warlike Maori took a similar approach, focusing mainly on wound herbs and external remedies with a limited range of internal treatments for fevers and digestive upsets. Before the European settlers arrived, life expectancy barely reached the mid-twenties, so many of the degenerative diseases of old age, common in the West, were unknown. Knowledge of healing herbs tended to be highly regionalized, with different plants used by various indigenous groups. European settlers took little, if any, interest in these native remedies, preferring to import and cultivate familiar Old World species, which now dominate herbal traditions in both countries. Over the past few years, interest has belatedly revived in native healing arts and several traditional remedies are being investigated. Tea tree and eucalyptus are probably the best known of the Aboriginal remedies – used as cure-alls for infections and injuries – and two of the few adopted by the early settlers. Others are proving significant: kangaroo apple (*Solanum aviculare*), for example, provides a precursor for the production of synthetic sex hormones and corticosteroids, while the bark of Moreton Bay chestnut (*Castanospermum australe*), a native poison, has been used in AIDS treatments and shows strong antiviral activity to HIV.

Acacia spp. – **Australian wattle**

Various acacia or wattle trees were an important source of Aboriginal medicines. Australian acacias vary from small shrubs, only a few centimeters high, to large trees reaching 15 meters or more. *A. ancistrocarpa*, was used to treat headaches, *A. holosericea* for coughs, colds, and laryngitis, and *A. decurrens* as a potent astringent for bleeding and mucus discharges. Ashes of certain *Acacia* spp. were also used in poultices for arthritic pains, and some studies suggest they contain salicylates – anti-inflammatory chemicals found in many European herbs used for similar disorders.

Parts used: Bark, roots.

Key uses: Acacia extracts are used in infusions and decoctions for a wide range of common ailments including common colds, diarrhea, and sore throats.

Pittosporum spp. – **lemonwood**

Traditionally, infusions of *P. phylliraeoides* were taken for colds. cramps and to encourage milk flow in nursing mothers; *P. venulosum* was one of a number of plants used by the Aborigines as aphrodisiacs. In New Zealand, *kohukohu* (*P. tenuifolium*) was largely used externally for skin irritations and eczema in the scalp, while gum extracted from the bark of *P. eugenioides* (*tarata*) was eaten for bad breath.

Parts used: Leaves, oleo-gum-resin, flowers.

Key uses: Research suggests that the essential oils for *Pittospermum* spp. are likely to be antimicrobial so may be useful remedies for infections and minor ailments; some anti-inflammatory activity also seems likely, and poultices of the leaves were effective for sores.

Melaleuca spp. – **paperbarks**

As well as tea tree (*Melaleuca alternifolia*) the Australian Aborigines used several other members of the genus for colds and sickness. In the Groote Islands, *M. symphocarpa* was known as "liniment tree" or *mawilyaburma* and used as a chest rub for respiratory problems or applied to the forehead for headaches. A maceration of the leaves was used as a wash for wounds and sores. Crushed leaves from the broad-leaved paperbark or *yinukwamba* (*M. viridiflora*) were also macerated as an internal remedy for coughs. Leaves from white paperbark or *yirarrnganja* (*M. leucadendron*) were used for coughs, rheumatic aches and pains, stomach upsets, and toothache. Leaves from the small-leaved paperbark *M. cajuputi*, made liniment for aches and pains and were used in steam inhalations for headaches.

Parts used: Leaves, bark, essential oil.

Key uses: In the West, cajeput (*M. cajeputi*) and niaouli (*M. viridiflora*) oils are used in chest rubs (5 drops per 5 ml of almond or vegetable oil) for coughs and colds or can be added to steam inhalants for nasal catarrh and sinus headaches.

Caution: The essential oils can cause skin irritation in sensitive individuals and should never be taken internally.

Grewia retusifolia – **emu berry**

Several members of the *Grewia* genus, a distant relative of the European linden, were used by Australian aborigines both as food sources and medicine. Fruits of the emu berry are eaten as food, while the root and bark are used medicinally as astringents and anti-inflammatories. The Aboriginals of the Northern Groote Islands, called the tree *mamurrinya* and roasted the roots before hammering them between stones and making a decoction for diarrhea. The same process of baking and crushing the root was used to make a maceration for treating sore eyes.

Parts used: Root, outer bark, fruit

Key uses: Root or bark decoctions and macerations can be used for diarrhea, inflammations and discharges.

Euphorbia spp. – **spurge**

Several varieties of spurge are used throughout the South Pacific, mainly for respiratory problems and skin sores. Pill-bearing spurge (*E. hirta*) was used in Australia for coughs and bronchial disorders and also to relieve asthma attacks. In the Philippines, decoctions of the plant were a traditional eye remedy, and in Hawaii it was used for poultices and gargles. *E. glauca*, Maori spurge, was used in infusions in New Zealand as a wash for skin sores. The nectar from the flowers of *E. atoto* was used in Australia for sore throats, while the leaves were used as a breast poultice to encourage milk production in nursing mothers.

Parts used: Aerial parts.

Key uses: Pill-bearing spurge is still used as an asthma remedy in the West in infusions and decoctions. The infusion is also worth trying as a wash for skin sores.

Leptospermum scoparium/Kunzea ericoides – New Zealand tea tree

The leaves of *kahikatoa* or *manuka* (*L. scoparium*) and *kanuka* (*K. ericoides*, formerly *L. ericoides*) were once used as a substitute for tea and were named "tea plant" by Captain Cook. The leaves were also used in steam inhalations by the Maori for colds, while the decoction made a lotion for muscular aches and pains and for urinary complaints. The seeds were used in Hawaii for diarrhea. A bark infusion of *kanuka* was taken as a calming sedative, while a bark decoction was preferred for diarrhea and dysentery. Young shoots and an infusion of the seed capsules were both used to treat dysentery.

Parts used: Leaves, seeds, seed capsules, bark, shoots.

Key uses: New Zealand tea trees are astringent and antimicrobial. *L. scoparium* contains an insecticide (leptospermone) which is also anthelmintic. Extracts are astringent and antiseptic and can be used for sores, infections and fevers.

FUNGI

MEDICINAL MUSHROOMS

Although we tend to associate healing, fungi-based remedies with modern antibiotic molds such as penicillin – identified in 1928 by Sir Alexander Fleming – they have been used medicinally since ancient times. Bracket fungi, such as agaric (*Polyporus officinalis*), collected from larch trees, were used by Dioscorides for a lengthy list of ills ranging from ague and "falling sickness" (epilepsy) to consumption, asthma, digestive upsets, and "the stinging of serpents and the biting of the same." Hoof fungus (*Fomes fomentarius*), another bracket variety, most common in Northern England and Scotland on birch and beech trees, makes an effective emergency styptic poultice for cuts and grazes. Many mushrooms have been used for their psychoactive properties – fly agaric (*Amanita muscaria*) extracts, for example, were eaten by Siberian shaman to induce the trance-like state needed for spirit traveling.

The edible wild mushrooms that make a seasonal appearance on supermarket shelves also have their therapeutic properties. Wood blewits (*Lepista nuda*), for example, have demonstrated antitumor activity in trials and will help to regulate sugar metabolism, so may be helpful in late-onset diabetes. St George's mushroom (*Calocybe gambosa*) is another effective remedy for diabetics. These cream-colored mushrooms traditionally appear around St. George's Day (April 23) in many parts of Europe and can be found in fields and downland throughout late spring and early summer.

Ganoderma lucidem – reishi mushroom

Known as *ling zhi* in China, reishi was highly regarded by the ancient Taoists as a spiritual tonic to enhance longevity by strengthening the disciple's determination to follow the path of virtue, central to Taoist belief. On a physical level, the fungus has been shown to stimulate the immune system, lower blood sugar and cholesterol levels, and is sedative and expectorant. It contains a number of polysaccharides, which have potent antitumor properties, and will lower blood pressure and act as a heart tonic. Reishi was once rare and only gathered from the wild, but commercial cultivation began in Japan in the 1970s and it is now widely available.

Parts used: Fruiting body.

Key uses: Reishi is a calming sedative for anxiety, insomnia, and nervousness, as well as a useful tonic for debility and exhaustion. It has been recommended in AIDS therapy, and it is used in Asia for degenerative diseases associated with aging such as chronic bronchitis, coronary heart disease, high blood pressure, and cancer. The usual dose is up to 1 g daily.

Cautions: Hemophiliacs are generally advised to avoid reishi, although research studies have shown conflicting results.

Lentinus edodes – shiitake

Shiitake is the second most commonly produced mushroom in the world. Shiitake is the Japanese name, and the mushrooms are known as *hua gu* and *xiang gu* in China; *edodes* in the botanical name means "edible." Research has shown that it is an effective tonic for the immune system and is strongly antiviral: it has been used in AIDS treatments and is effective against the polio virus, mumps, measles, herpes simplex I and II, and equine encephalitis. Shiitake is also antitumor, lowers cholesterol levels, and acts as an immune stimulant and liver tonic. Shiitake extracts have been used in Japan to help support patients undergoing chemotherapy and are also believed to improve the immune and endocrine function in the elderly.

Parts used: Fruiting body.

Key uses: Shiitake can be used in cooking to help stimulate the immune system, combat common colds, influenza and other viral infections and make a useful addition to anticancer diets. Unlike some fungi, they can also be helpful in candidiasis and will cleanse a sluggish liver and improve digestion. The traditional dose is about 90 g of fresh mushrooms or 15 g of dried in teas or soups. This is quite a significant amount and may lead to digestive upsets. For therapeutic use, concentrated extracts are available in capsules or tablets.

Wolfiporia cocos – tuckahoe or *fu ling*

Tuckahoe grows on the roots of pine trees and is known in both Chinese and Native American medicine. It is largely used in traditional Chinese medicine as a tonic for the spleen and stomach, to clear dampness and phlegm, treat jaundice and calm the spirit and dispel inappropriate behavior related to spiritual imbalance. In North America, tuckahoe is known as Indian bread and was an important food source. In China, various parts of the plant have different names: *fu ling* (the sclerotium), *fu ling pi* (the black outer skin), and *fu shen* (the tuber). These are used in subtly different ways, with *fu ling* mainly recommended as a diuretic and stomach tonic and *fu shen* regarded as a stronger sedative.

Parts used: Sclerotium, outer skin, tuber.

Key uses: Studies have shown tuckahoe to be antitumor, immune stimulant, antiviral, sedative, and analgesic. It is an effective diuretic used for such problems as scanty urination, edema, or painful urinary dysfunction, and is also helpful for palpitations and insomnia. Dosage is usually 9-15 g by decoction or 3-5 ml of tincture.

Cautions: *Fu ling* should be avoided in excessive urination or prolapse of the urogenital organs.

Cordyceps sinensis – caterpillar fungus

Caterpillar fungus, known as *dong chong xia cao* in China, is a parasite that grows on caterpillars of the moth *Hepialus armoricanus*, feeding on the animal and then fruiting in the spring. The traditional remedy used in China was a mixture of dead larvae complete with their fungal parasites, although today the fungus is cultivated on a grain base instead. In ancient China it was kept exclusively for use by the Emperor and his household and was always cooked with duck to increase its potency. Caterpillar fungus is an energy tonic, to strengthen lungs and kidney, and is helpful after chronic illness or exhaustion. It has been shown to have anticancer and antibacterial action and has been successfully used for patients with chronic kidney failure or hepatitis.

Parts used: Whole fungus.

Key uses: The fungus is used for asthma, bronchitis, persistent coughs, and other lung diseases. It is also used for irregular menstruation, traditionally taken in with chicken soup which, like duck, is believed to enhance its action. It also makes a restorative tonic in debility, weakness, and exhaustion associated with overwork. Typical dosage is 1 g of extract or up to 9 g of the crude herb twice a day.

WILD MUSHROOMS

Ceps (*Boletus edulis*), **chanterelles** (*Cantharellus cibarius*), **morels** (*Morchella esculenta*), and **oyster mushrooms** (*Pleurotus ostreatus*)

The autumn harvest of wild mushrooms is not only delicious to eat but also therapeutic. Wild ceps – generally found growing under conifers – are used in China as remedies for lumbago, leg pains and aching bones and tendons. Traditionally they are cooked with Siberian ginseng as a fertility remedy for women or with pork to combat vaginal discharges. The French regard them as a good source of minerals to combat fatigue and anemia. Ceps are known to contain eight essential amino acids so may act as a general metabolic tonic. Chanterelles contain a similar mix of amino acids but are also rich in vitamin A so make an important contribution to the diet and can help strengthen the retina and combat night blindness. They are used in European folk medicine as a remedy for colds and infections, suggesting antiviral activity. Highly prized and expensive, morels are used in China as a digestive tonic and are rich in amino acids and sterols. Oyster mushrooms are also a rich source of amino acids and B vitamins and display antitumor properties in laboratory studies. They also lower cholesterol levels, and the Chinese use them in remedies for lumbago and tendon pains.

Parts used: Fruiting bodies.

Key uses: Eat ceps, chanterelles, morels, and oyster mushrooms as a seasonal autumn tonic to combat colds and infections.

SOUTH AMERICAN HERBS

RAINFOREST REMEDIES

Healing plants from South America have been arriving in Europe since the fifteenth century and the days of the Spanish *conquistadors*. Many rapidly gained "cure-all" status and several have proved important sources of powerful drugs. Jesuit's bark (*Cinchona pubescens*) was first "discovered" by missionaries in Lima, Peru, in the 1630s, and became an important remedy for malaria and the original source of the drug quinine. *Lignum vitae* (*Guaiacum officinale*) was introduced by the Spaniards in 1508 as a remedy for syphilis; today, it is used by herbalists for treating gout and arthritis. Coca leaves (*Erythroxylum coca*) were chewed to combat fatigue, while extracts made a ritual psychoactive narcotic for South American tribes from at least 500 A.D. before finding their way to the West, first as an anesthetic and later as a much abused "recreational" drug. Chocolate (*Theobroma cacao*) was so highly esteemed by the Aztecs that the beans were used as currency. Cocoa powder was used for treating high blood pressure and angina pectoris, while cocoa butter is still used as a soothing ointment for burns and skin sores and as a base for pessaries. Today, new "wonder drugs" are still being discovered in the jungles of South America: many have been investigated by pharmaceutical companies in the hopes of finding powerful new chemicals while the plants themselves often become fashionable favorites in the health food market.

Caution: Many recently introduced South American plants have yet to be fully researched. As a precaution, it is best to avoid them in pregnancy and breastfeeding and take for limited periods only (up to four weeks followed by a break of two weeks).

Uncaria spp. – **Peruvian cat's claw**

Cat's claw, woody vine-like plant covered with thorns resembling the claws of a cat, has been used for centuries by the Ashaninka tribe in Peru as a cure-all. It was first identified by Western researchers in the 1960s, and by 1995 over-the-counter products were readily available. Two species are used: *U. tomentosa* and *U. guianensis*, which share many common properties: *U. guianensis* is said to be more specific for cancer of the female urinary tract and more suitable for digestive problems, while *U. tomentosa* is better for gynecological problems (including use as a post-childbirth tonic) and to combat the side effects of chemotherapy.

Parts used: Inner bark, although roots and leaves are also used in folk medicine.

Key uses: Traditional uses include arthritis, asthma, gastritis, diabetes, gonorrhea, cirrhosis of the liver, cancer and as a contraceptive. Research suggests that finely powdered bark or root needs to be decocted for at least 45 minutes to extract the active chemicals with a typical effective dose of 20 g of the herb to 1 liter of water taken in 60 ml doses daily.

Caution: Cat's claw is a traditional contraceptive so is best avoided by women trying to conceive.

Anemopaegma arvense – **catuaba**

Catuaba may be either *Erythroxylum catuaba* or *Anemopaegma arvense* depending on where in South America it originates. The plant is mainly regarded as a potent aphrodisiac – in Brazil, there is a saying that "until a father reaches 60, the son is his, after that the son is *catuaba*'s." A World Health Organization survey has identified the plant as worthy of further study for its possible antidepressant action. It is traditionally used in a decoction sweetened with cane sugar brandy or extracts of *Stevia rebaudiana* (a natural sweetener used in Brazil).

Parts used: Bark.

Key uses: Traditionally a male aphrodisiac, studies suggest that catuaba can be effective in treating male impotence. The Tupi Indians use the herb as a stimulant for the nervous system and as an invigorating tonic for both men and women. In the West, it is marketed in capsules with a recommended dose of 1 g morning and evening.

Paullinia cupana – **guarana**

Guarana has been known in the West as an energy-giving elixir since the seventeenth century when missionaries reported that members of the Maués-Sateré tribe carried it on journeys to combat hunger, fatigue, fevers, headaches, and muscle cramps. It is a popular drink in Brazil, much preferred to coffee, and is believed to stimulate the nervous system, improve concentration, and speed recovery after illness. It is also used as a diuretic and analgesic for menstrual problems and to relieve the discomfort of extreme heat. Guarana contains a caffeine-like compound called guaranine, which is slower to metabolize so gives a gentler, more sustained stimulating effect.

Parts used: Seeds.

Key uses: Usually described in the West as an energy-giving tonic, guarana can be helpful in chronic fatigue syndrome and is sometimes suggested for seasonal affective disorder (SAD) – tiredness and depression usually in the winter months. Usual dose is 1-2 g daily, in capsules.

Caution: Avoid in high blood pressure and heart disease.

Pfaffia paniculato – **paratudo**

Paratudo takes its name from *paro todo* – Portuguese meaning "for everything." The plant is known as Brazilian ginseng and is regarded in the Amazonian rain forests, where it grows, as a general cure-all and aphrodisiac. It was first described by the botanist Carl von Martius in 1891, but only became known in the West in the 1970s. Since then research has shown that paratudo is rich in steroidal compounds and saponins (similar to Korean ginseng), while pfaffic acid derived from the plant has been patented as an antitumor drug. The alternative common name "*suma*" is a recent invention for the U.S. health food market.

Parts used: Root

Key uses: Traditionally *paratudo* was used as an aphrodisiac, wound herb, for diabetes, and in cancer treatments. Since the 1970s the herb has been used effectively for cancer, chronic fatigue syndromes, arthritis, gout, to control cholesterol levels as a preventive for heart disease, and to reverse arterial damage caused by arteriosclerosis. Studies have also shown that it is rich in stigmasterol, which is a natural precursor for estrogen, and studies suggest it can be an effective treatment for menopausal problems and potentially a natural alternative to hormone replacement therapy. It is usually marketed in capsules with a recommended dosage of 1-4 g daily.

Tabebuia impetiginosa – **pau d'arco**

Pau d'arco, or *lapacho*, has been recognized as an antitumor and antimicrobial remedy since the 1860s. *Tabebuia* spp. are traditionally used by Amazonian tribes for treating asthma, diabetes, bronchitis, cancer, rabies, stomach ulcers, syphilis, and various infections. Pau d'arco is generally *T. impetiginosa* (syn. *T. avellenedae*) although, as always with wild-crafted South American herbs, contamination with other species is almost inevitable. Research in the early 1990s confirmed that *pau d'arco* extracts are effective for both cancer and candida infections, while Japanese studies suggest that it can be effective against leukemia and stomach cancer. Studies at the University of São Paulo have identified potent antibacterial, anti-inflammatory, and antifungal components, and the herb has also been used in treating breast and prostate cancers.

Parts used: Inner bark.

Key uses: In the West *pau d'arco* is often marketed as an anticandida remedy but is also effective for colds, flu and fevers. High doses have been used in experimental cancer treatments and it is also given for ulcers, rheumatism, high blood pressure, skin infections, urinary inflammations and pelvic inflammatory disease. The herb is generally sold in capsules with a typical recommended dose of 2-3 g daily. Traditionally the decoction is preferred although studies suggest that finely powdered bark is more effective.

Persea americana – **avocado**

The avocado originates in Central America, although it is now cultivated worldwide as a food plant. Oil, extracted from the seeds, is used as a base for massage oils in aromatherapy and also for minor skin irritations and blemishes. Traditionally the leaves and bark of the plant were used by Guatemalan tribes as a remedy for diarrhea and digestive upsets. Extracts were also taken to stimulate menstruation and as a cleansing remedy for skin diseases and gout. The fruit pulp is used in poultices for skin problems while the fruit skin acts as an anthelmintic to expel parasitic worms.

Parts used: Fruit, leaves, bark, seed oil.

Key uses: Avocados are readily available from food stores. Use the mashed pulp on skin sores and minor wounds. The oil can be used in skin lotions and massage rubs. Leaf and bark extracts are less readily available, although in areas where the plants grow can be gathered fresh for using in decoctions for diarrhea and abdominal bloating.

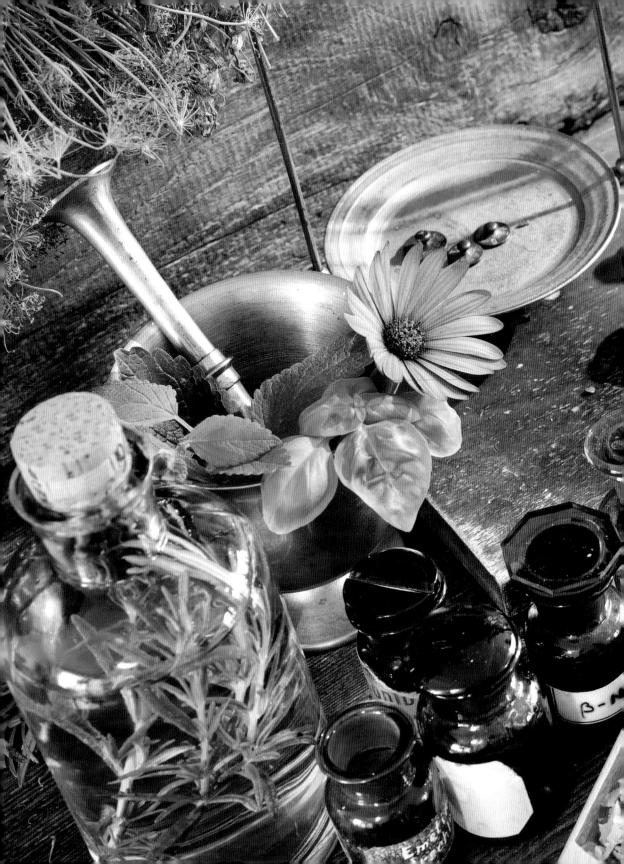

HERBAL REMEDIES

In many parts of the world herbs are the only option for all types of health problems. While professional herbalists in the West may use herbs for severe health problems, there is also a wide range of gentler remedies suitable for home treatment of common ailments. This section includes instructions on preparing remedies and an ailment-by-ailment guide. The focus is on herbs that can be safely used at home as an alternative to over-the-counter drugs. Other herbs that are commonly prescribed are included where appropriate.

HARVESTING & DRYING HERBS

When and where herbs are gathered can significantly affect the constituent chemicals and thus the therapeutic properties. In the past complex rituals where followed so that herbs were gathered at their most potent: at a particular phase of the moon, when the Dog Star could be seen, or during particular signs of the zodiac.

These traditions survive most obviously today in Tibetan medicine where herbs are often collected at times that are astrologically significant for the patient. The main considerations for most herb gatherers, however, are to collect the herbs on a dry day, when the plant is at the peak of maturity and the concentration of active ingredients is highest.

Herbs need to be dried as quickly as possible and away from bright sunlight to preserve the aromatic ingredients and prevent oxidation of other chemicals. A good circulation of air is also needed, so tie in small bunches and ensure a good circulation of air. Using an airing cupboard with the door left open, spare room, or a dry garden shed with a low-powered fan running can be effective. Avoid drying herbs in garages as they become contaminated with gasoline fumes. It is possible to dry herbs completely within a few days; the longer the plant takes to dry, the more likely it is to discolor and lose its flavor. Ideally the temperature in the drying room should be between 20–32°C/70–90°F and should never go above 38°C/100°F.

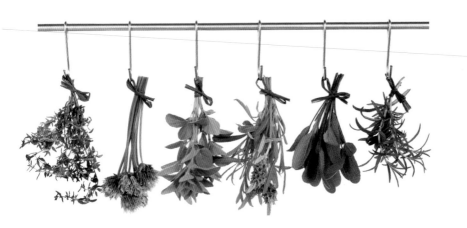

When the herbs are dry, store in clean, dry, dark glass or pottery jars with an airtight lid away from direct sunlight. If the herbs are stored when still slightly damp, they will go moldy. Label dried herbs with the variety, source, and date. Most should keep for 12–18 months without significant deterioration if they are dried and stored correctly.

FLOWERS

Harvest when fully open and the morning dew has evaporated. Handle carefully as they are easily damaged. Large flowers should be cut from their stems. Small flowers (such as lavender) can be dried on their stems although if the stem is fleshy, as with mullein, the flowers must be removed and dried individually.

Remove obvious dirt, grit, or insects and spread the flower heads on newspaper or trays and place in the airing cupboard or in a warm sunny spare bedroom to dry. When dry, store in dark glass or pottery containers, or in cupboards, as sunlight causes rapid deterioration of flower petals. Small flowers can be left intact but marigold petals are best pulled from the flower heads when dried and the central part of the flower discarded. Lavender flowers are best treated like seeds and dried in a paper bag or over a tray.

AERIAL PARTS AND LEAVES

Large leaves (such as burdock) can be gathered and dried individually but smaller ones (like lemon balm) are best collected with the stem. Generally, leaves of deciduous herbs should be harvested just before flowering while evergreen ones such rosemary can be gathered throughout the year. Coltsfoot leaves appear after the flowers so should be gathered then. If using all the aerial parts then the best time to collect is in the midst of flowering giving a mixture of leaves, stem, flowers, and seed heads.

Tie in small bunches of about 6–10 stems, depending on size, and hang upside down. When the leaves are brittle, but not so dry that they turn to powder when touched, the herb is ready. Rub from the stem onto paper or into a basin and discard any large pieces of stem. If all aerial parts of a plant are being used, then just crumble together. Pour or spoon the dried herbs into an airtight opaque container.

SEEDS

Harvest when ripe, or with large seed heads like fennel, when around two-thirds of the seeds on a particular head are ripe and before too many have been dispersed by birds or the wind. Large seed heads should be collected with about 15–25 cm of stem so that they can be dried in small bunches.

Either hang the bunch over paper or cover with a paper bag tied loosely to the bunch. The seeds will fall off when ripe and can be collected in the bag over the following couple of weeks. Store in an airtight, opaque container.

ROOT

Roots are generally harvested in the autumn when the aerial parts of the plant have died down and before the ground becomes hard enough to make digging difficult. An exception is dandelion, whose roots should be gathered in spring. Wash roots thoroughly to remove soil and dirt. Large roots should be chopped into small pieces when still fresh, as they can be difficult to cut when dry. Spread the pieces on trays and dry for 2–3 hours in a very cool oven (repeat this process two or three times for large roots but check regularly to avoid carbonizing the pieces), then transfer to an airing cupboard or quiet sunny room to complete drying undisturbed. Roots need to be stored in dry, airtight containers away from sunlight. Once dried, some tend to reabsorb moisture from the air and should be discarded if they become soft.

SAPS AND RESIN

These can be collected from trees by making a deep incision in the bark in autumn when the sap is falling and collecting the sap in a cup attached to the tree. A large bucket may be needed; copious amounts of birch sap, for example, can be collected overnight at certain times of year. Many saps can be corrosive so protective gloves should be worn. Sap from plants like lettuce and greater celandine can be collected by squeezing the leaf stems over a bowl, although usually the small amounts needed can simply be squeezed directly from the plant as required. Aloe sap can be collected by splitting open a leaf and scraping the gel it contains into a bowl using a palette knife or spatula.

FRUIT

Berries and other fruits should be gathered when just ripe and before they become too soft or pulpy to dry effectively. Spread on trays in an airing cupboard or warm place to dry. Fleshy fruits should be turned regularly to ensure even drying and any with signs of mold discarded.

BARK

Bark is generally best collected in the autumn when the sap is falling to minimize damage to the plant. Never remove all the bark – or a band of bark completely surrounding a tree – unless you want to sacrifice the plant to herbal medicine. Dust or wipe bark to remove moss or insects but avoid soaking in water. Break into manageable pieces (2–5 cm sq) and spread on trays in an airing cupboard or warm, dry, airy room and leave to dry.

BULBS AND CORMS

Harvest after the aerial parts have died down. Collect garlic corms quickly as they tend to move downwards once the leaves have wilted and can be difficult to find.

MAKING HERBAL REMEDIES

The instructions given here use standard quantities of herbs. Throughout the book, all quantities and doses are standard unless otherwise specified. In general, when using a combination of herbs the total quantity should be no more than the standard quantities suggested here. For example, an infusion for colds and flu could contain 10 g each of yarrow and elderflowers and 5 g of peppermint to give the usual proportion of 25 g to 500 ml of water. Doses for children and the elderly should be reduced depending on age and weight.

MEASURING REMEDIES

You can use standard spoons, droppers, or measuring cups for doses. The quantities given here for infusions and decoctions should be divided into three equal doses.

1 ml = 20 drops
5 ml = 1 teaspoon
20 ml = 1 tablespoon
1 sherry glass = approx. 65 ml
1 tea cup or wine glass = approx. 150 ml

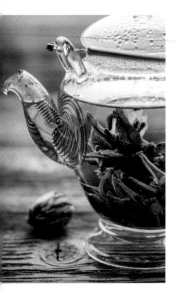

INFUSION

This is a very simple way of using herbs and can be made in much the same way as tea. The water should be just off the boil, rather than vigorously boiling, as otherwise valuable volatile oils would be lost in steam. This method can be used for flowers and the leafy parts of plants. The standard quantity should be made fresh each day and is sufficient for three doses; this can be strained and kept in a cool place for use later in the day. It may be drunk hot or cold.

Standard quantities
25 g dried herb or 75 g fresh herb to 500 ml water
Standard dose
One cup or wine glass three times a day
Equipment
Tea pot or tisane cup with lid
Kettle
Nylon sieve or strainer
Covered jug for storage

---

1. Put the required amount of fresh or dried herb into a lidded jug. Pour in 500 ml of boiling water and cover with the lid.
2. Infuse for 10 minutes, strain, and then drink the infusion in three wineglass doses during the day.

DECOCTION

Roots, barks, some berries, and twiggy parts of plants need more cooking to extract their active ingredients, and this is done by heating the herb in cold water and then simmering for up to 1 hour. As with infusions, the standard quantity should be made fresh each day and is sufficient for three doses; this can be strained and kept in a cool place for later use in the day. It may be drunk hot or cold.

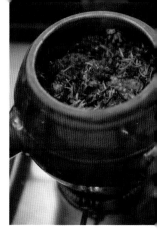

1. Put the required amount of herb into a saucepan and cover with 750 ml of cold water.
2. Bring to a boil and simmer until the volume has been reduced by one-third, usually about 20 minutes. Chinese decoctions are usually simmered for up to an hour to produce a very concentrated brew.
3. Strain into a jug with a lid, cover, and allow to cool slightly before taking in three wineglass doses during the day.

TINCTURE

This is made by steeping the herb in a mixture of alcohol or water: as well as extracting the active ingredients, the alcohol acts as a preservative and many tinctures will keep for up to two years. Single herbs are always used and then the prepared tinctured combined as required. Commercial tinctures use ethyl alcohol but for home use diluted spirits are suitable. Vodka is ideal as it contains fewer flavorings or herbal ingredients although rum can be useful for disguising the flavor of the less palatable herbs.

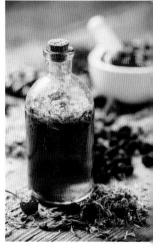

A 25% alcohol/water mixture is usually suitable with most based on a 1:5 ratio of herb to liquid (i.e. 100 g of herb to 500 ml of the alcohol/water mix). Commercially some tinctures are made with 45% or even 95% alcohol but such concentrations cannot easily be achieved for home production. Tinctures will general last for two years or more without deterioration, although Ayurvedic medicine argues that the tinctures increase in potency as they age.

1. Put the herb into a large jar then cover with the alcohol/water mixture.
2. Store in a cool place for two weeks.
3. Press the mixture through a wine press and store the resulting liquid in clean, dark glass containers. (The herbal residue is an ideal addition to the compost heap.)

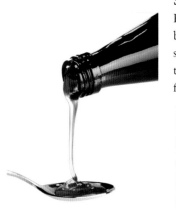

SYRUP

Honey or unrefined sugar can be used to preserve infusions and decoctions by making syrups, which are ideal for coughs; honey can be especially soothing. The added sweetness also disguises the flavor of more unpleasant tasting herbs, such as motherwort. Syrups can be used to flavor medicines for children.

Standard quantities
500 ml infusion or decoction
500 g honey or unrefined sugar
Standard dose
For coughs: 5–10 ml every 2–3 hours
Equipment
Saucepan
Wooden spoon
Dark glass bottles with cork stoppers for storage
Funnel (optional)

1. Heat 500 ml of a standard strained decoction or infusion with 500 g of honey or sugar.
2. Stir constantly until the sugar has dissolved. Bring to a boil and allow to boil gently for 1–2 minutes to sterilize the brew.
3. Cool and pour into dark glass bottles. Use cork stoppers on large containers, as syrups can ferment and cause screw-top bottles to explode. If making a small quantity for immediate use a screw-top bottle is acceptable.

INFUSED OILS

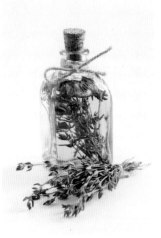

Active plant ingredients can also be extracted with oil for external use. The mixture will generally keep for about a year if kept cool and away from direct sunlight, although smaller quantities made fresh are more potent. The oils can also be used in ointments or creams. There are two techniques: hot infusion and cold infusion. The hot method is suitable for comfrey, chickweed (dried), rosemary or lavender. The cold method is suitable for flowers such as marigold, nettles or St. John's wort, and soft fresh leaves, such as chickweed or basil. Because the oil will not be heated in this second method, good quality, cold pressed, or unrefined seed oils rich in essential fatty acids, such as gamma-linolenic or cis-linoleic, which have significant therapeutic properties, can be used. If possible, "double infuse" oils made by the cold method by re-infusing the oil with a fresh batch of herb. Infused oils will generally last for at least a year, often longer.

HOT INFUSION

Standard quantities
Approx. 50 g of dried herb or up to 150 g of fresh to 500 ml of sunflower (or similar) oil
Equipment
Double saucepan
Wine press or muslin jelly bag
Large jug
Muslin or jelly bag for straining
Airtight storage bottle.

1. Put the required amount of herb into the top half of the double saucepan and cover with oil. If using bulky fresh herb additional oil may be needed to cover the material. Fill the lower half of the pan with water, bring to the boil and simmer for up to three hours.
2. Press out the oil through a muslin jelly bag or use a wine press.
3. Store in clean, airtight bottles.

COLD INFUSION

Standard quantities
Use enough fresh herb to tightly pack a storage jar.
Approx. 1 liter of sunflower or walnut oil depending on size of jar.
Equipment
Large jar
Jug
Muslin or jelly bag for straining
Airtight storage bottle

1. Fill a large jar with dried herb and completely cover with the oil. Put on the lid and leave on a sunny windowsill or in the greenhouse for two to three weeks.
2. Strain the oil through a jelly bag or wine press into a jug and if possible repeat the whole process using fresh herb and the once-infused oil leaving in a sunny place for an additional two or three weeks.
3. Finally, strain and store in clean, airtight bottles.

CREAM

A cream is a mixture of water with fats or oils and is "miscible" to soften or blend into the skin. It can easily be made using emulsifying ointment (available from most pharmacies), which is a mixture of oils and waxes that will blend with a given amount of water to make a cream. Homemade preparations like this will generally keep for several months, but the shelf life can be prolonged by storing in a cool larder or refrigerator. A few drops of benzoin can also be added to the mixture as a preservative. Creams made from organic oils and fats will deteriorate more quickly. The method described below is suitable for marigold petals, comfrey, chickweed, cleavers, lemon balm, chamomile flowers, elderflowers, and wood sage.

> **Standard quantities**
> 150 g emulsifying ointment
> 70 ml glycerol
> 80 ml water
> 30 g dried herb
> **Equipment**
> Double saucepan
> Wooden spoon
> Wine press and jelly bag
> Bowl
> Palette knife
> Glass jars with lids

1. Melt the emulsifying ointment in a double saucepan or a basin heated over a saucepan of boiling water.
2. Add the glycerin and water and then the dried herb, stirring to ensure the herb is covered by the liquid.
3. Continue heating for 2–3 hours, then pour the mixture into a wine press lined with muslin or a jelly bag and collect the melted cream mixture in a basin.
4. Stir the mixture until it sets, then use a palette knife to fill the jars. Start by filling around the edges and work towards the center to avoid trapping air bubbles in the jar.

OINTMENT

An ointment contains only oils or fats, not water, and unlike cream it will not soften or blend with the skin but forms a separate layer over it. Ointments are suitable where the skin is already weak or soft, or where some protection is needed from additional moisture, as in diaper rash. Traditionally ointments were made using animal fats such as lard, but soft paraffin wax (also called petroleum jelly) is also suitable.

> **Standard quantities**
> 500 g soft paraffin wax
> 60 g dried herb
> **Equipment**
> Double saucepan
> Wooden spoon
> Fine sieve or jelly bag
> Jug
> Palette knife
> Glass jars with lids

1. Melt the wax in the double saucepan or in a basin over a pan of boiling water.
2. Add the herb and stir to ensure it is covered by the melted wax.
3. Heat for about two hours or until the herb seems crisp, and then strain through a fine sieve or squeeze in a jelly bag into a jug.
4. Immediately pour the liquid into clean ointment pots and allow to set before closing the lids.

POWDERS AND CAPSULES

Herbs can also be taken as powders stirred into a little water or sprinkled on food or made into capsules: this can be ideal for the more unpalatable plants but is also convenient when traveling or at work. It is best to use commercially prepared powders which are available from specialist suppliers. Grinding herbs in a coffee grinder is possible, but usually generates heat, which can cause chemical changes within the plant, while hard roots can also damage the grinder. Two-part gelatin capsule cases are available from pharmacists and specialist suppliers.

1. To fill capsules, simply put some of the herb powder on a saucer, open the gelatin capsule, and bring the two halves together again, scooping up powder as you do so.
2. Store in a cool place; gelatin capsules do not respond well to heat and sunlight.

COMPRESS

Compresses are often used to accelerate healing, as with wounds or muscle injuries. They are basically cloth pads soaked in herbal extracts and usually applied when hot to painful limbs, swellings, strains, etc.

Standard application
Use a standard infusion, decoction or 5–20 ml of tincture in 500 ml of hot water (depending on herb).

1. Soak a clean piece of cotton, cotton wool, linen, or surgical gauze soaked in a hot, strained infusion, decoction, or tincture (diluted with hot water).
2. Apply to the affected area. When the compress cools or dries, repeat using hot mixture. Occasionally a cold compress may be used, as with some types of headaches when a cool pad soaked in lavender infusion may be suitable.

POULTICE

Poultices have a very similar action to compresses but involve applying the whole herb to an affected area directly rather than using a liquid extract. Poultices are usually applied hot for swellings, sprains, or to draw pus, but cold pastes/poultices can be useful, as with comfrey root applied to varicose ulcers. As with hot compresses, renew the hot poultice as it cools.

Standard application
Use sufficient herb to cover the affected area. Replace the poultice every 2–4 hours or earlier as needed.
Equipment
Saucepan
Bowl
Gauze/cotton strips
Hot water bottle

Fresh herbs
1. Bruise fresh herbs, mix in a food processor for a few seconds or sweat them in a pan.
2. spread the mixture onto gauze and apply to the affected area.

Dried herbs
1. Mix dried herbs with a little hot water to make a paste, squeeze out any surplus liquid, and then spread the residue on gauze or apply directly to the area affected.
2. Place a hot water bottle on top to keep the poultice hot.

OTHER HERBAL REMEDIES

MASSAGE OILS

As most essential oils will irritate the skin, they should be diluted before using for massage. Almond or wheatgerm oils are usually used as the "carrier" but sunflower or basic vegetable cooking oil can be substituted. Infused oil – such as comfrey or St. John's wort – can also be used. Once diluted in this way essential oils soon deteriorate so prepare mixtures as required. Generally a 5% solution of the essential oil in the base is adequate (e.g. 5 drops to 5 ml of carrier oil). Good massage needs skill and practice, but the oils can be suitable in home use for localized problems such as aching joints or chesty coughs. Pour about 2–5 ml of oil onto your hand and rub this gently into the affected area. Infused comfrey oil makes a good base for sprains, St. John's wort oil for inflammations, and bladderwrack for arthritic conditions.

CREAMS AND OINTMENTS FROM INFUSED OILS

Both hot and cold infused oils can be thickened with various fats and waxes, such as beeswax, cocoa butter, shea butter, and anhydrous lanolin to make ointments or creams.

Ointment: Use 100 ml of infused oil, 15 g beeswax, 20 g cocoa butter. Melt the wax and fat in a double saucepan and add the infused oil. Pour into clean glass jars while still warm and allow to cool.

Cream: Use 100 ml infused oil, 20 g beeswax, 20 g anhydrous lanolin and 50 ml herbal tincture. Melt the wax and fat in a double saucepan, add the infused oil and stir to ensure all is melted and remove from the heat. Warm the tincture to a similar temperature and then very slowly add the tincture to the melted mixture, stirring all the time. One can make various combination creams using different oil and herb/tincture combinations: comfrey and rosemary for arthritic pain, for example, or chamomile and St. John's wort for inflammations.

A NATURAL ALTERNATIVE TO EMULSIFYING OINTMENT

Instead of using emulsifying ointment for making cream, a combination of organic oils and waxes can be used. Follow the instructions given on p. 146, but melt 25 g of white beeswax and 25 g of anhydrous lanolin instead of the emulsifying ointment and then add 100 g sunflower oil, 25 ml glycerol, 75 ml water, and 50 g dried herb. Heat and strain as before, but stir 5 drops of benzoin into the cooling mixture as a preservative.

STEAM INHALANTS

These are ideal for catarrh, asthma, sinusitis, hay fever, or other forms of nasal congestion.
- Place the herb (usually 1 tablespoon of dried herb is sufficient) in a mixing bowl.
- Pour boiling water over the herb and mix well.
- Cover your head and the bowl with a towel and inhale for as long as you can bear the heat or until the mixture cools.
- Avoid going into a cold atmosphere for at least 30 minutes after the inhalation.

REDUCED ALCOHOL TINCTURES

In some cases a tincture based on ethyl alcohol may be unsuitable, such as for children, in pregnancy, in gastric or liver inflammation, or when treating reformed alcoholics. Adding a small amount (25–50 ml) of almost boiling water to the tincture dose (usually 5 ml) in a cup and allowing it to cool will effectively evaporate off most of the alcohol. Alternatively, it is possible to make tinctures using glycerol, wine, or cider vinegar. These are made in the same way as alcohol-based tinctures given on p. 143. A disadvantage of glycerol is that it is not a particularly effective solvent for oily or resinous herbs that may be incompletely extracted. Vinegar-based tinctures (known as acetracts) can taste extremely unpleasant and were traditionally sweetened with honey to make an oxymel. Vinegar itself is an expectorant and acetracts can sometimes be suitable as cough remedies. However, as vinegar also reacts chemically with some plant constituents, and may have additional side-effects, prolonged use or large doses of acetracts are not advisable.

FLUID EXTRACTS

These are made commercially and require special equipment that is not available for home use. They are more concentrated than tinctures – 1:1 weight:volume – so can be used in smaller quantities.

TONIC WINES

This is a delightful way to take your medicine and is especially suitable for roots, such as *he shou wu, dang gui,* or ginseng. Put 500 g of herb into a vat or large jug and add 2 liters of good quality wine (preferably red) so the herb is completely covered, otherwise it will go moldy. Cover the vat and leave for at least two weeks. Take one sherry-glass size dose daily.

MACERATIONS

Some herbs, such as marshmallow and valerian roots, are best macerated rather than infused or decocted, with the maceration then being used in the same way. Pour 500 ml of water onto 30 g of dried root and simply leave the mixture in a cool place overnight. Strain before use.

CHINESE DECOCTIONS

In China, herbs are mainly given in decoctions or soups (*teng*). Much larger quantities are used than in the West with up to 150 g of dried herb in 1 liter of water reduced down to 300–400 ml for three doses. The resulting mixture is very concentrated and may need to be diluted with water to suit Western palates.

LOTIONS

A lotion is a water-based mixture that is applied to the skin as a cooling or soothing remedy to relieve irritation or inflammation. It can also be used as a wash. Alcohol-based mixtures, such as tinctures, can be added to the lotion to increase the cooling effect. Typically, a lotion to relive skin irritation, for example, might include 40 ml rosewater, 20 ml borage juice, 20 ml distilled witch hazel and 20 ml chickweed tincture. A little of the lotion should be applied on cotton wool or absorbent gauze two or three times a day. If a small local area is being treated, then it can be useful to cover the area with a bandage afterward.

WASHES

Infusions or diluted tincture can be used to bathe wounds, sores, skin rashes, ulcers, etc. Use cotton wool to apply the wash bathing from the center of the wound or sore outwards. A plastic atomizer can be useful to spray rashes or varicose ulcers with the mixture.

PESSARIES AND SUPPOSITORIES

Special molds are available which will hold up to 24 pessaries or suppositories of various sizes. Homemade molds can be shaped from cooking foil – you need a small sausage shape, about 1 cm in diameter and 2 cm long, or shape your foil over a thimble. First lubricate the molds by filling them with a little lubricant (made from a mixture of 20 ml soft soap, 100 ml glycerin and 80 ml of industrial alcohol or methylated spirits). After a few minutes pour off the lubricant, drain well, and then fill with the pessary mixture. This is made by melting 20 g cocoa butter in a double saucepan, then stir in 10–20 drops (0.5–1 ml) essential oil. The unused pessary lubricant can be stored in a clean glass bottle for future use. Alternatively, melt 15 gm of gelatin with 20 gm of glycerin and 30 ml of herb infusions or tinctures diluted in water.

When set (about 2 hours) open the mold and remove the pessaries, which should be stored in a cool place.

JUICES

Herb juices can be prepared by using a domestic juicer or food processor to pulp the plant. Squeeze the mixture through a jelly bag to obtain the juice. Large quantities of herb are needed (a 2-gallon bucket full of fresh herb may yield only 100 ml or less of juice).

Herbal First Aid

In a domestic emergency, we are more inclined to reach for the standard over-the-counter remedies that fill the average first aid box than turn to herbal medicines. Yet herbs can provide effective alternatives to many pharmacy offerings and may be available when the standard first aid kit is not, such as using yarrow to stop a sudden nosebleed while in the depths of the countryside. For home use a selection of proprietary herbal preparations can be used to supplement fresh alternatives.

REMEDIES TO BUY

Herbal remedies are available in a variety of different formats such as creams, essential oils, flower remedies, and capsules. Shown here are some of the most useful herbal remedies to keep at home in the first aid box.

ARNICA TABLETS (6X)
Essential for any domestic shocks or accidents. The tablets can be taken at 30-minute intervals until the patient feels more settled.

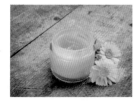

RESCUE REMEDY
The Bach Flower Remedies have a potent effect on the emotions. Rescue Remedy (also available as a cream) is good for shocks and nervous upsets.

ARNICA CREAM
Ideal for bruises and sprains but do not use on broken skin as it can be irritant. An alternative is to use a compress soaked in arnica tincture – 1 teaspoon to 500 ml of water.

COMFREY OINTMENT
This speeds healing by encouraging cell growth. Use only on clean cuts as otherwise the rapid healing may trap dirt in the wound.

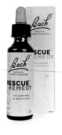

MARIGOLD CREAM
Often sold as *Calendula*. This is antiseptic and antifungal so is useful for athlete's foot or thrush as well as cuts, grazes, and patches of dry skin or eczema.

CHICKWEED CREAM
Generally used for eczema, but also a valuable first aid remedy for burns, scalds, and as a drawing ointment for removing toxins from boils and abscesses, insect stings, and stubborn splinters.

TEA TREE OIL
This is highly antiseptic and antifungal for cuts, grazes, and other skin infections. A cream is available for vaginal thrush. A few drops of the oil can be used neat on warts and cold sores.

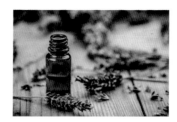

LAVENDER OIL
Add 2–3 drops to a teaspoon of vegetable oil and massage into the nape of the neck and temples at the first hint of an approaching headache or migraine. Use the same mix to soothe minor burns, scalds, sunburn, and cold sores.

THYME OIL
Also an effective antiseptic: use 2–3 drops in a teaspoon of vegetable oil as a chest rub for coughs and chesty colds.

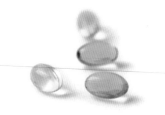

EVENING PRIMROSE CAPSULES
These can be used as a hangover cure. A large dose (2–3 g) on "the morning after" brings rapid relief.

DISTILLED WITCH HAZEL
This can be used for minor burns and sunburn while a swab soaked in distilled witch-hazel staunches the flow of blood from wounds, eases varicose veins, and soothes insect bites. For bruises and sprains a useful option is to keep an ice cube tray of distilled witch-hazel in the freezer – ensuring, of course, that they are clearly labeled!

SYRUP
Numerous patent herbal cough syrups are available – look for thyme and licorice, horehound and aniseed, or blends containing mousear, hyssop, elecampane, or Iceland moss.

HOMEMADE REMEDIES

Raw ingredients in the kitchen cupboard, such as garlic, ginger, and herbal teas, provide some of the most useful first aid remedies. In addition, infused oils can be made when the plants are in season and used throughout the year.

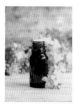

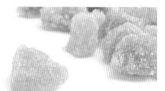

INFUSED OILS

Use St. John's wort oil for burns and sunburn; marigold oil for fungal infections (like athlete's foot), dry skin and grazes; comfrey oil for bruises, sprains, or arthritic joints; rosemary oil for rheumatic aches, and pains and lemon balm oil for insect bites and as an insect deterrent.

GARLIC

Use the highly antiseptic cloves rubbed on acne pustules and other infected spots or use crushed garlic to draw corns.

DRIED HERBS

Keep an assortment of dried herbs or herbal tea-bags handy: use chamomile flowers as a steam inhalation (1 tablespoon of flowers in a large basin of boiling water) for catarrh, hay fever, or mild asthma attacks, or drink as an infusion for shock and nervous upsets. Use a strong infusion of sage as a mouthwash for mouth ulcers and gargle for sore throats. Drink fennel or peppermint for indigestion, elderflower for colds and catarrh, lavender for headaches.

GINGER

Make a decoction of fresh root with a pinch of powdered cinnamon for chills or chew crystallised ginger or ginger cookies to prevent travel sickness.

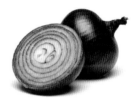

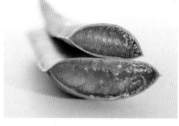

HONEY

Use runny honey for drying-up wounds or drawing pus from infected cuts.

ALOE

To soothe minor burns, scalds or sunburn break off a leaf from an *Aloe vera* plant, split it open and apply the thick sap to the affected area immediately.

ONIONS

Use fresh slices on insect stings. Home made cough syrup can be made by layering slices of onion with brown sugar or honey, leave overnight, collect the thick brown syrup and take 5–10 ml three or four times daily as required.

IN THE FIELD

In a countryside emergency look for yarrow for wounds and nosebleeds; crushed daisies for bruises and sprains; shepherd's purse, self-heal, woundwort, wild geranium, or herb Robert to stop bleeding; fresh plantain or lemon balm for insect bites, and dock leaves for nettle stings.

HOME REMEDIES

Herbalism has always been regarded as the "medicine of the people" – simple remedies that can be used at home, both for a wide range of minor ills or to supplement more potent remedies prescribed by professionals for chronic and acute conditions. Herbs can be taken quite simply as teas, although more complex preparations can be made at home (see pp. 142–147) or are available from health food shops and pharmacies as patent medicines. Although most herbs are intrinsically quite safe they do need to be treated with respect. Do not exceed stated doses or continue with home remedies if conditions are persistent, are worsening, or if the true diagnosis is in doubt.

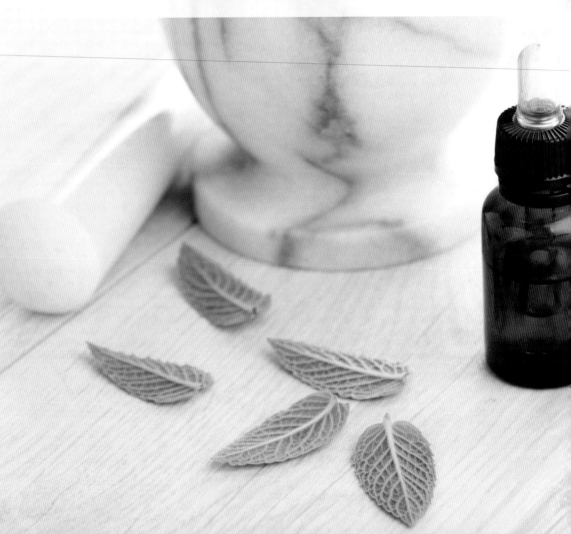

How to use this section

In this section, ailments are grouped according to body systems, life stages, or action. The complaints covered are those where home remedies are most appropriate, although herbs can, of course, be used for many more ailments than are included here. The list of complaints is not intended to be comprehensive nor exhaustive, and the herbs given for each ailment represent only a small cross-section of the many plants that could be suitable in each case. Selection of individual remedies will often depend on availability, but in selecting herbs for particular ailments choose those that appear to have the most relevant actions for a particular case. For example, for coughs, do you need an expectorant to clear phlegm, a suppressant to ease a persistent irritating tickle, an antibacterial to combat infection, or a tonic to strengthen weak lungs?

Herbs can work very quickly, especially in acute conditions. However, long-standing, chronic disorders may require treatment for several months before significant results are achieved. Traditionally it was said that one needed to take a remedy for one month for every year that the condition had persisted. Cyclical disorders, like menstrual disturbances, generally improve after two or three months. Generally, symptoms will change as the weeks progress, so be prepared to review the remedy at least once a month, and make changes to reflect new conditions. Professional herbalists will generally make adjustments to remedies every few weeks as health and energy balance change.

For ailments not covered in this section, or for persistent conditions, then consult a professional (see *Consulting an Herbalist*, p. 257). If gathering herbs in the wild or from gardens, consult a good plant key or field herbal to ensure that the correct plants are selected in each case.

Important notes
- In any acute condition – fevers, coughs, digestive upsets, severe headaches, etc. – seek professional help if there is no improvement within a few days or if the condition appears to be worsening.
- If taking medication for any particular complaint always consult your GP or other professional medical practitioner before changing dosages. Some herbs do interact with orthodox drugs so care is needed in some circumstances.
- Children should be given a fraction of the full adult dose depending on their ages. See p. 229 for details.
- In the elderly, metabolism gradually slows down so standard adult doses should be reduced with increasing frailty and loss of body weight.
- Essential oils are extremely potent and many can irritate mucous membranes. Unless otherwise clearly stated in the remedy charts, do not take essential oils internally without professional medical supervision. Before using externally, dilute essential oils in a carrier oil – wheatgerm, almond, or avocado are best but sunflower, olive, or safflower are acceptable if that is all you have. Because essential oils are so expensive, many synthetic chemical substitutes are offered for sale. Always buy a reputable brand, guaranteed to be pure and unadulterated; do not be mislead by low-cost products.

ACHES & PAINS

The usual reaction to muscular pain is to reach for the painkillers – aspirin, paracetamol, codeine – which very quickly lull the body back into pain-free comfort. Pain, however, is only a symptom: a reminder that something is not quite right. Pulled muscles and strained tendons need restricted movement to heal and those painful twinges remind us to keep physical exertion to a minimum while the body heals itself.

Herbal remedies can often do more than just deaden pain: many plants act as muscle relaxants and antispasmodics, as anti-inflammatories, or cell proliferants, actually repairing the damage of traumatic injury or degenerative disease like osteoarthritis. Essential oils can be the most effective for muscular or joint pains. Diluted rosemary essence can bring fast symptomatic relief when massaged into arthritic joints or used on hot compresses.

But while symptomatic relief can be valuable it doesn't always solve the problem: an herbal approach to osteoarthritis may involve the use of comfrey ointment to encourage the repair of damaged and degenerating bone, anti-inflammatory herbs like willow, devil's claw, or meadowsweet to help relieve pain and cleansing plants, such as yellow dock, burdock, or celery seed, to rid the body of toxins that can collect in the joints and contribute to the discomfort.

In traditional Chinese medicine, arthritis and rheumatic pains are termed "*bi* syndrome" and are attributed to the same "external evils" – wind, damp, cold, or heat – that are blamed for colds and fevers. A "cold" type of *bi* syndrome might be treated with warming diaphoretic herbs like *ma huang* or *gui zhi* while others, such as *bai zhu* or *bai shao yao*, could be used to strengthen the body's vital energies and improve *qi* circulation, helping to prevent future attack from other "evils."

CASE HISTORY

ARTHRITIC PAINS

Patient: Mary, a retired school secretary, age 66, an enthusiastic lace maker and gardener.

History and presenting complaint: Mary had a history of nervous problems and had taken regular antidepressants and sleeping pills for more than five years. For the past three years, she had suffered pains and stiffness in her hands, knees and hips. Hospital tests had ruled out rheumatoid arthritis but X-rays had revealed some wear and tear on the joints. A family bereavement had exacerbated the problem. She also reported breathlessness, palpitations, and sore, irritated eyes.

Treatment: Mary's regular antidepressant carried the risk of liver damage as a side effect and her symptoms suggested some liver congestion and weakness, so herbal medication included tinctures of *bai shao*, *huai niu xi*, and bogbean, as well as angelica root, willow bark, and *fang feng* (total 5 ml three times daily). A few drops of the Bach Flower Remedy, Star of Bethlehem, were added to help her cope with the shock of her recent loss. Mary was also given devil's claw capsules (two to three times a day) to take while symptoms were particularly acute and a massage oil containing 1 ml each of rosemary and juniper essence in 50 ml of infused comfrey oil to give symptomatic relief for painful joints.

Outcome: A month later Mary was back at her lace making class, the painful knees and sore eyes were back to normal, and her hands were no longer stiff. Medication, with a few changes, continued for a further two months gradually reducing the dose to 5 ml a day as her symptoms eased. Over the following months, Mary gradually switched to herbal remedies for insomnia and was able to wean herself off the sleeping pills. Her GP has found an alternative antidepressant with less harmful side effects and she is now slowly reducing the dosage with the help of herbal nervines.

SPRAINS AND STRAINS

Accidental injuries to joints and muscles including back strains. If fractures are a possibility or suspected or if symptoms persist beyond a few days without improvement seek urgent professional help.

KEY SYMPTOMS:

- Pain following obvious injury or exertion.
- Swollen joints or limbs.
- Bruising.

REMEDIES:

Arnica montana—ARNICA

FLOWERS

Actions: Wound herb and antibacterial, causes reabsorption of internal bleeding for bruises and sprains.

How to use: Externally use cream or dilute tincture as compress; take Arnica 6X every 1–2 hours.

Combinations: Use as a simple.

Precautions: Do not use on broken skin; only take homoeopathic arnica internally.

Symphytum officinale—COMFREY

INFUSED OIL

Actions: Encourages cell growth of connective tissues and bones; breaks down red blood cells in bruising.

How to use: Use ointment or infused oil frequently as required.

Combinations: Add 5–10 drops of essential oils, such as thyme, lavender, or juniper to 25 ml infused oil.

Precautions: Only use if the injury is clean; not advisable for long-term internal use.

Thymus vulgaris—THYME

ESSENTIAL OIL

Actions: Antispasmodic and stimulant encouraging blood flow to the tissue to encourage repair.

How to use: Use 10 drops of oil to 25 ml water in a compress, or 10 drops in a hot bath.

Combinations: With other essential oils, such as lavender, rosemary, or sage, in an almond or sunflower base as a massage oil.

Precautions: Massage can be damaging if given too soon after injury.

ARTHRITIS AND RHEUMATISM

Osteoarthritis (OA) is generally due to "wear and tear" on the joints but can be linked to cold and damp conditions. Rheumatoid arthritis (RA) involves inflammation in many joints, usually symmetrically, and requires professional treatment. Rheumatism is a general description for any muscle or joint pain, while lumbago refers to low back pains.

KEY SYMPTOMS:

- Stiffness and joint pain.
- Creaking sounds in joints.
- Joint deformities and swellings.
- Joints may feel hot or burning in RA.
- Symmetric joint swellings in RA.
- Symptoms are often worse in damp weather in OA.
- Frozen shoulder (chronic stiffness and pain in the shoulder joint) can be treated as for OA.

REMEDIES:

Harpagophytum procumbens—DEVIL'S CLAW

ROOT

Actions: Potent anti-inflammatory; action has been compared with cortisone. Better for OA and degenerative conditions.

How to use: Use 1–3 g powder daily in capsule form in acute phase; up to 15 ml tincture daily or in combinations.

Combinations: Often taken as a simple but can be combined with tinctures of angelica, St. John's wort, bogbean or celery seed.

Salix alba—WILLOW

BARK

Actions: Rich in salicylates, which are anti-inflammatory and cooling for hot joints; useful in acute phases.

How to use: Up to 5 ml of fluid extract three times daily or with other tinctures in combinations.

Combinations: Can be used with tinctures of angelica, black cohosh, *lignum vitae*, yellow dock, or burdock.

Precautions: Avoid in cases of salicylate allergy.

Menyanthes trifoliata—BOGBEAN

LEAVES

Actions: Cleansing, cooling, and anti-inflammatory: a useful herb for "hotter" types of arthritis and muscle pain.

How to use: Up to 8 ml of tincture three times daily; also as a infusion or macerate 10 g in 100 ml red wine.

Combinations: In decoctions with black cohosh or celery seeds; in tinctures with St. John's wort, meadowsweet or prickly ash bark.

Angelica archangelica—ANGELICA

ROOT

Actions: Good for "cold" type arthritis: warming and stimulating.

How to use: Dilute tincture or infusion as compress or internally as standard decoction.

Combinations: Add celery seed or prickly ash to decoctions.

Precautions: Avoid in pregnancy.

GOUT

Generally associated with build up of uric acid in joints; may be linked to dietary excess.

KEY SYMPTOMS:
- Swollen, inflamed and very painful joints.
- Toes or foot joints often affected.

REMEDIES:

Apium graveolens—CELERY

SEED

Actions: Clears uric acid from joints; useful in both gout and arthritic problems.

How to use: In infusions (1 teaspoon to 500 ml water) or combined with other tinctures.

Combinations: With *lignum vitae* in infusions; tincture with yarrow, gravel root or burdock.

Precautions: Use only seeds intended for medicinal use; avoid in pregnancy.

Teucrium chamaedrys—WALL GERMANDER

AERIAL PARTS

Actions: Bitter digestive tonic and diuretic.

How to use: Standard infusion or up to 15 ml of tincture daily.

Combinations: Combine with yarrow and celery seed in infusions or with burdock and gravel root in tincture.

RHEUMATISM OR MYALGIA

Rheumatism is a very non-precise term used to describe a range of muscular pains (myalgia). It can include fibrositis (inflammation of the muscle and muscle sheath) often affecting the back, or may simply be due to overexertion.

KEY SYMPTOMS:
- Painful, sore, aching muscles.
- May be associated with traumatic injury or food intolerance.

REMEDIES:

Actaea racemosa—BLACK COHOSH

ROOT

Actions: Analgesic, cooling and soothing; contains salicylic acid to reduce inflammation and ease stiffness.

How to use: Take a decoction or 10–40 drops of tincture per dose, three times daily; take 1 x 200 mg capsule up to three times a day.

Combinations: Combine with bogbean in decoctions or anti-inflammatories like devil's claw in capsules.

Rosmarinus officinalis—ROSEMARY

ESSENTIAL OIL

Actions: Stimulating, analgesic and antirheumatic; warms muscles by encouraging blood flow to the area.

How to use: Use 10 drops of oil in 5 ml of infused bladderwrack oil as a massage as required. Also helpful for arthritic pains.

Combinations: Use infused St. John's wort as an alternative base or add additional warming and analgesic essential oils such as eucalyptus, juniper, hyssop, or thyme.

BACKACHE & LUMBAGO

Common and often nonspecific, backache may be due to pulled muscles, damaged discs, nerve problems, strains or kidney weakness. Lumbago refers to low back ache in the lumbar region.

KEY SYMPTOMS:

• Pain which can be chronic, debilitating, and restrict movement.

Important: Seek professional help for any persistent back pain of unknown cause.

REMEDIES:

Berberis vulgaris—BARBERRY

STEM BARK

Actions: Anti-inflammatory, cleansing, can be especially helpful for low back pains.

How to use: Take in decoction, half a cup per dose, or up to 5 ml of tincture, three times daily.

Combinations: With diuretics like celery seed, buchu and horsetail for back pain associated with kidney problems; with anti-inflammatories, such as black cohosh and devil's claw for muscle or joint inflammations.

Precautions: Avoid in pregnancy.

Juniperis communis—JUNIPER

BERRIES & ESSENTIAL OIL

Actions: Antirheumatic, stimulating, clears excess lactic acid from muscles.

How to use: Take 10–20 drops of tincture per dose; use half a teaspoon of crushed berries per cup of infusion; use 10 drops essential oil per 5 ml almond oil as external massage.

Combinations: Use with analgesics and anti-inflammatories such as valerian, devil's claw, white willow, and black cohosh in tinctures or capsules (2 x 200 mg capsules per dose).

Precautions: Avoid in pregnancy; do not take internally for longer than six weeks without a break; do not take if there is any kidney damage or disease.

TENNIS ELBOW & TENOSYNOVITIS

Tenosynovitis is an inflammation of the tendon sheaths and commonly affects wrist, elbow, or fingers, while tennis or golfer's elbow involves inflammation of the bursa – a small sac filled with fluid that forms part of the joint.

KEY SYMPTOMS:

• Pain and difficulty in moving the affected joint.
• Numbness or tingling in the fingers.
• Worse when twisting the joint.

REMEDIES:

Guaiacum officinalis—LIGNUM VITAE

HEARTWOOD

Actions: Anti-inflammatory and cooling suitable for any muscle or joint inflammations including tendon problems.

How to use: Take half a cup of decoction made from half a teaspoon of chippings per cup; take up to 10 ml of tincture per day.

Combinations: With antispasmodics and anti-inflammatories like guelder rose, prickly ash bark, and black cohosh in tinctures or decoctions.

Achillea millefolium—YARROW

AERIAL PARTS & ESSENTIAL OIL

Actions: Reduces inflammation in joints, tendons and muscles to give pain relief and improve movement.

How to use: Use 10 drops of essential oil in 20 ml of infused St. John's wort oil as a massage; use a cold, chilled infusion for soaking a compress to relieve pain and stiffness.

Combinations: Use with lavender oil in external massage or combine with stinging nettle and arnica infusions in a compress.

Precautions: Prolonged use may case skin rashes or increase photosensitivity in rare cases.

REPETITIVE STRAIN INJURY (RSI)

Painful spasms and weakness in hands, arms, shoulders neck or back associated with repetitive physical actions that lead to gradual tissue damage.

KEY SYMPTOMS:
- Extreme pain in moving or manipulating the limbs or fingers.
- Sudden onset may be preceded by numbness and tingling.
- Limbs may be extremely sensitive and excruciating to touch.

REMEDIES:

Lentinus edodes—SHIITAKE

MUSHROOMS

Actions: Tonics like shiitake can help to improve the body's ability to cope with physical stress while reducing the inflammation associated with the symptoms.

How to use: Take up to 10 g of dried shiitake powder per dose with water; decoction use 90 g of fresh mushrooms in a daily soup.

Combinations: Add Siberian ginseng or *huang qi* powders, or add a piece of either root to the soup and simmer for at least 50 minutes to increase resistance to stress and tonify the system.

Filipendula ulmaria—MEADOWSWEET

AERIAL PARTS

Actions: Contains salicylates to reduce inflammation and ease pain; gentle digestive stimulate to improve metabolism.

How to use: Use in infusion or tincture.

Combinations: With nervines such as St. John's wort and vervain in infusions; with white willow and valerian in tinctures.

Precautions: Avoid in cases of salicylate allergy.

SCIATICA

Nerve pain caused by irritation or pressure on the sciatic nerve, which runs from the spine along the back and outer thigh to the foot. Often caused by damage to discs. The label is applied to general backache but should only refer to problems associated with the sciatic nerve.

KEY SYMPTOMS:
- Back pain and stiffness; pain travels along the path of the nerve.
- Pain on bending or picking up items from the floor.

REMEDIES:

Zanthoxylum americanum—PRICKLY ASH

BARK

Actions: Stimulates circulation to supply nutrients to tissue and help repair and remove wastes; eases spasmodic pains.

How to use: Use in decoctions (half a teaspoon per cup) or take up to 10 ml of tincture daily.

Combinations: In decoctions with anti-inflammatories and nervines such as *lignum vitae*, black cohosh, and valerian; in tinctures with St. John's wort, white willow, and black cohosh.

Capsicum frutescens—CAYENNE

FRUIT

Actions: Stimulates blood flow, strengthens the nerves and relieves nerve pains.

How to use: Use the infused oil in massage or take 5 drops of tincture in water per dose.

Combinations: Add 2–5 drops of juniper or rosemary oil to the infused oil as additional circulatory stimulants; add up to 5 ml of nervines like St. John's wort or valerian tincture per dose.

Precautions: Prolonged or excessive topical use may lead to blistering.

CRAMP

Muscle spasm which can be painful and prolonged. Can be associated with imbalance of salts or stress and fatigue.

KEY SYMPTOMS:
- Sharp, severe pain in the legs.
- Affected muscle feels hard and rigid to touch.

REMEDIES:

Viburnum opulus —GUELDER ROSE

BARK
Action: Effective relaxant for both smooth and skeletal muscle; anti-inflammatory.

How to use: Use 25% tincture in rosewater as a lotion or in creams.

Combinations: Combines well with Indian tobacco in cramp creams.

Dioscorea villosa—WILD YAM

RHIZOME
Action: Muscle relaxant and mild peripheral vasodilator.

How to use: Sip a standard decoction or take 20 drops of tincture and repeat every 15 minutes if symptoms persist.

Combinations: As a simple or with guelder rose tincture.

Precautions: Avoid in pregnancy unless under professional guidance.

HEADACHES & MIGRAINES

Headaches and migraines need to be regarded as symptoms of *disease* rather than identifiable illnesses in their own right, and a holistic approach to health care always looks for underlying causes of discomfort. Headaches can, of course, be associated with stress or tension, in which case calming, sedating herbs (known as nervines) could be suitable. Persistent stress headaches could signify a need for a radical reappraisal of lifestyle, or simply a need to learn basic relaxation techniques to cope with day-to-day stresses. Nasal catarrh and sinusitis can also cause head pain – usually around the frontal sinuses over the nose and below the eyes. There are many decongestant herbs to clear the upper respiratory tract that can be used here, such as elderflower, marshmallow leaf, golden rod, hyssop, or bistort. Fresh air and a diet free of mucus-forming foods (dairy products, alcohol, and an excess of sugars and refined carbohydrates) can also help.

Migraines are generally associated with visual disturbances, such as flashing lights zig-zagging across the visual field, and these headaches can be related to food intolerance or pollutants. Some migraines are "hot" – relieved by ice-packs – while others are "cold" and can be helped by a hot towel on the forehead. "Cold" migraines respond to warming, stimulating herbs such as rosemary, ginger, or *gui zhi*, while the "hot" types are best treated with cooling, bitter remedies like lavender and vervain. Digestive remedies, especially cleansing liver herbs like dandelion or agrimony, can also be helpful; in traditional Chinese medicine, the eyes are closely associated with liver function and migraines, with their visual upsets and light sensitivity, can be identified with over-exuberant liver *qi* or pathogenic "wind" affecting the liver.

Note: *Consult a professional practitioner for sudden persistent headaches or any change in the pattern of regular headaches.*

Cross references
Anxiety and Tension, p. 201; PMS, p. 209; Sinusitis p. 167.

CASE HISTORY

TENSION HEADACHES

Patient: Vera, 45, a part-time secretary with a husband, two teenage children, and an elderly mother-in-law living with them.

History and presenting complaint: Frequent headaches – for which Vera took patent analgesics – once or twice a week, always localized over her right eye and often persisting for two or three days. Vera had suffered from headaches since her teens and also complained of a "nervous tummy" with frequent bouts of diarrhea, a tendency for depression, and extreme tiredness. Medical tests had been unable to detect any abnormalities contributing to the condition. Her teenage daughters were "difficult" and Vera found her mother-in-law's constant presence increasingly irksome. Shortage of money was a constant worry.

Treatment: Like many highly stressed, working women with families, Vera never managed to find time for herself – the prescription therefore included a little self-indulgence: lavender oil for the bath and five minutes with her feet up when she got home from work. Medication focused mainly on relaxing and tonic nervines to improve stress tolerance and ease the depression, in addition to remedies that were also helpful for liver and stomach tensions. Internally, tinctures included wood betony, vervain, lemon balm, oats, and pasque flower (in total 5 ml three times daily), with capsules of Siberian ginseng as a tonic.

Outcome: Over the next couple of months there was a significant improvement in the headaches, which were less frequent or severe. A bout of family arguments brought them back, but Vera began to realize how closely linked her headaches were to the stresses at home and her own emotions – when her mother-in-law went on holiday for two weeks, Vera had a happy pain-free fortnight. In an ideal world, an in-law apartment or nearby residential home for her mother-in-law might have easily solved Vera's problems; as it was, Bach Flower Remedies (impatiens, willow, and beech to encourage a little tolerance) had to do the job instead.

TENSION HEADACHES

May be caused by tightening of the neck muscles due to stress or anxiety. Symptoms may resolve with relaxation.

KEY SYMPTOMS:
• Pain, generally frontal.

REMEDIES:

Stachys officinalis—WOOD BETONY

AERIAL PARTS
Actions: Sedative and stimulant for cerebral circulation; useful nervine for anxiety and worries.

How to use: Standard infusion or tincture.

Combination: Add lavender, vervain, St. John's wort, skullcap to infusion or tincture.

Precautions: Avoid high doses in pregnancy.

Scutellaria lateriflora—SKULLCAP

AERIAL PARTS
Actions: Relaxant and restorative for the central nervous system; sedative and antispasmodic.

How to use: Standard infusion or tincture.

Combination: Mix 45 ml of skullcap tincture and 5 ml of lemon balm and take in 5 ml doses (up to four times daily).

MIGRAINE

Can be linked to food sensitivity, menstrual cycle, or other stresses. Associated with tension changes in the arteries of the brain. Untreated symptoms may last for a few minutes or several days.

KEY SYMPTOMS:
- Characteristic visual disturbances always precede pain.
- Pins and needles in limbs.
- Sickness and nausea.
- Light sensitivity.

REMEDIES:

Tanacetum parthenium—FEVERFEW

AERIAL PARTS

Actions: Anti-inflammatory, dilates cerebral blood vessels so helpful for migraines associated with constriction.

How to use: Eat one leaf daily as a prophylactic or use 10 drops of tincture every 30 minutes while symptoms persist.

Combination: Combine with valerian or Jamaican dogwood tincture in drop doses.

Precautions: Side-effects can include mouth ulceration; avoid if taking anti-coagulant drugs such as warfarin.

Lavandula spp.—LAVENDER

FLOWERS & ESSENTIAL OIL

Actions: Sedative and analgesic with antispasmodic action.

How to use: Massage lavender oil (neat or diluted 50:50 with carrier oil) into temples at the first hint of symptoms.

Combination: Follow massage treatment by drinking lavender flower and vervain infusion.

Precautions: Do not take lavender oil internally without professional guidance.

Gelsemium sempervirens—YELLOW JASMINE

ROOT

Actions: Potent analgesic and sedative that can be used for migraine and neuralgia.

How to use: 5 drops of 1:10 tincture in water; repeat up to four times daily while pain persists. Maximum dose 5 ml per week.

Combination: Best as a simple in acute phase; can combine with Jamaican dogwood or lavender.

Precautions: Use is restricted to professional practitioners in some geographies. Overdose can cause nausea and double vision.

FACIAL OR TRIGEMINAL NEURALGIA

Severe burning of stabbing pain often following the course of the facial or trigeminal nerves. Can follow injury or exposure to cold and draughts.

KEY SYMPTOMS:
- Very localized pain that is severe.
- Related skin areas highly sensitive to touch.
- May recur regularly.

REMEDIES:

Citrus x *limon*—LEMON

FRUIT & ESSENTIAL OIL

Actions: Cooling, astringent, reputed nerve tonic, and anti-inflammatory

Combinations: Gently rub a slice of fresh lemon or a little juice on the affected area or use well-diluted lemon oil.

How to use: Use as a simple for symptomatic relief.

Precautions: Lemon oil can be irritant; use no more than 5 drops in 25 ml of carrier oil.

Hypericum perforatum—ST. JOHN'S WORT

AERIAL PARTS

Actions: Trophorestorative for the nervous system and anti-inflammatory.

Combinations: Standard infusion internally plus infused oil applied externally to affected area.

How to use: Add lavender and skullcap to infusion.

Precautions: Avoid internal use if taking prescription medicine; seek professional advice.

Verbena officinalis—VERVAIN

AERIAL PARTS
Actions: Sedative, antispasmodic and restorative for the nervous system.

How to use: Use as a poultice of fresh leaves or an infusion as a compress on affected area and take the standard infusion or tincture internally.

Combinations: Add lavender or St. John's wort to tincture or infusion or up to 20 drops of Jamaican dogwood tincture.

Precautions: Avoid high doses in pregnancy.

INFECTIONS

Modern science attributes infections to a range of bacteria and obscure viruses; previous generations blamed "flying venom," "elf-shot," or the "evil eye," while Chinese medicine has its "six evils" related to climatic factors (wind, cold, heat, dampness, dryness, and fire) to account for many chills and fevers, with "pestilence" to blame for severe epidemics.

Many of the herbs that were traditionally used to counter these assorted ills have now been identified as potent antibiotics and immune system stimulants. *Huang qi*, for example, is an important Chinese tonic herb used to strengthen the *wei qi* or defense energy – the energy that protects the exterior of the body from attack by those six evils. Modern science now labels it as both antibacterial, inhibiting the growth of *Streptococci*, *Staphylococci* and other bugs, and an immunostimulant – increasing the body's production of macrophages (scavenger cells that devour invading bacteria) and generally strengthening the defense mechanisms. Unlike wide-spectrum antibiotics, these antibacterial herbs tend to be specific to certain microbes that they attack, so unlike wide-spectrum orthodox antibiotics, they have less impact on the friendly bacteria that inhabit our guts, and the digestive upsets that can follow orthodox medication are therefore less likely.

Herbs can also be used to control the course of an illness as the body works to restore balance. Common colds can be "hot" or "cold" in character – sometimes tending to alternate between the two as the illness progresses. "Cold" conditions need warming herbs like ginger, *gui zhi*, or angelica. "Hot" infections can be cooled with diaphoretics and the many febrifuges that once played an important role in fever management: herbs like boneset, catmint, peppermint, or mulberry leaf, for example.

Cross references
Candidiasis, p. 195; Catarrh, p. 167; Coughs, p. 166; Fungal Skin Infections, p. 178.

CASE HISTORY

RECURRENT INFECTIONS
Patient: Lucy, age 35, the mother of an active three-year-old, busily engaged in renovating an old farmhouse with her husband.

History and presenting complaint: For the past four years, Lucy had suffered from constant colds and miscellaneous "viruses" – if her daughter or husband so much as sneezed, Lucy would go down with a severe head cold. The repeated "infections" left her exhausted, "down," and lethargic. For two years she had been prescribed antidepressants – as well as fairly constant antibiotics – by her GP. Her diet was good and she took regular exercise.

Treatment: The problem had started with Lucy's pregnancy as she exhausted her energies trying to cope with a high-powered job in publishing and making the transition from career woman to full-time mom. Herbal remedies focussed on immune stimulants and uplifting tonic herbs – *ling zhi*, *huang qi*, vervain, lemon balm, and echinacea. Capsules of purple coneflower were also used as an additional boost when incipient cold symptoms began to appear. *Lactobacillus acidophilus* and other friendly bacteria were used as supplements to help the digestive system recover from the excessive use of antibiotics. Cold symptoms were treated as need be with elderflower, yarrow and peppermint tea, sage gargles, and by white horehound, thyme, and licorice cough syrups.

Outcome: After four months, the recurrent colds had disappeared and Lucy felt more energetic. After discussion with her GP Lucy stopped the antidepressants, and when her daughter started nursery school – and got a bad cold – a few months later, Lucy remained symptom-free.

COLDS AND FLU

Generally considered to be due to bacterial or viral infections, although often associated with external stresses, fatigue, depression, excess cold or heat.

KEY SYMPTOMS:

- Fever.
- Muscle pain and/or headache.
- Nasal catarrh, stuffiness.
- Coughs.
- Sore throat.

REMEDIES:

Eupatorium perfoliatum—BONESET

AERIAL PARTS

Actions: Diaphoretic, febrifuge and expectorant useful in hot, feverish colds and flu with joint or muscle pain.

How to use: Standard dose of infusion or tincture 3–4 times daily.

Combinations: Use with arrow, elderflowers, and peppermint in flu and feverish colds.

Precautions: High doses are emetic.

Allium sativa—GARLIC

CLOVE

Actions: Effective antimicrobial and antifungal suitable for wide range of infectious conditions.

How to use: Up to 5 fresh cloves daily in acute conditions; or use prepared capsules.

Combinations: Best as a simple. Eat parsley if concerned about garlic smells.

Precautions: Can be stomach irritant; if so, use ginger or fennel tea to reduce symptoms. Avoid therapeutic doses in pregnancy/lactation.

Nepeta cataria—CATMINT

AERIAL PARTS

Actions: Cooling in fevers, encourages sweating, and is astringent in catarrhal congestion.

How to use: Standard dose of infusion or tincture 3–4 times daily.

Combinations: For feverish colds add yarrow, elderflower, boneset, ground ivy, or mulberry leaf.

Cinnamomum cassia—CINNAMON

TWIGS

Actions: Warming for cold conditions, diaphoretic with antibacterial action.

How to use: Standard decoction or tincture; use cinnamon bark if twigs unavailable.

Combinations: With fresh ginger root in chills.

Precautions: Avoid in pregnancy. Not suitable for hot feverish colds.

BOILS AND ABSCESSES

Localized infection often due to *Staphylococcus aureus* entering hair follicle or to infected wound. Often indicates a weakened immune system.

KEY SYMPTOMS:
- Tender, inflamed area of skin – although abscesses may be found in other parts of the body.
- Boils contain obvious pus which may need surgical incision.
- Can be painful.

REMEDIES:

Forsythia suspensa—LIAN QIAO

BERRIES
Actions: Broad spectrum antibacterial, anti-inflammatory and antipyretic to resolve abscesses and boils; also for fevers.

How to use: Standard decoction.

Combinations: Combine with honeysuckle flowers, burdock seeds, or *huang qin*, and take echinacea in capsules.

Precautions: Use before boils start to suppurate; Avoid in diarrhea.

Scrophularia spp.—FIGWORT

AERIAL PARTS AND XUAN SHEN ROOT
Actions: Anti-inflammatory and antibacterial. Cleansing herbs for toxic conditions.

How to use: Use figwort leaves as a poultice; take a standard decoction or tincture of *xuan shen*.

Combinations: Add *lian qiao*, honeysuckle flowers, goldenseal, *huang qin*, or echinacea to the decoction.

Precautions: Heart stimulant – avoid in heartbeat abnormalities (tachycardia).

IMMUNE STIMULANTS

A weak immune system may be associated with chronic exhaustion or depression or more serious underlying illness.

KEY SYMPTOMS:
- Persistent colds or flu.
- Regular fungal or skin infections.
- Chronic fatigue.

REMEDIES:

Astragalus membranaceus—HUANG QI

RHIZOME
Actions: Increases production of white blood cells and strengthens immune response; also antibacterial and energy tonic.

How to use: Standard decoction or tincture.

Combinations: With other energy tonics – licorice, *dang gui*, *bai zhu* in debilitated conditions.

Precautions: Avoid if condition involves excess heat or *yin* deficiency.

Echinacea spp.—ECHINACEA

ROOT OR LEAVES
Actions: Important antibacterial and antiviral, also strengthens resistance to infections; for all septic or infectious conditions.

How to use: Take 500 mg of powdered root in capsules or 10 ml of tincture. Repeat up to four times daily.

Combinations: Effective as a simple or add elderflower, yarrow, or catmint tinctures.

RESPIRATORY PROBLEMS

A holistic approach to health requires that illness is not just tackled on a physical level, but that the emotional and spiritual factors are considered as well. To define chest problems in terms of infection, industrial pollution or ailing heart is only a part of the problem. In Chinese medicine, the lung is associated with the emotion grief and chest problems can often follow a bereavement or other sorrow; chesty colds, bronchitis, and other apparent "infections" can also strike when we're feeling down – in a job we dislike, unhappy at home, or at crisis points in family life. Herbs cannot solve these sorrows, but strengthening lung tonics like elecampane or cowslip, which also acts on the nervous system, can help.

Breath also has greater significance than simply an intake of air. In Ayurvedic medicine it is the life force, *prana*, and breath control (*pranayama*) is an important Yogic art. Good breath control increases energy and strength and is a therapeutic tool to heal the lungs. Breathing in through the left nostril and out through the right is believed to help inflammatory lung conditions, while the opposite routine is warming for cold, damp disorders.

In Chinese medicine, too, breath is equated with vital energy and controls the flow of *qi*. Their equivalent of *pranayama* is *qi gong*, which is taught in Chinese hospitals to chronically ill patients with impressive results. Breathing problems are seen as not only damaging to the vital energy, but also signifying *qi* weakness or imbalance. Asthma, for example, can, in Chinese theory, be related to a lack of kidney energy, hindering its action in drawing *qi* downwards as part of the inhalation process, so treatment focuses on herbs to strengthen the kidney rather than simply lung remedies.

Note: *Always seek professional help for any persistent cough of unknown cause. Chronic asthmatics should seek professional advice before interrupting regular orthodox medication.*

Cross references

Hay Fever, p. 195; Sore Throats, p. 173; Tonsillitis, p. 174.

CASE HISTORY

PERSISTENT COUGH

Patient: John, 52, an export manager with an engineering company whose work involved a reasonable amount of overseas travel. Married with two teenage sons.

History and presenting complaint: John had been suffering from an irritating dry cough for "at least seven years." It had started after a severe cold, which trailed off into a persistent cough – worse at night – which kept both him and his wife awake. Countless hospital tests had all proved negative and the latest theory from his GP had been that the cough was being caused by too much acid in the stomach for which Zantac was prescribed. Three months of this treatment failed to bring improvements and John's wife persuaded him to try alternative medicine.

Treatment: Neither hospital tests nor medical history suggested a major problem with stomach acid, although John did tend to feel hot and thirsty. Herbal remedies in this case included moistening herbs such as ribwort plantain, *sang bai pi*, and white horehound with wild cherry bark to suppress the cough and elecampane as a lung tonic. Wild lettuce was added to the mixture at night as an even stronger cough suppressant.

Outcome: Within three weeks, the coughing bouts were reduced from a nightly interruption to only once or twice a week. The wild cherry bark was dropped from the medicine as the other herbs took over strengthening and restoring the lungs and after two further months John's irritating cough finally cleared.

COUGHS

Reaction to irritation or blockage in the bronchial tubes.

KEY SYMPTOMS:

- Productive cough may vary from thin watery mucous to thick yellow or green phlegm.
- Unproductive cough can be very dry and irritating.
- Often associated with infections – such as colds and influenza.
- May be associated with nervous tension and without pathological cause.
  NB Always seek professional help for any persistent cough of unknown cause.

REMEDIES:

Althaea officinalis—MARSHMALLOW

LEAF OR FLOWER

Actions: Demulcent and expectorant; soothing for inflamed respiratory mucosa.

How to use: Standard infusion or tincture; syrup of leaves or flowers in 5 ml dose.

Combinations: Combine with anti-catarrhals such as ground ivy or additional expectorants such as licorice, mulberry bark, or white horehound.

Hyssopus officinalis—HYSSOP

AERIAL PARTS OR ESSENTIAL OIL

Actions: Warming and expectorant, antispasmodic helpful for bronchitis; also useful for thin, watery phlegm.

How to use: Standard infusion or tincture; essential oil in chest rubs (5 ml to 20 ml carrier oil).

Combinations: Can be combined with restoratives such as elecampane and white horehound in chronic conditions. Use 2 parts hyssop to 1 part of other herb.

Precautions: Do not take essential oils internally.

Morus alba—MULBERRY (*Sang Bai Pi*)

BARK

Actions: Cooling expectorant and antitussive – good for "hot" conditions.

How to use: Standard decoction or tincture.

Combinations: Combine with other soothing or cooling herbs such as marshmallow leaf, ribwort plantain, or with thyme if there is infection.

Phyllostachys nigra—ZHU LI

SAP OR ZHU RU/VAMSHA ROCHANA SHAVING

Actions: Antimicrobial, cooling and expectorant to clear the thick, infected yellow sputum or productive coughs.

How to use: Use 1 teaspoon of shavings per dose in decoctions; 250 mg in capsules or up to 50 drops of tincture; use 5 ml of the fresh sap diluted in water.

Combinations: Add an equal amount of ginger juice to the sap; add cinnamon, cardamom, or black pepper to the powdered shavings with an equal amount of sugar or honey and take in teaspoon doses. Combine *zhu ru* with elecampane and ginger in decoctions.

Precautions: Avoid in diarrhea and coughs associated with cold.

Prunus serotina—WILD CHERRY

BARK

Actions: Cough suppressant; useful for dry, irritant, or nervous coughs.

How to use: Standard decoction; 2 ml tincture per dose.

Combinations: Combine with astringents such as mullein, tonics like elecampane, or additional cough suppressants like wild lettuce.

Precautions: Suppresses the cough reflex so should not be used for productive coughs or infections. Can cause sleepiness.

CATARRH

Excessive secretions from the respiratory mucosa. Can be "cold type," with copious watery secretions, or "hot," which is thick and yellow and can be difficult to shift. Cold type catarrh is often associated with excessive sweet foods and sluggish system while the hot type catarrh can be associated with tense, nervous personality.

KEY SYMPTOMS:
- Post-nasal drip with irritant cough.
- Hot type may involve pain in sinus areas.
- Inflammation of the nasal mucosa.
- May be associated with colds or allergic conditions.

REMEDIES:

Sambucus nigra —ELDER
FLOWERS
Actions: Anti-catarrhal, anti-inflammatory, and expectorant. For upper respiratory tract catarrh associated with colds and hay fever.

How to use: Standard infusion or tincture.

Combinations: Use with other drying and astringent herbs, such as yarrow, ground ivy, golden rod, agrimony, or bistort.

Gnaphthalium uliginosum—MARSH CUDWEED
LEAVES
Actions: Anti-inflammatory and tonifying to the respiratory mucosa.

How to use: Standard infusion or tincture.

Combinations: Use with other anti-catarrhal herbs such as elderflowers or golden rod using 2:1 marsh cudweed to the other herb.

Solidago virgaurea—GOLDEN ROD
AERIAL PARTS
Actions: Drying, astringent, and anti-catarrhal; anti-inflammatory for the mucosa.

How to use: Standard infusion or tincture.

Combinations: Can be used with additional anti-catarrhals such as march cudweed, wild indigo, or ribwort plantain.

Verbascum Thapsus—MULLEIN
LEAVES
Actions: Cooling, astringent, and soothing for thick or hot catarrh and nasal congestion.

How to use: Take in infusion or tincture.

Combinations: Combines well with anti-catarrhals like coltsfoot and elderflowers in infusions; add antimicrobials such as thyme or mulberry leaf in infections.

SINUSITIS

Inflammation or infection involving the sinus cavities of the skull. May follow a cold or be associated with dental problems such as deep-seated root abscesses.

KEY SYMPTOMS:
- Generally follows common cold.
- Pain affecting sinus areas—headaches that can be severe.
- Sinuses tender to the touch.
- Nasal discharge often streaked with blood.
- Often linked to tense, uptight personality with a tight rein on emotions—unwilling to cry.

REMEDIES:

Hydrastis Canadensis—GOLDENSEAL
RHIZOME
Actions: Powerful cooling astringent and anti-catarrhal.

How to use: Use two 200 mg powder in capsules three times daily or 20 drops of tincture per dose.

Combinations: Add eyebright powder to capsules.

Precautions: Avoid in pregnancy and high blood pressure; do not exceed stated dose.

Myrica cerifera—BAYBERRY

BARK

Actions: Warming and astringent; circulatory stimulant.

How to use: Use the powder as snuff or add 5 ml tincture to 20 ml emulsifying ointment and use as sinus massage.

Combinations: Add 2–3 drops of eucalyptus oil to ointment.

Precautions: Heating herb so avoid in very "hot" conditions.

Glechoma hederacea—GROUND IVY

AERIAL PARTS

Actions: Anti-catarrhal and astringent suitably drying for catarrh in both sinuses and bronchi.

How to use: Standard decoction or tincture.

Combinations: Can be used with other anti-catarrhal herbs such as elderflower, magnolia flowers, ribwort plantain, or yarrow.

Piper longum—PIPPALI/LONG PEPPER

FRUIT

Actions: Warming anti-catarrhal useful for sinus headaches and also allergic rhinitis.

How to use: Take in milk infusion, capsules (1–2 times, 200 mg per dose), or up to 40 drops tincture per dose.

Combinations: Generally used as a simple with milk, but support with antibacterials like thyme, _lian qiao_, or echinacea in tinctures or capsules where there is infection.

BRONCHITIS

Inflammation of the bronchi. May be acute due to infection or chronic – associated with smoking and pollution.

KEY SYMPTOMS:

- Productive cough, often purulent sputum.
- Fever, high temperature.

- Chronic bronchitis may involve chest pains and breathlessness and often follows a cold.

REMEDIES:

Inula helenium—ELECAMPANE

ROOT

Action: Lung tonic and expectorant; restorative and warming; good for weakened lungs and old coughs.

How to use: Standard decoction, tincture, or syrup.

Combinations: Use as a simple or add 10 ml horsetail juice to heal lung damage; or else add hyssop or white horehound to tinctures.

Primula veris—COWSLIP

ROOT

Actions: Potent expectorant good for loosening old phlegm and easing stubborn, dry coughs. Also helpful for asthma.

How to use: Standard decoction, tincture, or syrup.

Combinations: Can be combine with other strong expectorants such as gumplant and a soothing demulcent like licorice.

Thymus vulgaris—THYME

AERIAL PARTS OR ESSENTIAL OIL

Action: Antiseptic and expectorant; useful for thick, infected phlegm and dry, difficult coughs.

How to use: Herb in standard infusion syrup or tincture; 10 drops of essential oil in 25 ml almond oil as a chest rub.

Combinations: Add additional expectorants such as licorice, or mulberry bark to syrups and tinctures; add horsetail juice to repair damage or combine the essential oil with hyssop, pine, or peppermint oils in chest rubs.

Precautions: Do not take essential oils internally.

Marrubium vulgare—WHITE HOREHOUND

AERIAL PARTS

Action: Antispasmodic, demulcent, and expectorant relaxing the bronchi and easing congestion.

How to use: Standard infusion, tincture or syrup; horehound candy also available commercially.

Combinations: Combine with warming expectorants such as hyssop or angelica and tonics like elecampane.

Note: All the herbs listed under bronchitis can also be used in asthmatic conditions.

ASTHMA

Bronchospasm leading to wheezing and breathlessness.

KEY SYMPTOMS:

- Characteristic wheeze on expiration.
- May be associated with other allergic symptoms such as hay fever or eczema.
- May be family tendency.
- Great difficulty in breathing.
- May be associated with fever and infection.

Note: *Severe asthma can be life threatening and professional medical help may be required.*

REMEDIES:

Ephedra sinica—MA HUANG

AERAIL PARTS

Action: Bronchial relaxant and vasodilator; warming for all cold conditions of the chest.

How to use: 100 mg of dried stems to a cup of water as a decoction or as prescribed. The herb is restricted in some geographies with a maximum dosage in the UK of 2.5 ml of a 1:4 tincture three times daily.

Combinations: May be prescribed in combination with other herbs such as gumplant, angelica, white horehound, hyssop, or pill-bearing spurge.

Precautions: Not to be used by patients taking MAO inhibitors as antidepressants; avoid in severe hypertension.

Matricaria chamomilla—GERMAN CHAMOMILE

FLOWERS

Action: Anti-allergenic, anti-inflammatory, and antispasmodic – useful for allergic asthma.

How to use: Use a steam inhalation (1 tablespoon of dried flowers to a bowl of boiling water) at the first sign of an attack. The essential oil can be added to chest rubs and inhalants,

Combinations: Support with internal medication as for bronchitis above.

Grindelia camporum—GUMPLANT

AERIAL PARTS

Action: Antispasmodic and expectorant to ease bronchospasm.

How to use: 15 g herb to 500 ml water for infusions; up to 5 ml daily in doses of 1–2 ml.

Combinations: Can be combined with additional antispasmodics such as pill-bearing spurge or with expectorants such as cowslip root.

Precautions: Hypotensive, avoid in cases of low blood pressure. High doses can irritate the kidneys.

Eucalyptus globulus—EUCALYPTUS

ESSENTIAL OIL

Actions: Antiseptic, antispasmodic, and expectorant (also for bronchitis).

How to use: 40 drops of eucalyptus oil in 20 ml of carrier as a chest rub; use a few drops on a pillow or handkerchief as an inhalant.

Combinations: Add a total of 10–15 drops of thyme, peppermint, lemon balm, anise, or fennel oils to the chest rub.

Precautions: Do not take eucalyptus oil internally.

Ear, Eyes, Mouth & Throat

Modern medicine tends to isolate sight, sound, and speech from the rest of the body, but the health of the eyes, ears, and mouth can reflect the state of the whole person. Persistent problems with these organs can be indicative of other underlying systemic disorders. Glue ear (secretory otitis media) in children, for example, is now acknowledged – even by the orthodox – as often being connected with milk allergies, while all cold sore sufferers are only too well aware that the *Herpes simplex* virus flares up if they are feeling tired, stressed, or heading for a cold. Eye problem, in Chinese theory, can be related to liver imbalance; hearing difficulties and tinnitus can imply kidney weakness, and persistent mouth problems or sore lips may suggest excess heat in the spleen.

Although symptomatic remedies can bring relief, tackling the underlying cause is just as important. Tired, strained eyes, for example, can be helped by eye baths of rosewater or weak infusions of eyebright, pot marigold, cornflowers, or strawberry leaves. A longer-term solution may be to improve lighting levels, take frequent short breaks from VDU screens, or try cleansing liver herbs. Similarly, one stye may be treated with marigold compresses or bathing with marigold infusion, but if the condition is persistent and recurring then antimicrobial remedies or cleansing herbs to counter toxins may be needed – burdock, cleavers, echinacea, or garlic, for example. Similarly with mouth ulcers – one may simply be the result of local injury and infection and can be eased with herbs like purple sage and myrrh, but persistent ulcers can suggest a weak immune system or underlying yeast infections (candidiasis) and may need dietary changes or stimulant herbs as well.

Cross references

Candidiasis, see p. 195.

Case History

Deafness from excess catarrh

Patient: Robert, age 12, an active boy but becoming more withdrawn and silent and falling behind with his school work.

History and presenting complaint: Robert had suffered from constant catarrh since babyhood. As well as the running nose, his ears were always blocked and prone to infection. As a toddler he had suffered from persistent "glue ear" and had gone through three sets of grommets and was now into his third year of T-tubes. His hearing was getting worse and he complained of a permanent "buzzing" in his ears; whenever he went swimming, earache and infection followed. His diet was fairly typical of any 12-year-old – too few green vegetables and in excess of a pint of milk a day.

Treatment: As a trial his mother agreed to cut out all milk and milk products from his diet for a month, replacing these with soy milk – itself a reasonably good source of calcium – and adding more leafy green vegetables and fish to boost mineral and vitamin intake. Herbal medicines included golden rod, echinacea, and pasque flower in tincture form, with goldenseal in capsules as the taste is very bitter.

Outcome: After only two weeks of herbs and a milk-free diet, both Robert and his mother noticed improvements in his hearing, and a month later he was able to go swimming and not get an ear infection. The constant catarrh also cleared. Herbal medicine was continued for three months, by which time Robert had been totally free of ear-infections and catarrh for more than six weeks. He quite liked the taste of soya milk and was happy to continue on a low-milk diet indefinitely, with the occasional ice cream causing few problems. Three months later at his next hospital visit, Robert's ears and hearing had improved so much that the specialist decided to finally remove the T-tubes.

EARACHE

Can be associated with catarrhal conditions or infection. Note: Severe conditions can lead to deafness, so seek professional medical help if symptoms persist.

KEY SYMPTOMS:
- Pain in one or both ears that can be severe.
- Blocked sensation in the ears.
- Buzzing or ringing sounds.
- Excessive waxy discharge.
- Fever.
- Vertigo, nausea if inner ear is affected.

REMEDIES:

Verbascum thapsus—MULLEIN

FLOWERS

Action: Demulcent and mildly sedative wound herb.

How to use: Cold infused oil of the flowers can be used as ear drops.

Combinations: Support with antibiotic herbs like echinacea and anti-catarrhals such as elderflower or goldenseal taken internally.

Precautions: Do not put anything in the ear if there is a risk that the ear drum has perforated.

Pulsatilla vulgaris—PASQUE FLOWER

AERIAL PARTS

Action: Sedative and analgesic; directionally acting on ears and reproductive system.

How to use: Take 1–2 ml tincture, three times daily.

Combinations: Combine with anti-catarrhals such as goldenseal or eyebright tinctures.

Hydrastis canadensis—GOLDENSEAL

RHIZOME

Action: Powerful cooling astringent and anti-catarrhal.

How to use: Use two 200 mg powder in capsules three times daily or 20 drops of tincture per dose.

Combinations: Add eyebright powder to capsules.

Precautions: Avoid in pregnancy and high blood pressure; do not exceed stated dose.

Plantago lanceolata—RIBWORT PLANTAIN

LEAVES

Action: Tonifies mucous membranes and controls catarrh. Useful for catarrhal conditions of the middle ear.

How to use: Standard infusion or tincture.

Combinations: Combine with elderflower tincture and add 10 drops of pasque flower tincture to enhance focus on the ears.

CONJUNCTIVITIS & BLEPHARITIS

Conjunctivitis is an inflammation of the conjunctiva (the membrane covering the eyeball and lid) and blepharitis is an inflammation of the eyelids. Both may be caused by caused by infection, allergy, or physical/chemical irritants.

KEY SYMPTOMS:
- Gritty feeling in the eye.
- Increased light sensitivity.
- Pain, soreness and swelling.
- Obvious red or pink eye.
- Discharge that may be watery or contain pus if there is an infection.

REMEDIES:

Euphrasia officinalis—EYEBRIGHT

AERIAL PARTS

Actions: Astringent, anti-catarrhal, and anti-inflammatory.

How to use: Use a compress soaked in standard infusion for eyes or 5–10 drops of tincture in an eye bath of boiled and cooled water.

Combinations: Support with internal antibacterials, such as echinacea, if there is infection.

Agrimonia eupatoria—AGRIMONY

AERIAL PARTS

Actions: Astringent and healing for mucosa; also liver tonic which may help the eyes.

How to use: Use weak infusion (10 g to 500 ml of water) well-strained as an eye bath.

Combinations: Support with internal antibacterials, such as echinacea, if there is infection.

Calendula officinalis—POT MARIGOLD

FLOWER PETALS

Actions: Anti-inflammatory, astringent, wound herb, antiseptic. Helpful for local irritation.

How to use: Use a compress soaked in well diluted tincture; also for bathing styes (5 ml to 50 ml water).

Dendranthema x grandiflorum—JU HUA

FLOWERS

Actions: Antibacterial, anti-inflammatory and liver herb. Good for persistent eye problems.

How to use: Standard infusion or tincture internally.

Combinations: Combine with eyebright, elderflower, agrimony, self-heal to reduce inflammation and support the liver.

MOUTH ULCERS (aphthous stomatitis)

Painful white ulcers on cheeks, tongue, or gums, often related to fungal or bacterial infection. They may be related to excessive consumption of sugar or other foods that encourage fungal proliferation. Associated split or cracked lips may indicate a vitamin deficiency.

KEY SYMPTOMS:
- Ulcer is obvious on visual inspection.
- Can be very painful and persistent.

REMEDIES:

Commiphora molmol—MYRRH

RESIN

Actions: Antimicrobial, astringent, wound herb.

How to use: 5–10 drops of oil or 5 ml tincture in a glass of warm water as a mouthwash.

Combinations: Add 5 ml sage or rosemary tincture to the mouthwash or chew bilberries afterwards to help disguise the flavor.

Precautions: Avoid high doses internally in pregnancy.

Salvia officinalis Purpurescens Group or *Salvia officinalis*—PURPLE or GREEN SAGE

LEAVES

Actions: Antiseptic and astringent; also suitable for gingivitis, and other mouth/gum disorders.

How to use: Standard infusion as mouthwash or 10 ml tincture in a glass of water.

Combinations: Add self-heal, echinacea or rosemary tincture to mouthwash.

Precautions: Avoid high doses internally in pregnancy.

Polygonum bistorta—BISTORT

ROOT

Actions: Astringent, demulcent and anti-inflammatory; also for other mouth inflammations.

How to use: Standard decoction or 5 ml tincture to a glass of water as mouthwash.

Combinations: Add self-heal, rosemary, bilberry, wild indigo to mouthwash. For persistent problems take echinacea or garlic internally (see Infections).

COLD SORES

Small collection of blisters usually on the mouth or face due to *Herpes simplex* virus. Once infected with the virus, sores may recur when the system is weakened by infection, stress, or fatigue.

KEY SYMPTOMS:
- Painful with characteristic appearance.

Melaleuca alternifolia—TEA TREE

ESSENTIAL OIL

Actions: Antibiotic and immune stimulant.

How to use: Use 10 drops of essential oil in 5 ml of carrier oil and dab onto the affected area as soon as "tingle" of developing sore starts.

Combinations: Use as a simple. If sore are recurrent use immune stimulants, such as *huang qi*, or Siberian ginseng to improve stress tolerance. If the sore heralds a cold take echinacea or garlic internally.

Precautions: Do not take essential oils internally without professional advice. May cause allergic dermatitis in some people; if in doubt do a skin test before using medicinally.

Lavandula officinalis—LAVENDER

ESSENTIAL OIL

Actions: Topically antiseptic

How to use: use a drop of neat oil directly to the affected area as soon as "tingle" of developing sore starts.

Combinations: Use as a simple. If sore are recurrent use immune stimulants, such as *huang qi*, or Siberian ginseng to improve stress tolerance. If the sore heralds a cold take echinacea or garlic internally.

Precautions: Do not take essential oils internally without professional advice.

SORE THROATS

Pain at the back of the mouth associated with infection or chemical irritants; may be linked with tonsillitis, pharyngitis, or laryngitis.

KEY SYMPTOMS:

* Pain.
* Difficulty in swallowing.
* Voice may be affected – hoarse or croaking.
* Related fever or cold may be present or starting.
* Inflammation apparent on inspection.

Agrimonia eupatoria—AGRIMONY

AERIAL PARTS

Action: Astringent and healing for the mucosa.

How to use: Standard infusion as a gargle or use 10 ml tincture in a glass of warm water.

Combinations: Add 5 ml of echinacea, purple sage, or rosemary tincture to the gargle.

Alchemilla vulgaris—LADY'S MANTLE

LEAVES

Action: Astringent and reduces inflammation; helpful for laryngitis.

How to use: Standard infusion as a gargle or use 10 ml tincture in a glass of warm water.

Combinations: Add 5 ml of rosemary or purple sage tincture or no more than 5 drops of cayenne tincture to the gargle.

Precautions: Avoid large internal doses in pregnancy.

Echinacea spp.—ECHINACEA

ROOT OR LEAVES

Action: Antibacterial and astringent; useful for all throat problems including tonsillitis.

How to use: Use 5 ml of tincture in a glass of warm water as a gargle. Swallow the gargle to help combat infection.

Terminalia belerica—BIBHITAKI

FRUIT

Actions: Closely associated in Ayurvedic tradition with both the throat and voice, bibhitaki fruits are astringent, antiseptic, and cooling.

How to use: Take 1 teaspoon of powder in honey for sore throats and vocal problems; use the infusion or juice as a gargle

Combinations: Use as a simple or add antimicrobials such as 5 ml of echinacea infusion to the gargle to combat infection.

Precautions: Avoid in pregnancy and severe exhaustion.

Tonsillitis

Inflammation of the tonsils usually associated with bacterial or viral infection. May be complicated by quinsy (peritonsillar abscess), which can need surgical incision to release pus.

Key Symptoms:
- Sore throat.
- Difficulty swallowing.
- Fever.
- Tonsils may be enlarged or suppurating on inspection.

Remedies:

Galium aparine—CLEAVERS
Aerial Parts
Action: Lymphatic cleanser and alterative; useful lymphatic problems including glandular fever and adenoids.

How to use: Use 10 ml of fresh juice, three times daily or standard infusion internally.

Combinations: Add additional antibacterial tinctures such as 10 drops of goldenseal or poke root, or up to 10 ml of echinacea to the juice internally; use gargles as suggested for "sore throat" above.

Phytolacca Americana—POKE ROOT
Dried Root
Action: Anti-catarrhal and cleansing for lymphatic system; reduces lymphatic swellings.

How to use: 10–20 drops of tincture made from dried root, three times daily.

Combinations: Use with 10 ml of cleavers juice or add additional antibacterial tinctures such as 10 ml echinacea.

Precautions: Large doses are emetic and purgative – do not exceed stated dose. Do not use any part of the fresh plant which is toxic.

Baptisia tinctorial—WILD INDIGO
Leaves and Root
Action: Anti-microbial, anti-catarrhal, cleansing for lymphatics; good for persistent infection.

How to use: 10–20 drops of tincture, three times daily taken internally.

Combinations: Combine with cleavers juice or echinacea tincture to enhance action.

Precautions: Large doses can cause nausea—do not exceed stated dose.

Gnaphalium uliginosum—MARSH CUDWEED
Leaves
Action: Anti-inflammatory and tonifying for the mucosa; also for laryngitis, pharyngitis, and quinsy.

How to use: Take a standard infusion or tincture internally and also use as a gargle.

Combinations: Combine with cleavers juice or echinacea tincture to enhance action.

Skin & Hair

While modern medicine often depends on hydrocortisone creams to treat skin problems, a herbal approach focuses instead on restoring internal balance, often with cleansing or cooling herbs rather than using external remedies which may alleviate the symptoms but do little to treat the cause of the problem. The same need for re-balancing is adopted in Ayurvedic medicine; too much *pitta* (fire) causes the blood to over-heat and poison the skin; too much *vata* (wind) causes dryness and itching, while excess *kapha* (damp) leads to weeping or oozing sores. Treatment is with the relevant cooling, drying, or moistening herbs and appropriate diet.

The Chinese associate skin with the lung, *wei qi* (defense energy) and body fluids, so dry, flaking eczema, for example, would be treated with herbs to cool and increase body fluids. Trials at a London hospital adopting this approach have had impressive results. Fungal or parasitic skin conditions are regarded as a weakness of the *wei qi* and are treated with immunostimulants and antimicrobials. Western herbalism adopts a similar with persistent fungal infections suggesting some systemic weakness to be treated with tonic herbs and immunostimulants rather than simply persistent use of symptomatic antifungals.

Hair problems, too, can be a sign of other physical weaknesses. In Chinese medicine, hair is associated with the kidneys, so premature graying of the hair is associated with weakening in kidney energy, to be treated with tonics rather than colorants.

Cross references
Head Lice, see p. 232; Vaginal Thrush, see p. 212; Candidiasis, see p. 195.

CASE HISTORY

TEENAGE ACNE

Patient: Edward, 17, a typical teenage acne sufferer with pustules around his nose and cheeks.

History and presenting complaint: The problem had started 18 months previously and Edward had also suffered from heavy catarrh and recurrent colds for the best part of a year. Like many teenagers, his diet was far from perfect with an excess of chocolates, chips, and fizzy drinks. He admitted to a "very sweet tooth" which his mother translated as at least two chocolate bars a day and as many cookies as he could find when he got home from school.

Treatment: Like most teenagers, Edward did not relish the prospect of rubbing his face with garlic each evening or washing in cabbage water, so tea tree oil in rosewater was used as a lotion instead. Internal herbal remedies focused on clearing dampness and heat from the system and improving immunity. Spots around the nose suggested excess lung heat so *huang qin* and *sang bai pi* were included with *chi shao yao*, heartsease, yellow dock, and echinacea. Edward also promised to try very hard to cut down on the chocolates.

Outcome: After six weeks, the acne was considerably reduced and the catarrh had disappeared along with the sweet mucus-forming foods from his diet. Then came exams. In between bouts of revision, Edward binged on chocolate bars and before long the spots and heavy catarrh were back. Fortunately, Edward realized his sweet tooth was a contributing factor and after a further course of herbs is managing to avoid excess chocolates.

ECZEMA

Skin inflammation may be associated with allergies, nervous stress, or chemical/metal irritants. It may be highly localized if a local irritant (e.g., a metal watch strap) is involved, but allergic eczema can affect all parts of the body. Creases of skin – for example, folds of elbows or under breasts – may often be affected.

KEY SYMPTOMS:
- Red, inflamed patches on the skin.
- Can be itchy.
- May start oozing serum from raw surface.
- Crusts of serum can be formed.
- Lesions may bleed in acute conditions.

REMEDIES:

Stellaria media—CHICKWEED

AERIAL PARTS

Actions: Soothing and slightly astringent wound herb to ease irritation and help heal lesions.

How to use: Apply ointment or cream as required; add infused oil to bathwater.

Combinations: Use externally as a simple.

Oenothera biennis—EVENING PRIMROSE

SEED OIL

Actions: Contains essential fatty acids that are needed to maintain healthy tissues.

How to use: In capsules: 1–2 g daily for children; 3 g for adults.

Combinations: Use as a simple.

Paeonia lactiflora—RED PEONY (*Chi Shao Yao*)

ROOT

Actions: Cools and stimulates blood flow; useful for "hot" conditions.

How to use: Standard decoction or tincture: best combined with other herbs.

Combinations: Combine with additional cooling remedies such as *sheng di huang*, heartsease, *mu dan pi*, *fang feng*, and *mu tong*.

Arctium lappa—BURDOCK

LEAF

Actions: Cleansing, diuretic, and laxative. Good for any toxic skin condition especially dry, scaling eczema.

How to use: Standard decoction of root or up to 4 ml of tincture, three times daily.

Combinations: Combine with other cleansing remedies such as yellow dock, figwort cleavers, heartsease, and red clover tinctures.

Urtica dioica—STINGING NETTLE

AERIAL PARTS

Actions: Astringent, tonic and circulatory stimulant; useful if eczema is associated with poor circulation.

How to use: Standard infusion or tincture. Also as cream or ointment.

Combinations: Use as a simple of combine with other cleansing herbs such as heartsease, red clover, figwort, and cleavers tinctures.

ACNE

Inflammation of sebaceous glands in the skin, which may start with blackheads; especially common among teenagers.

KEY SYMPTOMS:
* Inflamed pustules.
* Often excessive oiliness of skin.
* In severe cases there may be infected cysts and scarring.

REMEDIES:

Allium sativa—GARLIC

CLOVE

Actions: Antibacterial and antifungal; good antiseptic action for infected skin conditions

How to use: Rub the affected area directly with a cut clove.

Combinations: Use as a simple; eat parsley to limit garlic odour – and use garlic in cooking.

Precautions: Because of the odour this is best done at night.

Melaleuca alternifolia—TEA TREE

ESSENTIAL OIL

Actions: Potent antibacterial for infected skin conditions.

How to use: Use 10 ml of tea tree oil in 100 ml of water or a 50:50 mixture of rosewater and distilled witch-hazel as a lotion.

Combinations: Use as a simple and take tinctures of cleavers, yellow dock, burdock, or echinacea internally.

Precautions: Do not take essential oils internally without professional advice. May cause allergic dermatitis in some people; if in doubt do a skin test before using medicinally.

Brassica oleracea —CABBAGE

LEAF

Actions: Antibacterial and anti-inflammatory; nutritive and healing.

How to use: Mix 250 g of fresh leaves and 250 ml of distilled witch hazel in a blender; strain and add 2 drops of lemon oil and use as a lotion.

Combinations: Use as a simple and take tinctures of cleavers, yellow dock, burdock, or echinacea internally.

VERRUCAS AND WARTS

Growth in the outer layer of the skin due to a virus.

KEY SYMPTOMS:
- Obvious growth.
- Can spread by contact.
- May be persistent.

REMEDIES:

Thuja occidentalis—ARBOR VITAE
LEAF TIPS
Actions: Volatile oil contains thujone which is strongly antiseptic and effective against many topical fungal and viral infections.

How to use: Use drops of the tincture neat on verrucas or warts; can also be made into ointment. Repeat often.

Precautions: Avoid in pregnancy.

Chelidonium majus—GREATER CELANDINE
SAP
Actions: Potent antiviral to destroy warts.

How to use: Squeeze the fresh sap from the stems directly to the wart; repeat at least twice a day and even longstanding warts will generally clear in 2–3 weeks.

Combinations: Use as a simple; dandelion stem sap can be used in a similar way.

Precautions: Do not take internally or use any part of the plant in pregnancy; avoid touching surrounding skin with too much sap.

PSORIASIS

Due to an overproduction of skin keratinocytes that fail to mature into normal keratin; it can be associated with immune dysfunction and may follow streptococcal infection or skin injury. It can also be aggravated by stress and worry and linked to a tense, isolated personality unwilling to get close to other people. A tendency for psoriasis often runs in families.

KEY SYMPTOMS:
- Red skin patches often with silver-colored scales.
- Cycle of remission and reoccurrence.

REMEDIES:

Galium aparine—CLEAVERS
AERIAL PARTS
Actions: Cleansing, diuretic, and astringent useful for many types of skin problems.

How to use: Use 10 ml fresh juice three times daily or standard infusion. Also externally as ointment or cream.

Combinations: Combines well with red clover to help overproduction of cells and with cleansing stimulants such as figwort or stinging nettles in the infusion.

Iris versicolor—BLUE FLAG
RHIZOME
Actions: Anti-inflammatory and cleansing of both blood and lymphatic systems; a favorite with the physiomedicalists and stimulating for the liver.

How to use: Use in decoction (half a teaspoon per cup in half cup doses) or tincture.

Combinations: With cleansing remedies such as poke root and yellow dock; add valerian to the decoction if stress or anxiety are significant factors, use aloe vera sap or slippery elm powder as a topical treatment.

Scrophularia nodosa—FIGWORT

AERIAL PARTS

Actions: Anti-inflammatory, cleansing, and circulatory stimulant: good for many chronic skin conditions.

How to use: Standard infusion or tincture.

Combinations: Use with red clover or heartsease to help normalize skin growth or with cleansing herbs such as cleavers and yellow dock.

Precautions: Avoid in certain heart conditions such as tachycardia.

Trifolium pratense—RED CLOVER

FLOWERS

Actions: Cleansing and diuretic useful for many skin problems including eczema.

How to use: Standard infusion or tincture also externally in creams and ointments

Combinations: Combine with cleavers in infusion or add 2 ml yellow dock or 10 drops *arbor vitae* to tinctures.

Rumex crispus—YELLOW DOCK

ROOT

Actions: Cleansing diuretic and laxative; stimulates bile flow and clears toxins.

How to use: Standard decoction or tincture.

Combinations: Combine with burdock and figwort tinctures.

Precautions: Avoid high does in pregnancy.

FUNGAL INFECTIONS

Ringworm, athlete's foot, and other fungal infections are caused by micro organisms such as *Microsporum*, *Trichophyton* and *Epidermophyton* spp. They can affect any part of the body, commonly toes, nails and scalp.

KEY SYMPTOMS:

- Very irritant.
- Red patches.
- Skin may be scaly and peeling.

REMEDIES:

Calendula officinalis—POT MARIGOLD

FLOWER PETALS

Action: Antifungal and astringent; wound herb and soothing for dry or inflamed skin.

How to use: Use as cream or ointment or a standard infusion in a footbath or as a wash.

Combination: Add 5 ml of tea tree oil to 500 ml of pot marigold infusion used as a wash.

Commiphora molmol—MYRRH

RESIN OR ESSENTIAL OIL

Action: Antifungal, immune stimulant, and astringent

How to use: Use 10 drops of oil or 10 ml tincture to 100 ml water as a wash. Take up to 20 drops of tincture in water three times daily.

Combination: Pot marigold, echinacea, *arbor vitae* tincture three times daily internally

Precautions: Do not take essential oils internally. Avoid internally in pregnancy.

Aloe vera—ALOE VERA

GEL

Action: Demulcent, cooling for irritated skin, antiparasitic; also for infestations such as scabies.

How to use: Use the sap from a fresh leaf directly on affected area; aloe gel is available commercially.

HAIR LOSS – ALOPECIA

Alopecia can be total or localized to particular patches; mild hair loss problems can be linked to vitamin deficiency.

KEY SYMPTOMS:

- Excessive loose hairs; a small loss is quite normal.
- Bald patches.

REMEDIES:

Arnica montana—ARNICA

FLOWERS

Actions: Stimulates blood circulation.

How to use: Use as cream or ointment on affected areas of scalp; or use 5 ml of 1:10 tincture in 500 ml warm water as a rinse.

Combination: Support with nervines (see p. 200) taken internally to combat any stress and Vitamin B supplements. Drink cleansing infusions of burdock, stinging nettle, cleavers or red clover.

Precautions: Do not use on broken skin or take internally.

Artemisia abrotanum—SOUTHERNWOOD

AERIAL PARTS

Action: Traditional remedy to stimulate hair growth – although there is no scientific basis for this action.

How to use: Take 10–20 drops of tincture internally three times daily; use a standard infusion as a hair rinse.

Combination: Add stinging nettles, rosemary, or sage infusions to the hair rinse; take mineral supplements and vitamin B.

Precautions: Avoid completely in pregnancy or if trying to conceive.

PREMATURE GRAYING

Can be an inherited tendency, or associated with stress or a premature menopause.

KEY SYMPTOMS:

- Hair starts to lose its color in twenties or thirties.

REMEDIES:

Salvia officinalis Purpurescens group or *Salvia officinalis*—PURPLE or GREEN SAGE

LEAVES

Action: Traditionally used to restore color – possibly associated with general tonic and hormonal properties of sage.

How to use: Standard infusion internally and as a hair rinse.

Combination: Add rosemary and stinging nettles to the infusion or rinse.

Precautions: Avoid high doses internally in pregnancy.

Polygonum multiflorum—HE SHOU WU

ROOT

Action: Kidney tonic used in China for premature menopause early graying hair.

How to use: Standard decoction or tincture taken internally (up to 15 ml daily).

Combination: Can be used as a simple or combined with *nu zhen zi*, *shu di huang*, and licorice tinctures.

Precautions: Avoid if also suffering from diarrhea.

DANDRUFF

Small flakes of dead skin on the scalp; may be accompanied by seborrhoeic dermatitis and can be linked to underlying yeast infections.

KEY SYMPTOMS:

- Obvious scurf on collars and combs.
- Hair may be dry and brittle or greasy with yellow dandruff flakes.

REMEDIES:

Rosmarinus officinalis—ROSEMARY

AERIAL PARTS

Action: Astringent, antiseptic and circulatory stimulant; also useful for psoriasis affecting the scalp.

How to use: Standard infusion as a hair rinse; or macerate 15 g rosemary in 250 ml shampoo for 2 weeks; strain before using.

Combination: Add stinging nettle root to infusion for hair rinse.

Quillaja saponaria—SOAP BARK

BARK

Actions: Rich in saponins – cleansing and anti-inflammatory.

How to use: Mix 500 ml of standard decoction with 200 g of soft soap to use as shampoo.

Precautions: Large internal doses can cause digestive tract irritation and inflammations.

Heart, Blood & Circulation

Ancient medical traditions regarded the heart as much more than just an efficient pump to control the circulation of blood. In Ayurvedic medicine, it is the seat of the soul, the dwelling of *atman* – the divine self or spirit of immortal life – while to the Chinese, it stores *shén*: the spirit and sense of awareness. What modern Western medicine may regard as mental illness or nervous disorders, Chinese medicine blames on disharmonies of *shén* and may favor herbs such as *fu ling*, which is used as a sedative to "pacify the heart" in insomnia and palpitations.

Western heart herbs can boast a more conventional set of actions: ever since William Withering identified foxglove (*Digitalis purpurea*) as a potent heart remedy in 1768, scientists have been investigating herbal heart remedies. Some are extremely potent and significant in modern medicine but others are suitable for home use – hawthorn and linden flower tea, for example, which is safe enough to use for high blood pressure in pregnancy.

Herbal remedies for hypertension include vasodilators to relax and increase the size of blood vessels, diuretics to reduce the blood volume, and cardiac depressants to slow the heart rate. Chinese medicine takes a different standpoint, relating hypertension to excessive flaring of liver fire, for example. Herbs also have a role to play in controlling cholesterol levels and many will lower abnormally high serum lipid levels and help to prevent atherosclerosis – although good diet, healthy lifestyle, and a pollution-free environment would probably prevent this being a problem for many people.

Cross references
Heavy Menstrual Bleeding, p. 210; Wounds, pp. 150–151; Hemorrhoids, p. 193.

Case History

High blood pressure at menopause
Patient: Sarah, 52, divorced with a daughter at college to support, and dividing her time between caring for elderly parents and occasional engagements as a freelance musician.

History and presenting complaint: Sarah had been diagnosed as having slightly raised blood pressure during a routine insurance medical, 10 years previously, and had been prescribed beta-blockers. She disliked using "drugs" and soon abandoned the tablets for various patent herbal and homeopathic remedies. Eight years later another routine check revealed glaucoma and she was also experiencing menopausal symptoms. Her GP was urging a return to beta-blockers. Her blood pressure was 180/110 mm Hg and other symptoms included lower back pains, dizziness, a tendency for tinnitus, palpitations and "hot flushes" whenever she felt emotionally upset or did anything energetic.

Treatment: In Chinese medicine *jing* or vital essence is responsible for both reproductive and creative energies. A lifetime of professional music making and the menopause were taking their toll of Sarah's store of *jing*. Herbs to boost kidney energy and nourish the liver rather than drugs to slow down her heart were used. These included *shu di huang*, *shan zhu yu*, *mu dan pi*, and *he shou wu*. She was also given an herbal tea containing *ju hua*, hawthorn, and motherwort.

Outcome: Within a month Sarah's "hot flushes" had vanished, she had fewer palpitations and more energy with none of the dizzy feelings. Her blood pressure was down to 155/95 mm Hg. The herbs were continued for three months by which time Sarah's blood pressure had stabilized at 140/85 mm Hg, so she continued with only the herbal tea on a regular basis. Six months later at a routine check her blood pressure was still the same and her regular glaucoma test also showed improvements.

High Blood Pressure

Hypertension should really be regarded as a symptom of imbalance in the body rather than as a single disease. It may be related to other underlying disorders including atherosclerosis, heart disease, and liver problems.

Key Symptoms:
- Headaches.
- Eye problems.
- Dizziness or fainting spells.
- Raised blood pressure reading on repeated examination.
- Diastolic (lower reading) greater than 90–95 mm Hg.

Note: Do not replace orthodox medication with herbs without consulting your practitioner.

Remedies:

Viburnum opulus—GUELDER ROSE
Bark
Action: Smooth muscle relaxant for the vascular system; lowers the diastolic pressure.

How to use: Standard decoction or tincture.

Combinations: Combines with linden flowers if there is atherosclerosis, or valerian or passion flower is stress is involved; add hawthorn as a heart tonic if required.

Stachys officinalis—WOOD BETONY
Aerial Parts
Action: Circulatory tonic, relaxant, and sedative; calms the heart.

How to use: Standard infusion or tincture.

Combinations: Combines with linden flowers if there is atherosclerosis, or with guelder rose to relax blood vessels; add valerian or passion flower is stress is involved.

Precautions: Uterine stimulant so avoid high doses in pregnancy.

Dendranthema x grandiflorum—JU HUA
Flowers
Action: Dilates the coronary artery and increases blood flow; also clears liver heat which can cause hypertension.

How to use: Standard infusion or tincture.

Combinations: Combine with liver herbs such as *gou qi zi* and diuretics like dandelion leaf and *fu ling*.

Crataegus spp.—HAWTHORN
Berries or Flowering Tops
Action: Improves coronary circulation and strengthens heart muscles; useful tincture for angina pectoris. Helps stabilize BP as cardiac function improves.

How to use: Standard infusion or tincture.

Combinations: Combines well in teas with linden flowers and yarrow, or with guelder rose to relax blood vessels; add valerian or passion flower if stress is involved.

Tilia x europaea—LINDEN
Flowers
Action: Peripheral vasodilator with healing effect on blood vessels; reputed prophylactic against arteriosclerosis.

How to use: Standard infusion or up to 10 ml tincture daily.

Combinations: Combine with hawthorn as a cardiac tonic or with ginkgo and linden flowers if arteriosclerosis is significant.

Low Blood Pressure

Often not considered serious by doctors, but hypotension can be a significant health problem.

Key Symptoms:
- General tiredness.
- Weak constitution.
- Dizziness and/or fainting spells.
- Palpitations and cardiac arrhythmias.

- Can be serious if the systolic (upper) reading is consistently below 110 mm Hg, in which case seek professional help.

REMEDIES:

Cytisus scoparius—BROOM

FLOWERING TOPS

Action: Regulates heartbeat steadying the arrhythmias that can be associated with low BP and heart failure.

How to use: Use 15 g to 500 ml water for infusions or up to 5 ml tincture daily.

Combinations: Use with tonics such as hawthorn.

Precautions: Avoid in pregnancy.

Convallaria majalis—LILY-OF-THE-VALLEY

LEAVES

Action: Stimulates heart contractions and improves efficiency; useful for weak, failing, and elderly hearts.

How to use: Restricted to professional use in some geographies. Maximum dose in the UK is 20 drops of a 1:5 tincture three times daily.

Combinations: Always combined with a diuretic such as dandelion leaf; heart tonics such as hawthorn often added.

Precautions: High doses are emetic and purgative; take only as prescribed.

Leonurus cardiac—MOTHERWORT

LEAVES

Action: Relaxing for palpitations and arrhythmias; also has a stimulating action on the heart.

How to use: Standard infusion or tincture.

Combinations: Combine with rosemary as a tonic or add sedatives such as passion flower for stress-related problems.

Precautions: Avoid in pregnancy.

VARICOSE VEINS

Swollen or stretched veins in the legs associated with poor venous return or raised abdominal pressure (as in obesity and pregnancy).

KEY SYMPTOMS:
- Obvious enlarged and stretched veins.
- Pain in the legs.

REMEDIES:

Melilotus officinale—KING'S CLOVER

AERIAL PARTS

Actions: A good venous tonic, rich in coumarin-like compounds; anti-coagulant and anti-inflammatory.

How to use: Use a standard infusion; up to 3 ml of tincture three times a day; externally as cream; or use 10% tincture in witch-hazel or rosewater.

Combinations: Use with liver herbs (like goldenseal) if sluggish digestion is a contributing factor; add pot marigold to creams and compresses.

Precautions: Do not use with warfarin or similar anti-coagulant drugs to thin the blood or if there is any problem with the blood's ability to clot.

Aesculus hippocastanum—HORSE CHESTNUT

SEED

Action: Astringent and internally strengthening to the blood vessels possibly due to the presence of aescine.

How to use: Take up to 2.5 ml of tincture three times a day; use dilute tincture for compresses.

Combinations: Use with liver herbs (like goldenseal) if sluggish digestion is a contributing factor; add distilled witch-hazel to compresses.

Precautions: Seed coatings of horse chestnut can be toxic; peel before use if using large quantities.

POOR CIRCULATION

May be a sign of more serious heart disorder but is often simply an inherited tendency and not a major problem.

KEY SYMPTOMS:
- Exceptionally cold hands and feet.

- Tendency for chilblains.
- Raynaud's phenomenon ("dead" or white fingers).

REMEDIES:

Zanthoxyllum americanum—PRICKLY ASH

BARK

Action: Diaphoretic and circulatory stimulant; warming for all cold conditions.

How to use: Use 15 g to 600 ml water for decoctions; take up to 5 ml tincture daily.

Combinations: Add angelica root or a pinch of cinnamon powder to decoctions; or combine with rosemary tincture.

Cinnamomum cassia—GUI ZHI

TWIGS

Action: Warming, diaphoretic; encourages both blood and *qi* circulation.

How to use: Standard decoction or tincture.

Combinations: Combines well with ginger in decoction or add rosemary or ginkgo to tinctures.

Precautions: Avoid high doses in pregnancy.

Capsicum frutescens—CAYENNE

FRUIT

Action: Heating, diaphoretic, and a strong circulatory stimulant.

How to use: Use 30–50 mg to 500 ml of water for infusions; up to 1 ml of a 1:20 tincture three times daily; externally as infused oil in massage.

Combinations: Combine with other warming stimulants such as angelica root or bayberry decoctions.

Precautions: Do not exceed stated dose.

Zingiber officinale—GINGER

ROOT

Action: Strong circulatory stimulant, diaphoretic and vasodilator; very warming.

How to use: Use up to 10 g fresh root to 600 ml water for decoctions and footbaths; up to 2 ml of a 1:20 tincture three times daily.

Combinations: Add rosemary or *gui zhi* to decoctions or take a circulatory stimulant such as ginkgo.

PALPITATIONS & ANGINA PECTORIS

Palpitations are simply an awareness of the heartbeat which may be associated with shock, exercise, alcohol, or excitement. Angina pectoris is associated with narrowing of the coronary artery restricting blood supply to the heart – palpitations may herald an attack.

KEY SYMPTOMS:
- Angina attacks usually involve a heavy, pressing pain in the chest which may radiate to the jaw or left arm.
- Breathlessness, panic.

Important: Angina pectoris always requires professional treatment.

REMEDIES:

Alpinia galangal—GALANGAL

ROOT

Actions: Traditional heart remedy, now known to ease heart pains, dizziness, and fatigue, and reduce the symptoms of angina pectoris.

How to use: Take in tablets, tinctures, or decoction; a few drops of neat tincture on the tongue may help avert an angina attack.

Combinations: Use with hawthorn berries, *khella*, and prickly ash in decoctions and tinctures.

Leonurus cardiac—MOTHERWORT

AERIAL PARTS

Actions: Heart tonic and relaxant to combat feelings of panic and normalize heartbeat in palpitations.

How to use: Take in tinctures or infusions.

Combinations: Use with hawthorn flowers and linden in infusions; add rose petals or skullcap for feelings of panic or shock causing palpitations.

Precautions: Avoid in pregnancy.

Passiflora incarnate—PASSION FLOWER

AERIAL PARTS

Actions: Sedative and calming, heart tonic, and relaxant for blood vessels.

How to use: Take in infusions, tablets, and tinctures.

Combinations: Use with hawthorn and linden as an infusion for everyday drinking in angina pectoris; add skullcap or wood betony for palpitations associated with shock or emotional upsets.

Precautions: Use only low doses in pregnancy; may cause drowsiness.

IRON DEFICIENT ANEMIA

Low hemoglobin levels which can be due to poor diet, hemorrhage (or heavy menstrual bleeding) or digestive disorders.

KEY SYMPTOMS:
- Breathlessness.
- Very pale finger nails and inner eyelids.
- Rheumatic-type pains.
- Palpitations.

REMEDIES:

Urtica dioica—STINGING NETTLES

AERIAL PARTS

Actions: Rich in iron, other minerals and vitamins; highly nutritious.

How to use: 10 ml of juice three times daily; use a standard infusion or make nettle soup.

Combinations: Use as a simple but add other iron-rich foods to the diet, such as liver, parsley, watercress, or apricots. Supplements of *ashwaghanda* can also help.

Angelica polyphorma var. *sinensis*—DANG GUI

ROOT

Actions: Nourishes the blood and invigorates the circulation; contains vitamin B12 and folic acid so can also help pernicious anemia.

How to use: Standard decoction and tincture.

Combinations: Can combine with *shu di huang* and *he shou wu*. Add other iron-rich foods to the diet,

such as liver, parsley, watercress, or apricots. Supplements of *ashwaghanda* can also help.

Precautions: Avoid in pregnancy.

HIGH CHOLESTEROL

Excessive levels of lipids (e.g. cholesterol) in the blood which can lead to atherosclerosis and increased risk of heart attack. Often associated with excess saturated fat in the diet; your family history is important. Cholesterol is needed for various body transport mechanisms and is not intrinsically harmful. If dietary cholesterol is very low, then the body will tend to manufacture more to maintain balance.

KEY SYMPTOMS:
- Generally only diagnosed after blood tests.

REMEDIES:

Camellia sinensis—GREEN or OOLONG TEA

LEAF

Actions: Phenols inhibit cholesterol absorption; circulatory stimulant and tonic for blood vessels helping to prevent atherosclerosis.

How to use: 1–2 teaspoons per cup of boiling water as infusion.

Combinations: Use as a simple. *Pu erh* is the most effective variety of oolong tea for reducing cholesterol levels.

Precautions: Limit to 2 cups daily in hypertension and pregnancy.

Allium sativa—GARLIC

CLOVE

Actions: Reduces serum cholesterol levels and has been shown to help prevent repeat heart attacks and atherosclerosis.

How to use: 1 clove daily; 2 g powdered garlic in capsules if there is a high risk of heart attacks.

Combinations: Use as a simple or in cooking. Limit intake of high cholesterol foods and saturated fats.

Avena sativa—OATS

SEED

Actions: Effectively reduces serum cholesterol levels, particularly low-density lipoproteins.

How to use: Make oatmeal porridge or add 25 g of oat bran to breakfast cereal.

Combinations: Use as a simple. Limit intake of high cholesterol foods and saturated fats.

CAPILLARY FRAGILITY

Weakness in the blood vessel walls.

KEY SYMPTOMS:
- Tendency to bruise easily.
- Retinal haemorrhages.
- Petechiae (flat dark red spots caused by bleeding into the skin).

REMEDIES:

Fagopyrum esculentum—BUCKWHEAT

SEED

Action: Rich in rutin which tonifies and repairs the arteriole walls; specific for retinal haemorrhage.

How to use: Standard infusion or tincture; commercial tablets also available.

Combinations: Use with 10 ml of horsetail juice per dose.

Viola tricolor—HEARTSEASE

AERIAL PARTS

Actions: Contains flavonoids, which strengthen the capillary walls.

How to use: Standard infusion or tincture.

Combinations: Use with 10 ml of horsetail juice per dose or add yarrow or ribwort plantain to infusions.

DIGESTIVE PROBLEMS

Good digestion is central to good health; dysfunction here not only starves the body of the right nutrients, but leads to a build-up of toxic excretion products. Ayurvedic theory argues that these excretion products are the source of the three humors – *pitta*, *vata*, and *kapha* – which can account, if out of balance, for most disease states. Ayurvedic theory therefore believes that health depends on the *agni* or digestive fire remaining strong and vigorous.

In Chinese five element theory (see pp. 5–8) the liver is associated with the eyes, vision, energy circulation, blood supply, tendons, nails, menstrual disorders, and mental activity, while the spleen and stomach are associated not only with digestion but also with the blood vessels, muscles, mouth, memory, and intention. Imbalances in the digestive organs can therefore be associated with a wide range of apparently disparate physical and emotional symptoms.

In the West, too, herbal medicine has long focused on digestive function, echoing, perhaps, the medieval maxim that "death dwells in the bowels." Herbs can provide an impressive array of tonics, stimulants, carminatives, and relaxants to ensure healthy function. Bitter remedies like gentian or barberry stimulate digestive activity, while liver tonics like milk thistle can stimulate cell production to repair damage. The strong purgatives of orthodox medicine, such as senna and cascara, are also herbal in origin, although often gentler laxatives are preferable.

Good digestion also depends on the nervous system to stimulate acid or enzyme production, peristaltic gut contractions (which move the food and faeces along), and blood flow to collect the extracted nutrients. Many of the most popular herbal digestive remedies, such as lemon balm, chamomile, hops, rosemary, guelder rose, vervain, and lavender, thus also act on the nervous system and can be useful for stress-related problems like colitis or hyperacidity.

Note: Seek professional advice for any change in normal bowel pattern that lasts for more than two or three days or occurs suddenly.

Cross references
Mouth Ulcers and Gum Disorder, p. 172; Intestinal Worms, p. 232.

CASE HISTORY

IRRITABLE BOWEL SYNDROME

Patient: Louise, a secretary, age 24; an only child still living with her parents but leading an active social life and fond of overseas travel.

History and presenting complaint: She had suffered from "irritable bowel syndrome" for three years, which had started with a bout of food poisoning on a trip to France. Main symptoms were diarrhea (up to five times a day) and vomiting (copious phlegm produced after each meal). Endoscopies, stool analyses, and barium meal tests had all proved negative, and she had been variously prescribed antidepressants, antibiotics, tranquilizers, and bulking laxatives. Louise's diet was far from ideal with far too many cakes, cookies, sweets, and milky drinks. She sucked fruit sweets constantly to suppress feelings of nausea.

Treatment: A priority was to improve Louise's diet. She had recently cut out chocolate, which she had found led to catarrhal problems, and agreed to limit dairy products and carbohydrates, which were producing so much mucus that her system was literally flooded with phlegm. Soya milk and whole grain products were recommended as alternatives. Herbs to help regulate body fluids, tonify the stomach, and astringe the system were prescribed including *ban xia*, *bai zhu*, cinnamon, and agrimony. She was also given *Lactobacillus acidophilus* bacteria in capsules to restore the natural gut flora. Capsules of dried ginger were recommended as an alternative to sucking fruit drops for nausea.

Outcome: After battling with her sweet tooth and fondness for milky drinks, Louise began to improve, but it took around three months before she was able to eat without immediately throwing up. Her stools became firmer, with motions passed on average twice a day. After six months, the herbs were gradually phased out. Louise still avoids too many refined carbohydrates, sugars, and milk products, but is otherwise eating normally.

CONSTIPATION

Generally a symptom of other health problems and may be associated with poor diet, sluggish digestive function or muscle tone, or may be due to nervous tension inhibiting normal bowel action.

KEY SYMPTOMS:

- Lack of bowel motions for more than 24 hours.
- Low abdominal pain or griping.
- Difficulty in passing stool.

REMEDIES:

Rheum palmatum—RHUBARB

ROOT

Actions: Contains anthraquinones, which irritate the gut, increasing peristalsis.

How to use: 10–15 g to 600 ml water as decoction; 2 ml tincture up to three times a day.

Combinations: Add 1–2 ml of fennel, lemon balm, or chamomile tincture per dose or to decoctions to combat any griping; enhance with mild laxatives such as butternut, yellow dock, or licorice, or add senna pods in more severe cases.

Precautions: Avoid in pregnancy, arthritic conditions, or gout.

Viburnum opulus—GUELDER ROSE

BARK

Actions: Smooth muscle relaxant; useful if constipation is linked to visceral tension.

How to use: Standard decoction or tincture.

Combinations: Add 1–2 ml of fennel, lemon balm, or chamomile tincture per dose or to decoctions to combat any griping; enhance with mild laxatives such as butternut, yellow dock, or licorice, or add senna pods in more severe cases.

Plantago psyllium and *Plantago ovata*—PSYLLIUM and ISPHAGULA

SEED

Actions: Mucilaginous and bulking laxative which lubricates the bowel; useful if the stool is dry.

How to use: Use 1 teaspoon of seeds to a cup of boiling water; allow to cool and then drink (inc. seeds), repeat once or twice a day.

Combinations: Use as a simple or mix 2:1 with linseed.

DIARRHEA

Often a symptom of other imbalances in the digestive system but may be caused by obvious food poisoning or infection. Suspect food usually apparent in food poisoning with others sharing the same meal also affected, while an infection can easily be caught by other household members.

KEY SYMPTOMS:

- Loose and frequent stools.
- Abdominal cramps or griping pains.

REMEDIES:

Potentilla erecta—TORMENTIL

ROOT

Action: Contains up to 20% tannins, making the herb very astringent and reducing the inflammation and irritation associated with diarrhea.

How to use: 20 g to 600 ml water as decoction; 2–3 ml of tincture up to three times a day.

Combinations: Add soothing herbs such as ribwort plantain or marshmallow root to ease any inflammation of the gut.

Agrimonia eupatoria—AGRIMONY

AERIAL PARTS

Action: Stringent and healing for any intestinal tract inflammation; especially suitable for children.

How to use: Standard infusion or tincture.

Combinations: Add soothing herbs such as ribwort plantain or marshmallow root to ease any inflammation of the gut; use bilberry or bistort to increase astringency.

Geranium maculatum—AMERICAN CRANESBILL

HERB OR ROOT

Actions: Astringent, but gentle enough for children, the elderly and debilitated.

How to use: Leaf: standard infusion or tincture. Root: 20 g to 600 ml water for decoction; 2–3 ml of tincture three times a day.

Combinations: Add soothing herbs such as ribwort plantain, meadowsweet, or marshmallow root to ease any inflammation of the gut; use bilberry or bistort to increase astringency.

GASTRITIS

Inflammation of the gastric mucosa which if persistent can lead to ulceration eventually. May be due to dietary factors.

KEY SYMPTOMS:

- Heartburn and acid reflux.
- Persistent vomiting in acute gastritis.
- Diarrhea and abdominal discomfort.

REMEDIES:

Athaea officinalis—MARSHMALLOW

ROOT

Actions: Soothing and demulcent for irritated mucus membranes; healing for damaged tissue.

How to use: Use a maceration or tincture made from fresh herb or powder.

Combinations: Use with meadowsweet with a pinch of cinnamon; combine with carminatives such as fennel and peppermint infusions.

Ulmus fulva—SLIPPERY ELM

BARK

Actions: Demulcent to sooth irritated mucosa; also nutritive for debilitated conditions.

How to use: Up to 5 g of powdered bark in capsules or mixed with water, before meals.

Combinations: Can be combined with an equal amount of powdered marshmallow root.

Filipendula ulmaria—MEADOWSWEET

AERIAL PARTS

Actions: Anti-inflammatory, reduces stomach acid secretions and is soothing and healing for gastric mucosa.

How to use: Standard infusion, fluid extract or tincture 5 ml tincture daily.

Combinations: Increase astringency with 10 drops of bistort or American cranesbill tincture or soothe with 10 drops of licorice per dose. Add extra anti-inflammatories, such as pot marigold, if desired.

Precautions: Avoid in cases of salicylate sensitivity.

PEPTIC/DUODENAL ULCERS

Ulceration of the stomach or duodenal mucous membranes now associated with the *Heliobacter pylorii* bacterium; also associated with stress and dietary abuse.

KEY SYMPTOMS:

- Easily located pain in the upper abdomen.
- Pain often worse at night or when hungry.
- Possible nausea, heartburn, flatulence, and weight loss.

REMEDIES:

Leptospermum scoparium—NEW ZEALAND TEA TREE (MANUKA or KAHIKATOA)

POLLEN, FLOWERS, LEAVES, OR BARK

Actions: Studies in New Zealand suggest that anti-microbial manuka honey is very effective at killing the *Heliobacter* bacterium.

How to use: Take 1½ teaspoons of manuka honey twice a day or use the flowers and leaves in infusions or the bark in decoctions.

Combinations: Add other antibacterials such as echinacea, blue flag, or thyme; add soothing demulcents such as marshmallow root or licorice as decoctions.

Glycyrrhiza glabra—LICORICE

ROOT

Actions: Anti-inflammatory; produces a viscous mucus which coats and protects the stomach wall and limits acid production.

How to use: Standard decoction, tincture of fluid extract; juice sticks can be sucked like sweets.

Combinations: In severe cases add extra soothing herbs such as marshmallow root or slippery elm or add anti-inflammatories such as meadowsweet or pot marigold.

Precautions: Avoid in cases of high blood pressure or if taking digoxin-based drugs.

INFLAMED GALLBLADDER

Cholecystitis may be chronic or acute and is often linked to high fat consumption.

KEY SYMPTOMS:

- Constant, severe upper abdominal pain often radiating to the shoulder.
- Sweating, nausea, erratic breathing.

REMEDIES:

Berberis vulgaris—BARBERRY

BARK

Actions: Stimulates bile flow and eases liver congestion; bitter and laxative.

How to use: 15 g of herb to 600 ml water for decoctions or up to 8 ml tincture daily.

Combinations: Combine with anti-inflammatories such as goldenseal (5 drops of tincture per dose) and add liver tonics such as vervain infusion or globe artichoke juice.

Precautions: Avoid in pregnancy.

Chionanthus virginicus—FRINGE TREE

BARK

Actions: Stimulates bile flow and liver function; laxative and cleansing.

How to use: Use a standard decoction in tablespoon doses or up to 5 ml tincture daily.

Combinations: Combine with bitters, liver tonics or stimulants such as dandelion root, milk thistle, chicory, globe artichoke, or centaury, plus anti-inflammatories like pot marigold.

GALLSTONES

Made of bile pigment and/or cholesterol that becomes lodged in the bile duct.

KEY SYMPTOMS:

- Brief attacks of severe upper abdominal pain.
- Most common in the "fair, fat, forty, female, and flatulent."
- Jaundice, indigestion, vomiting.

REMEDIES:

Peumus boldo—BOLDO

LEAVES

Actions: Stimulates bile flow and liver activity; reduces inflammation and helps protect the liver.

How to use: Use 10–30 drops of tincture per dose or half a teaspoon of dried leaves to two cups of infusion taken in half-cup doses.

Combinations: Traditionally combined with barberry and fringe tree for gall stones; add guelder rose or wild yam to help relieve spasmodic pain.

Precautions: Avoid in pregnancy.

Citrus x limon—LEMON

JUICE

Actions: Used in traditional treatments with olive oil to break down and encourage excretion of gallstones; liver tonic and restorative.

How to use: After fasting for the day, take 50 ml of olive oil and the juice of 2 lemons in water at 6 p.m. Repeat three times over the next hour. Bile sand is passed in stools over the following three days.

Combinations: With olive oil (see "*How to use*").

INDIGESTION & ACIDITY

Usually due to eating too much, too quickly, missing meals, or anxiety. Antacids actually encourage further stomach acid secretion and can worsen the condition.

KEY SYMPTOMS:

- Bloating and feelings of abdominal fullness.
- Heartburn or acid reflux.
- Stomach pain.

REMEDIES:

Mentha x piperita—PEPPERMINT

AERIAL PARTS

Actions: Cooling carminative to ease flatulence and heartburn; stimulates bile flow; good for nervous tummies and nausea.

How to use: 15 g of dried herb to 500 ml water in infusions; up to 2.5 ml tincture per dose.

Combinations: Use as a simple; add American cranesbill to reduce acid secretions; add marshmallow root or licorice for inflammation.

Precautions: May reduce milk flow; use with caution if breastfeeding.

Melissa officinalis—LEMON BALM

AERIAL PARTS

Actions: Carminative and relaxing; sedative action so useful for nervous tummies.

How to use: Standard infusion or tincture.

Combinations: Add chamomile or fennel as anti-inflammatories or 10–20 drops of hop tincture as a bitter stimulant.

Foeniculum vulgare—FENNEL

SEEDS

Actions: Carminative and anti-inflammatory, effective for griping pains.

How to use: Standard infusion or tincture useful as an after-dinner tisane.

Combinations: Use as a simple; add American cranesbill to reduce acid secretions; add marshmallow root or licorice for inflammation.

IRRITABLE BOWEL SYNDROME & COLITIS

A convenient medical label for a variety of digestive symptoms often associated with anxiety, food intolerance, or infection.

KEY SYMPTOMS:
- Alternating bouts of diarrhea and constipation.
- Characteristic "rabbit dropping" stools.
- Bloating and flatulence.
- Mucous in stools.

REMEDIES:

Dioscorea villosa—WILD YAM

RHIZOME

Actions: Visceral relaxant and antispasmodic, anti-inflammatory and bile stimulant.

How to use: In decoctions (1 teaspoon to 500 m water) or combined with other tinctures.

Combinations: Add meadowsweet to soothe gastric mucosa; chamomile or lemon balm if stress is an issue; or a few drops of fresh ginger tincture to help regulate bowel activity.

Precautions: Avoid in pregnancy or if trying to conceive.

Matricaria chamomilla—GERMAN CHAMOMILE

FLOWERS

Actions: Sedative, anti-inflammatory and carminative; good for nervous dyspepsia.

How to use: Standard infusion or tincture.

Combinations: Add a few drops of peppermint or fresh ginger tincture to relieve abdominal bloating and regulate bowel activity. Combine with lemon balm or passion flower if stress is a factor.

Iberis amaria—BITTER CANDYTUFT

AERIAL PARTS

Actions: antispasmodic, relaxant, tonifies the digestive tract; carminative.

How to use: Take up to 2 ml tincture per dose or an infusion made of 5 g herb to 500 ml water.

Combinations: Add angelica root and milk thistle seeds as liver tonics; add chamomile or lemon balm if stress is an issue.

Precautions: High doses may cause nausea.

LIVER DISORDERS

In our polluted society liver congestion is very common; can manifest as pathological disorders but often simply involves feelings of anger and stagnation.

KEY SYMPTOMS:
- Tendency for constipation.
- Abdominal bloating.
- Emotional lability.
- Menstrual disorders in women.
- Red, itching palms.
- Small petechiae on the abdomen.
- Sore, itching eyes.

REMEDIES:

Bupleurum chinense—CHAI HU

ROOT

Actions: Bitter liver tonic; stimulates bile flow, energy tonic, anti-inflammatory and antibacterial.

How to use: 10 g to 600 ml water for decoctions or up to 6 ml tincture daily.

Combinations: Combine with *bai shao yao, chuan xiong,* goldenseal, or dandelion in decoctions to improve liver function.

Silybum marianum—MILK THISTLE

SEEDS

Actions: Encourages liver cell renewal and repair; effective liver healer in degenerative conditions, including alcohol abuse.

How to use: Standard infusion or up to 10 ml tincture daily.

Combinations: Use as a simple or add vervain, gentian, dandelion root, or globe artichoke as additional liver tonics.

Picrorrhiza kurroa—KATUKA

ROOT

Actions: A traditional bitter Ayurvedic digestive remedy that protects the liver from a variety of toxins and stimulates bile flow to help cleanse the gallbladder.

How to use: Take 1 g per dose as powder in capsules or mixed with ghee, or use half a teaspoon of crushed root for three doses of decoction.

Combinations: Use with other bitter digestive or liver stimulants such as turmeric, barberry, gotu kola, and cardamom.

Precautions: High doses may cause diarrhea, abdominal griping and flatulence; cases of allergic skin reaction have been reported.

NAUSEA & VOMITING

A symptom, rather than an identifiable disease; can be associated with various factors including food poisoning, infections, fever, migraines or pregnancy.

Note: Projectile or prolonged vomiting requires urgent professional medical help.

REMEDIES:

Zingiber officinale—GINGER

ROOT

Action: Very effective antiemetic useful for travel sickness as well as digestive upsets.

How to use: Use standard tincture in drop doses on the tongue frequently while symptoms persist or chew crystallised ginger.

Combinations: Use as a simple or combine with black horehound or chamomile tinctures

Precautions: Use with care in early pregnancy.

Syzygium aromaticum—CLOVES

FLOWER BUDS OR ESSENTIAL OIL

Actions: Stimulant and carminative also locally antiseptic.

How to use: Standard infusion or use 1–2 drops of oil on a sugar lump internally; or sprinkle powdered spice on food.

Precautions: Do not exceed the stated dose of essential oil.

FLATULENCE & ABDOMINAL BLOATING

Often associated with minor digestive or liver problems, but can indicate serious illness.

KEY SYMPTOMS:

* Wind that may go up or down.
* Uncomfortable abdominal distention.

REMEDIES:

Elettaria cardamomum—CARDAMOM

SEED OR ESSENTIAL OIL

Actions: Carminative and soothing for the digestive system; relieves abdominal cramps and stimulates appetite.

How to use: Use the crushed seeds in infusions or tinctures; use 2–5 drops of essential oil in 5 ml of carrier oil for abdominal massage; use seeds in cooking.

Combinations: Use with soothing digestive remedies such as gotu kola, fennel, chamomile, or lemon balm in infusions; add a pinch of galangal, ginger, or black pepper.

Cnicus benedictus—HOLY THISTLE

FLOWER HEADS

Actions: A bitter digestive stimulant which encourages stomach secretions and normalizes function.

How to use: Use in infusions or tinctures.

Combinations: Add lemon balm or chamomile with teas or centaury as an additional bitter; add carminatives such as pinch of fennel seeds, black pepper, or cinnamon.

Precautions: May cause vomiting in excessive doses.

FOOD POISONING & GASTROENTERITIS

Gastric infection by viruses, bacteria, or protozoa, which may be due to pets, farm animals, or environmental hazards; food poisoning is a notifiable disease in some countries.

KEY SYMPTOMS:
- Sudden onset with abdominal pain, nausea, and vomiting.
- Diarrhea, general malaise and weakness.

REMEDIES:

Matricaria chamomilla—GERMAN CHAMOMILE

FLOWERS
Actions: Antimicrobial to combat infection, soothing and calming for the digestive system, reduces inflammation in the digestive tract.

How to use: Use in infusions.

Combinations: With astringents like agrimony or lady's mantle, soothing demulcents such as meadowsweet or marshmallow and digestive tonics such as gotu kola. Add a pinch of ginger or cinnamon to combat nausea.

Alchemilla xanthoclora—LADY'S MANTLE

LEAVES
Actions: Astringent digestive tonic to reduce inflammation and discomfort.

How to use: Use in infusions or tinctures.

Combinations: With milk thistle seeds and marshmallow root to soothe the digestive tract and normalize function; eat garlic or take echinacea to combat infection.

POOR APPETITE

Loss of appetite may be due to chronic illness, stress, or debility, all of which should also be treated.

KEY SYMPTOMS:
- No interest in meals or eating.
- Weight loss and absence of menstruation in severe cases.

Note: Poor appetite may suggest eating disorders such as anorexia nervosa; seek immediate professional help if this is suspected.

REMEDIES:

Trigonella foenum-graecum—FENUGREEK

SEEDS
Actions: Stimulating and tonifying for the whole digestive system; a traditional remedy for thin people hoping to put on weight.

How to use: Take the seeds in infusions or use drops of the tincture on the tongue half an hour before meals.

Combinations: Combine with milk thistle seeds or agrimony in infusions with a pinch of powdered ginger or galangal for additional stimulation. Add chamomile, vervain, or wood betony if stress is a factor.

Jateorhiza calumba—CALUMBA

ROOT
Actions: Bitter and stimulating for the digestive system; also helps to relieve indigestion and normalize digestive function; stimulates production of stomach acid.

How to use: Use in macerations – half a cup, half an hour before meals or take 20–40 drops of tincture in a little water before meals.

Combinations: Combine with mugwort tincture in menstrual disorders or mix the maceration with agrimony, lemon balm, and chamomile infusions to soothe the digestive tract.

Precautions: Avoid in pregnancy and gastric ulceration.

Halitosis/Bad Breath

Infections in the mouth, throat, lungs, or stomach can all contribute to bad breath; poor dental hygiene is often to blame.

Key Symptoms:

- Stale or offensive breath.

Remedies:

Levisticum officinale—LOVAGE

Seeds

Actions: A tonic to normalize both digestive and respiratory function and improve the appetite; eases flatulence and combats bacteria; the seeds also contain aromatic oils.

How to use: Chew a few seeds as required to freshen the breath and help normalize digestive function.

Combinations: Mix with dill or fennel seeds if preferred; gargle with 5–10 drops of myrrh tincture in a glass of water to help clear any mouth or gum infections; use appropriate remedies to treat any associated disorders contributing to the problem.

Iris versicolor—BLUE FLAG

Root

Actions: Cleansing and stimulating for sluggish digestion, lymphatics, and glandular systems.

How to use: Use powdered in capsules, 200 mg daily

Combinations: Combine with powdered goldenseal, licorice, and echinacea or myrrh to combat underlying infections and congestion.

Hemorrhoids/Piles

Anal varicose veins associated with poor muscle tone and often due to straining or constipation.

Key Symptoms:

- Palpable piles at anus.
- Bleeding on passing stool.

Remedies:

Sophora japonica—HUAI JIAO

Fruit

Actions: Cooling, anti-inflammatory, and hypotensive; clears liver heat, cools blood, and stops bleeding. Also helps constipation.

How to use: Standard decoction or tincture; powdered in capsules (400 mg, three times a day).

Combinations: Use as a simple or combine with liver tonics and digestive remedies such as dandelion root, barberry, *dang gui*, or *zhi ke*.

Precautions: Avoid in pregnancy.

Ranunculus ficaria—PILEWORT

Root or Leaves

Actions: Astringent to tonify blood vessels and stop bleeding.

How to use: Apply ointment frequently.

Combinations: Use as a simple but take supportive liver herbs or venous tonics such as king's clover. Take additional laxatives if need be to avoid constipation.

Precautions: Do not take internally.

Allergic Conditions

Allergies act as an additional stress on the body. When everything is ticking along happily, the system can cope with allergens, but if there is increased tension, infection, or fatigue, the arrival of an allergen tips the balance and an allergic response in the form of hay fever, gastric upsets, skin rashes, or other reaction results.

Food allergies often start in infancy when the immature gut has to cope with unknown proteins, such as cow's milk. The immune system is triggered to repel the invader with inflammations, mucus, and irritation. If the allergen continues to be ingested then after a while the response becomes muted or masked and while the allergen is still a stress on the body, there is no tell-tale rash or catarrh, only a general weakening of the immune system, which continues to battle with the allergen. This sort of masked allergy can manifest as vague arthritic pains, irritable bowel syndrome, or persistent sinusitis, and careful elimination diets may be needed to identify the troublemaker. Dairy products (usually cow's milk but sometimes goat's or sheep's as well) commonly cause problems as do wheat, gluten (found in wheat, barley, oats, and rye), and beef. Salicylates are found in many fresh fruits, vegetables, and herbs, and regular use of aspirin-based drugs does seem to increase sensitivity to salicylates. This can be a difficult allergy to identify, as affected children may produce a rash after such disparate foods as tomatoes, oranges, broccoli, mushrooms, tea, sweet corn, peanuts, and honey. With food intolerance one needs to totally eliminate the troublesome foods while the digestive system is soothed and repaired, and then reintroduce them slowly and on a rotation basis (no more than once every four days) so that there is no buildup of potential toxins.

Some allergens cannot be so easily avoided – house dust or pollen is troublesome and persistent. Again, the herbal approach concentrates on strengthening the respiratory and immune systems so that the allergen does not cause the characteristic response.

Cross references

Asthma, p. 169; Eczema, p. 175.

Case Studies

Hay fever

Patient: Jonathan, age 10, had suffered from hay fever each year since he was seven.

History and presenting complaint: An otherwise healthy boy (if a little overweight), Jonathan started sneezing when the flowering currants appeared in March and continued with increasing severity until August. Antihistamines were proving less and less effective and it was when the GP suggested that steroids might be necessary that his worried mother turned to alternative medicine.

Treatment: Treatment started in January with regular doses (5 ml per day) of an herbal brew containing elderflower, white horehound and ground ivy for the upper respiratory tract with self-heal, dandelion root, and gentian to cool and cleanse the liver. The taste was heavily disguised with licorice as, like many small boys, Jonathan was extremely reluctant to swallow the bitter mixture even once a day. That first year his hay fever symptoms did not really start until May and were kept in check with a combination of eyebright and goldenseal capsules. Antihistamines were only needed in late May when the oilseed rape crop peaked, but the severe symptoms soon abated. The following year, a similar regime was followed – again taking the strengthening herbal mixture from February to early April. Again, the symptoms were reduced still further (despite the added stresses of upper-school exams to cope with).

Outcome: Three year after starting treatment Jonathan survived a summer without recourse to antihistamine, steroids, or ventilators. For the first time in five years the repeat prescription for antihistamine remained unfilled even when the pollen count was highest using only eyebright capsules occasionally as needed.

HAY FEVER/ALLERGIC RHINITIS

Hay fever is generally triggered by grass or tree pollens and occurs when these are prevalent. Allergies to house dust, pets, etc., generally occur throughout the year without seasonal variation.

KEY SYMPTOMS:
- Copious nasal catarrh.
- Sore, irritated eyes.
- Sneezing.
- Severe cases can produce asthma-like symptoms.

REMEDIES:

Euphrasia officinalis—EYEBRIGHT

AERIAL PARTS
Actions: Decreases nasal secretions and soothes mucous membranes and conjunctiva.

How to use: Standard infusion, tincture, or two 200 mg capsules three times daily; also use 5 drops of tincture in an eye bath of water.

Combinations: Combine with goldenseal powder in capsules; with elderflower in infusions or tinctures. Often prescribed with *ma huang*, which is a restricted herb in some geographies.

Glechoma hederacea—GROUND IVY

AERIAL PARTS
Actions: Astringent and anti-catarrhal to dry secretions and inflammations.

How to use: Standard infusion or tincture.

Combinations: Combine with anti-catarrhals, such as marsh cudweed, in tinctures; take chamomile in infusions or use in steam inhalants.

Plantago lanceolata—RIBWORT PLANTAIN

LEAVES
Actions: Good for allergic rhinitis, toning mucous membranes, and healing inflammations.

How to use: Standard infusion or up to 4 ml of tincture three times daily.

Combinations: Add astringent anti-catarrhals such as marsh cudweed or ground ivy. Take chamomile in infusions or use in steam inhalants.

FOOD INTOLERANCE

Common food allergens include cow's milk, wheat, and beef and can be responsible for an enormous range of symptoms. Candidiasis due to overgrowth of yeasts in the gut, can also be related to food intolerance. Salicylate (aspirins, etc.) allergy is increasingly common. Coeliac disease (intolerance of gluten) can cause severe health problems.

KEY SYMPTOMS:
- Digestive upsets – often diarrhea and flatulence.
- Stiffness and joint pain.
- Skin rashes and eczema.
- Respiratory problems including asthma.
- Persistent urinary infections or vaginal thrush in candidiasis.
- Candidiasis can also be related to nervous disorders.

REMEDIES:

Calendula officinalis—POT MARIGOLD

FLOWER PETALS
Actions: Antifungal and useful for excess yeasts in the gut in candidiasis.

How to use: Use standard infusion or tincture well diluted in water.

Combinations: Combine with elder-flowers and agrimony or add antimicrobials such as echinacea in candidiasis or nervines if stress is an issue.

Hydrastis canadensis—GOLDENSEAL

ROOT

Actions: Good liver stimulant and helps to ease gastric sensitivity; astringent and healing for the mucosa.

How to use: Use in capsules – two 200 mg up to three times daily or in 2–4 ml tincture doses.

Combinations: With powdered fenugreek or agrimony in capsules; with licorice in tinctures to soothe and heal mucous membranes.

Precautions: Avoid in pregnancy and high blood pressure; do not exceed stated dose.

Allium sativa—GARLIC

CLOVES

Actions: Antifungal, useful for excess yeasts in the gut and supports recovery of gut flora.

How to use: Use 1 clove a day in cooking or take two 200 mg capsules.

Combinations: Best as a simple or with parsley to reduce the garlic odour.

Agrimonia eupatoria—AGRIMONY

AERIAL PARTS

Actions: Soothes gut irritation and inflammation and heals damaged mucosa.

How to use: Use standard infusion or up to 4 ml of tincture three times daily.

Combinations: Add lemon balm and chamomile to reduce stress. Combine with soothing demulcents such as marshmallow root and take garlic or echinacea as antifungals.

URTICA/HIVES

Skin blisters and rashes caused by particular allergens including foods, such as peanuts, or contact with chemicals. Rashes are generally transient but can be severe and persistent. May be associated with salicylate allergy.

KEY SYMPTOMS:
*   Irritant red swellings on the skin.

Note: Severe reactions and swelling may restrict breathing or lead to anaphylactic shock which can be fatal; seek urgent professional help.

Urtica dioica—STINGING NETTLE

AERIAL PARTS

Actions: Taking nettles for nettle rash may seem a contradiction, but it can reduce itching and act as an antihistamine.

How to use: Use in infusions, tincture or take two 200 mg capsules of powdered herb.

Combinations: Use with red clover, wood betony and meadowsweet in infusions; add 20 drops of *ma huang* tincture dose to reduce the allergic reaction.

Precautions: *Ma huang* is restricted in some geographies and may only be available on prescription.

Viola tricolor—HEARTSEASE

AERIAL PARTS

Actions: Anti-inflammatory and soothing for any skin inflammation.

How to use: Standard infusion or up to 15 ml of tincture daily, also as a wash or in ointments and creams.

Combinations: Add 1–2 drops of thyme oil to 20 ml heartsease cream or add stinging nettle to infusions and tinctures.

Brassica oleracea—CABBAGE

LEAVES

Actions: Anti-inflammatory and healing; useful standby for emergencies.

How to use: Apply a fresh leaf directly to the affected part or extract juice and use as a lotion.

Combinations: Use as a simple. Fresh slices of onion can be similarly used.

Urinary Disorders

The kidneys and urinary system often mirror the health of an individual – something that persistent cystitis sufferers know well, as their symptoms increase at times of stress or fatigue. Just as recurrent colds can indicate a weak immune system, so can repeated urinary infections; tonic herbs, immune stimulant herbs are often needed after the symptoms have been eased. Herbal remedies will generally include a urinary antiseptic, which often contains volatile oils that survive the digestion process, pass into the bloodstream, and are excreted via the kidneys. Soothing demulcent herbs are also added to remedies for the urinary tract to help reduce inflammation and repair damage to the mucosa. There will also be diuretics to increase the flow and flush out the toxins and dead bacteria.

In Chinese medicine, urinary inflammations are regarded as problems of heat and damp rather than "infections" due to bacteria, and are treated with cooling herbs such as *huang qin, zhi zie, ze xie, mu tong, sheng di huang*, or rhubarb root (*da huang*). In traditional Chinese theory the kidney and urinary bladder are associated organs so weak kidney energy (*qi*) may lead to bladder problems. Excessive or nocturnal urination, incontinence, the sort of dribbling after urination we regard as a classic prostate disorder could all be classified as signs of weak kidney energy so tonic herbs, including *huang qi, dang gui*, ginseng, or *bai zhu*, may be recommended.

Cross references:
Incontinence, p. 224; Bedwetting, p. 233; Vaginal Thrush, p. 212.

Case Study

Recurrent cystitis and thrush

Patient: Pamela, 48, married for the second time with a son in his 20s and a 10-year-old daughter, working full time in sales.

History and presenting complaint: Pamela had suffered from recurrent cystitis for 15 years that was treated with regular doses of antibiotics. Main symptoms included severe burning on passing urine and increased frequency, making her frequent travel to business appointments a nightmare. She was also prone to persistent thrush and tended to eat too many chocolates and Marmite sandwiches. She had been on antibiotics for two weeks after another flare-up of cystitis but these had had little effect and she was reluctant to return to her GP for more.

Treatment: Strictly curtailing sugar and yeast intake was an important factor in long-term control of the thrush and initial medication focused on the immediate symptoms with buchu, bearberry, echinacea, corn silk and couch grass. Capsules of buchu and couchgrass powder were also supplied for use during the day, as Pamela was "on the road" a lot and taking herbal tinctures or teas at work would be a problem. Tea tree pessaries were used for the thrush and *Lactobacillus acidophilus* capsules were also suggested to restore the gut flora after those antibiotics.

Outcome: Pamela's work and family commitments meant it was nearly six weeks before she managed a second appointment. By this time she had been completely free of cystitis for a month. A "twinge" had been quickly treated with echinacea capsules (two capsules, three times a day for two days) and she was continuing to drink a weak infusion of buchu and couchgrass tea on a daily basis as a preventative. Pamela took away a further supply of tea and capsules and promised to "try harder" to cut down on sugar to control the thrush. Two years later she has only one further bout of cystitis – again rapidly resolved with a similar remedy. However, binging on cream cakes and chocolates usually causes the thrush to flare up, although this is soon resolved with pessaries. Pamela maintains that this is a small price to pay for indulging her love of gooey cakes.

URINARY TRACT INFECTIONS & CYSTITIS/URETHRITIS

Infections in the urinary tract usually lead to bladder inflammation (cystitis) in women and urethritis in men. In some cases there can be kidney involvement, which may be severe.

KEY SYMPTOMS:
- Pain or burning sensation on passing water.
- Possible blood, mucus, or pus in the urine.
- Increased frequency of urination.
- Fever (more likely the higher up the urinary tract is the infection).
- Pain – may be located from groin to mid-back, depending on the site of infection.

NB: All cases of kidney involvement must be referred to a profession practitioner. If the origin is venereal, cases must in UK law be referred to a doctor.

REMEDIES:

Agathosma betulina—BUCHU
LEAVES

Actions: Diuretic and urinary antiseptic also has a warming and stimulant effect on the kidneys.

How to use: 15 g of herb to 500 ml in infusion or up to 2 ml of tincture, or three 200 mg capsules three times daily.

Combinations: Add couchgrass and yarrow to infusions or capsules. Add corn silk to soothe severe burning sensations.

Arctostaphylos uva-ursi—BEARBERRY
LEAVES

Actions: Produces potent antiseptic in the kidney tubules; effective with acid urine,

How to use: 5 g of herb to 500 ml in infusion or up to 2 ml of tincture three times daily.

Combinations: Add couchgrass and yarrow to infusions; use horsetail juice or pellitory if there is damage to the mucosa.

Precautions: High doses may cause nausea.

Apium graveolens—CELERY
SEED

Actions: Urinary antiseptic and cleanses uric acid from the system.

How to use: Standard infusion or up to 4 ml tincture three times daily.

Combinations: Use horsetail, corn silk, or couchgrass to soothe inflamed mucosa.

Precautions: Avoid in pregnancy; do not use seeds prepared for the garden trade.

Elymus repens—COUCHGRASS
RHIZOME

Actions: Contains mannitol, which is a diuretic, mucilages to soothe the mucosa, and is mildly anti-biotic.

How to use: Standard infusion or tincture.

Combinations: Use with buchu, bearberry, or juniper as more potent antiseptics.

URINARY GRAVEL

Deposits of insoluble material – usually calcium salts or small particles of uric acid – formed in the bladder, which can be associated with changes in the acidity or alkalinity of the urine

KEY SYMPTOMS:
- Sensation of "grittiness" on passing urine.
- Blood in urine in severe cases.
- Pain, which can be severe, between "loin and groin."

REMEDIES:

Eupatorium purpureum—GRAVELROOT
ROOT

Actions: Diuretic and soothing for the urinary mucosa useful for all irritations and inflammations.

How to use: Use 20 g to 600 ml water in decoctions or up to 3 ml of tincture three times daily.

Combinations: Can be combined with parsley piert, corn silk, couchgrass, or pellitory-of-the-wall to soothe and encourage healing.

Parietaria diffusa—PELLITORY-OF-THE-WALL

AERIAL PARTS

Actions: Diuretic and demulcent; useful for pain on urination; for kidney stones.

How to use: Standard infusion or tincture; the fresh juice in 20 ml doses is particularly effective.

Combinations: Add buchu or bearberry for infections; with couchgrass or corn silk to soothe and heal.

Juniperis communis—JUNIPER

BERRIES OR ESSENTIAL OIL

Actions: Urinary antiseptic and diuretic; good for clearing acid wastes.

How to use: Use 10 g of berries to 500 ml for infusions; up to 2 ml of tincture three times daily. Use the well-diluted oil as a abdominal massage.

Combinations: Use with parsley piert or hydrangea to help clear stones and add soothing remedies such as pellitory, cornsilk, or couchgrass.

Precautions: Avoid in pregnancy and do not use continuously for more than six weeks without a break.

KIDNEY STONES

Insoluble calcium or oxalates formed in the kidney leading to renal colic as they pass through the ureter to the bladder. Stones may be linked to excess calcium consumption.

KEY SYMPTOMS:

- Agonising "loin to groin" pain due to the passage of stones or gravel.
- Nausea, vomiting, blood in the urine.

Note: Always consult a professional practitioner.

REMEDIES:

Aphanes arvensis—PARSLEY PIERT

AERIAL PARTS

Actions: Also called parsley breakstone for its ability to break down stones in the kidney or bladder; diuretic, demulcent, and soothing for the urinary tract.

How to use: Use in infusions or tinctures (up to 10 ml per dose).

Combinations: Use with hydrangea, ginger, and gravel root in tinctures; with cornsilk, pellitory of the wall, and *khella* (restricted in Australia) in infusions. Apply a hot compress of ginger to the lower abdomen if possible.

Amni visnaga—KHELLA

SEEDS

Actions: Relieves spasmodic pain by relaxing the muscles in the ureter which helps ease the stone towards the bladder.

How to use: Use in infusions or tincture.

Combinations: Use with soothing demulcents such as cornsilk or marshmallow root; add shepherd's purse to help reduce any bleeding.

Precautions: Restricted herb in Australia; prolonged or excessive use may cause nausea, headaches, and insomnia.

NERVOUS DISORDERS

A holistic approach to medicine focuses on the needs of body, mind, and spirit, and this is especially true with any condition labeled as "nerves." Physical manifestations of "nervous disorders" may include insomnia, palpitations, or headaches; emotional aspects can include irritability, depression, and feelings of anger or guilt, while the lack of determination, emptiness, or sense of purpose felt by so many people can typify the spiritual vacuum at the center of so many modern lifestyles.

Herbs can be equally holistic, operating on the same three levels to improve well-being: vervain is a good example. It can be considered a good liver tonic and relaxing nervine. Taken in the form of a Bach Flower Remedy it is good for the perfectionist, slightly obsessional personality who tries to do too many jobs at once and runs each task to death, like a dog worrying a bone. On a spiritual level vervain can increase understanding and psychic awareness: it was once used to raise the consciousness in scrying and some maintain that it will repair holes in the human aura (a layer of psychic energy that surrounds all living things).

In Chinese and Ayurvedic medicine, emotional imbalance is well-accepted as a possible cause of physical disease: the Chinese associate fear with the kidneys, for example, so panic attacks could be a sign of kidney imbalance or contribute to kidney weakness. Herbs can also be used to strengthen the *chakras* – the body's spiritual centers in Eastern philosophy; basil, for example, is believed to reinforce the root, second, and third *charkas*.

Herbal nervines can thus work on several levels: they can be used in much the same way as orthodox sedatives, hypnotics, or antidepressants, but also have an emotional aspect familiar from the various flower and gem remedies now available. Modern science also has to accept that herbs can affect the mind and emotions in ways that we are only beginning to understand. Aromatic chemicals from essential oils, for example, travel through the olfactory system to reach parts of the limbic center in the inner brain – a center for emotions that also has a role in interpreting and recalling experiences and memory.

Cross references
Tension Headaches, p. 160; Neuralgia, p. 161; Hyperactivity, p. 233; Parkinson's Disease, p. 222; Forgetfulness/Confusion in the Elderly p. 225.

CASE STUDY

LACK OF SELF-DETERMINATION
Patient: Rosemary, 52, a reformed alcoholic in an unhappy marriage with a domineering husband.

History and presenting complaint: After years of finding solace in the bottle, Rosemary had started to take control of her own life again with the support of friends, her church, and Alcoholics Anonymous. But she felt unable to leave her husband, largely because of financial considerations, and was concerned that his constant nagging would force her to start drinking again. Physical symptoms included rheumatic-type pains in her legs and lower back, persistent colds, sleeplessness and general lack of enthusiasm for life. A hysterectomy three years earlier had been followed by hormone replacement therapy, which she had recently stopped, leading to hot flashes and night sweats. Rosemary had recently had a brief affair with a friend's husband which left her lonely and guilt ridden.

Treatment: A massage oil of lavender, basil and rosemary was suggested for the aches and pains while also easing the nervous problems while chaste-berry and goldenseal capsules were given for the menopausal symptoms. Wood betony, gotu kola, and skullcap were used to counter the depression, sense of loss, and lingering need for addiction with *ling zhi* to provide a spiritual boost and help Rosemary's self-determination. All herbs were prescribed in powders or teas as tinctures need to be avoided with reformed alcoholics.

Outcome: The aches and pains in the legs disappeared within a week – perhaps signifying that Rosemary no longer felt physically tied to her home and husband. She began to feel more cheerful and her sleep improved. The hot flushes eased. Over the following months, Rosemary began to feel that the alcohol problem was getting under her control and she took on a new part-time job in a local fashion shop, focusing her attentions on outside activities more. Her husband is still domineering, but she feels less threatened by his behavior and also acknowledges that leaving him is a possibility she might consider in future. She continues to drink wood betony tea and takes *ling zhi* periodically.

ANXIETY/TENSION

Excessive life stresses can lead to a variety of health problems, not always obviously linked to tension.

KEY SYMPTOMS:
- Inability to relax.
- Emotional lability – tendency to cry or be irritable for no obvious cause.
- Headaches.
- Sleeplessness.

REMEDIES:

Stachys officinalis—WOOD BETONY

AERIAL PARTS

Actions: Sedative and calming for the nervous system; good for nervous debility, fearfulness, and exhaustion.

How to use: Standard infusion or tincture. Can be used powdered in capsules.

Combinations: Good as a simple, or combine with chamomile, vervain, skullcap, or lavender to enhance tonic or sedative action.

Precautions: Very large doses can be emetic.

Scutellaria lateriflora—SKULLCAP

AERIAL PARTS

Actions: Relaxant and restorative for the central nervous system; good for nervous debility.

How to use: Standard infusion or tincture or powdered in capsules.

Combinations: Use as a simple or combine with wood betony, lavender, or lemon balm to increase calming, sedative action.

Tilia x *europaea*—LINDEN

FLOWERS

Actions: Reduces nervous tension and also helps prevent arteriosclerosis.

How to use: Standard infusion or up to 10 ml of tincture daily.

Combinations: Combines well with lemon balm and chamomile in infusions for an all-purpose relaxing tea.

Pulsatilla vulgaris—PASQUE FLOWER

AERIAL PARTS

Actions: Nervine and anodyne with sedative action; useful for nervous tension and sexual problems.

How to use: Up to 20 drops of tincture three times a day or use 5 g to 500 ml of water in infusions.

Combinations: Add Jamaican dogwood or passion flower tincture for additional calming action.

Precautions: Use only the dried plant as fresh is toxic.

Verbena officinalis—VERVAIN

AERIAL PARTS

Actions: Relaxing nervine with a tonic effect on the liver.

How to use: Use a standard infusion or tincture.

Combinations: Use as a simple of combine with wood betony, linden, chamomile or gotu kola to enhance sedative effect.

Precautions: Avoid high doses in pregnancy.

PANIC ATTACKS

Can be associated with excessive stress and also food intolerance. Severe cases may need psychiatric counselling.

KEY SYMPTOMS:

- Palpitations.
- Intense feeling of fear.
- Feelings of impending doom.

REMEDIES:

Rosa x damascena—DAMASK ROSE

ESSENTIAL OIL

Actions: Very soothing for the nerves, antidepressant and antiemetic; gentle sedative.

How to use: Add 5–10 drops of rose oil to 10 ml of carrier oil and use to massage temples or throat. Add 2–5 drops of essential oil to baths and use rosewater in lotions or cooking.

Combinations: Can combine with a few drops of sandalwood or lavender oils to enhance the calming effect.

Precautions: Do not take oils internally without professional advice. Rose oil is extremely expensive and synthetic substitutes are commonplace; buy only good quality genuine rose oil.

Citrus aurantium—NEROLI

ESSENTIAL OIL

Actions: Sedative and antidepressant, traditionally used for hysteria, panic and fearfulness. Eases palpitations and cardiac spasm.

How to use: Add 5–10 drops of rose oil to 10 ml of carrier oil and use to massage temples or throat. Add 5–10 drops of essential oil to baths and use orange flower water in lotions or cooking.

Combinations: Combine with 10 drops of lavender or benzoin oils to enhance calming action.

Precautions: Do not take oils internally without professional advice.

Piscidia erythrina—JAMAICAN DOGWOOD

BARK

Actions: Sedative and anodyne useful for severe nervous tension, insomnia, or nervous migraine.

How to use: Use up to 5 ml tincture daily or in decoction with other herbs (use 5 g of Jamaican dogwood and up to 15 g of others in 600 ml water).

Combinations: Add pasque flower, valerian or hop tinctures to give a combined total of up to 5 ml per dose for additional sedative action.

Precautions: Do not exceed stated doses.

Hyssopus officinalis—HYSSOP

AERIAL PARTS OR ESSENTIAL OIL

Actions: Antispasmodic and mildly analgesic, traditionally used for hysteria and some forms of epilepsy; it is also gentle enough for upsets in children.

How to use: Take an infusion or tincture; use 2–3 drops of essential oil in almond oil to massage temples and neck.

Combinations: Add skullcap, passionflower or wood betony to infusions to enhance sedating effect if desired.

Precautions: Do not take oils internally without professional advice.

DEPRESSION

Debility of the nervous system traditionally associated with a surfeit of the "melancholic" humor in Galenical medicine.

KEY SYMPTOMS:

- Poor digestive function with constipation.
- Misery, "feeling down."

- Inability to concentrate.
- Lack of interest in the present.
- Withdrawn, silent demeanour.

REMEDIES:

Ocimum basilicum—BASIL

LEAVES AND ESSENTIAL OIL

Action: Antidepressant and spiritually uplifting, especially effective for the lower *chakras* – useful to encourage earthing and groundedness.

How to use: Eat fresh leaves; use 5 drops of the oil in bath-water, or add to massage oils; take up to 3 ml of tincture per dose.

Combinations: Combine leaves with lemon balm or rose petals in infusion; add a few drops of geranium or rose oils to massage mix to increase uplifting effects.

Precautions: Do not take oils internally without professional advice; do not use the oil in pregnancy.

Avena sativa—OATS

STRAW AND SEEDS

Actions: Antidepressant and restorative nerve tonic.

How to use: Use 2–3 ml wild oat fluid extract or standard decoction; eat oatmeal as porridge.

Combinations: Combines well with vervain tincture or add 10 drops of lemon balm or St. John's wort tinctures per dose to enhance antidepressant action.

Precautions: If sensitive to gluten, see notes regarding decoction on p. 32.

Borago officinalis—BORAGE

LEAVES

Actions: Restorative for the adrenal cortex, eases depression.

How to use: Use 10 ml of juice three times daily.

Combinations: Use as a simple.

Precautions: Restricted herb in some geographies.

Turnera diffusa—DAMIANA

AERIAL PARTS

Actions: Stimulating nervine (especially good for the male hormonal system); antidepressant.

How to use: Use up to 2.5 ml of tincture. three times daily or 20 g to 500 ml water for infusions.

Combinations: Combine with oat tincture or fluid extract for general depression; add St. John's wort or wood betony tincture if anxiety is a problem to give a total combined dose of 5 ml.

INSOMNIA

Can be associated with over-excitement, anxiety and worries, or some physical cause (such as pain) that needs treating. In Chinese medicine can signify excessive "heart fire."

KEY SYMPTOMS:
- Inability to fall asleep.
- Frequent wakefulness during the night.
- Restlessness, vivid dreamy sleep.

REMEDIES:

Passiflora incarnates—PASSION FLOWER

LEAVES

Actions: Sedative, hypnotic and anodyne – calms the nervous system and promotes sleep.

How to use: Take 5 ml of tincture 30 minutes before retiring at night or drink an infusion with 2 teaspoons dried leaves per cup.

Combinations: Add lavender and chamomile to infusions if desired.

Precautions: Avoid high doses in pregnancy.

Lactuca virosa—WILD LETTUCE

LEAVES

Actions: Sedative – the latex was once known as "poor man's opium" – fresh herb is especially potent when it goes to seed (garden lettuce can have a similar but milder effect).

How to use: Drink a cup of a standard infusion or up to 5 ml of tincture 30 minutes before retiring at night

Combinations: Can be combined with additional calming herbs such as tinctures of passion flower, valerian or cowslip petals to give a total of 5 ml of the combined tinctures per dose.

Precautions: Large doses may cause confusion and stupor; may cause sudden sleepiness soon after ingestion so avoid if driving or using machinery.

Humulus lupulus—HOPS

STROBILES

Action: Sedative, hypnotic and anodyne – calms excess excitability.

How to use: Use up to 5 ml of tincture daily, or 10 g of dried herb with 500 ml water for infusions.

Combinations: Can be combined with additional calming herbs such as valerian or passionflower tinctures up to a maximum of 5 ml of the combined tinctures per dose.

Precautions: Hops rapidly oxidize and actions vary depending on the age of the herb.

Eschscholzia californica—CALIFORNIA POPPY

AERIAL PARTS

Actions: Gentle and non-addictive hypnotic, tranquilizer and anodyne. Safe for children.

How to use: Standard dose of infusion or tincture taken before retiring at night.

Combinations: Use as a simple of combine with passionflower or lavender; add cowslip petals if over-excitability is a problem.

INABILITY TO RELAX

Herbs have long been used to induce relaxation and, in traditional societies, trance-like states with altered levels of awareness: tobacco and cannabis are still used this way in the West.

KEY SYMPTOMS:

- Restlessness, cannot sit still.
- Irritability, poor attention span.
- Constant chatter.

REMEDIES:

Lavandula spp.—LAVENDER

FLOWERS & ESSENTIAL OIL

Actions: Sedative and analgesic with antispasmodic action.

How to use: Take a standard infusion, or up to 4 ml of tincture per dose. Massage diluted oil into temples.

Combinations: Use as a simple or combine with wood betony, linden flowers, or vervain in infusions to ease tensions and stress.

Precautions: Do not take lavender oil internally without professional guidance.

Chamaemelum nobile—ROMAN CHAMOMILE

FLOWERS & ESSENTIAL OIL

Actions: Sedative, carminative and antispasmodic. Good for excitement and nervous tummies.

How to use: Add 2–3 drops of essential oil or 500 ml of infusion to baths; drink chamomile tea regularly.

Combinations: Use as a simple or add lemon balm, skullcap or gotu kola to tinctures to relax and restore; combine with 2–3 drops of lavender oil in baths as an additional sedative.

Precautions: Do not take essential oils internally without professional guidance.

Centella asiatica—GOTU KOLA

AERIAL PARTS

Actions: Relaxing and restorative for the nervous system; good for neurotic disturbances.

How to use: Take a standard infusion or tincture.

Combinations: Use as a simple or mix with a little lavender or chamomile flowers in infusions to enhance calming action.

Precautions: Best taken for short periods (4–6 weeks) then give a two week break.

EMOTIONAL UPSETS

Temper tantrums, mood swings, irritability, grief – the emotional ups-and-downs of life are an everyday occurrence at all ages. Specific extracts (such as Bach Flower Remedies or Bush Essences) can often help.

KEY SYMPTOMS:
• Irrational tears or anger with no apparent cause.

REMEDIES:

Melissa officinalis—LEMON BALM

LEAVES

Actions: Antidepressant and restorative for the nervous system.

How to use: Drink an infusion of fresh herb as required or take up to 5 ml of tincture daily (it is more effective in low doses).

Combinations: Use as a simple or combine with wood betony, skullcap or vervain tinctures for sedative and restorative action.

Valeriana officinalis—VALERIAN

ROOT

Actions: Very potent tranquilizer, antispasmodic and mild anodyne.

How to use: Take a maceration or tincture, also available in 200 mg capsules or tablets.

Combinations: Use as a simple or add a small amount of hops if there is excitability. Support with massage using rose or lavender oils.

Precautions: Can lead to over-excitedness in some individuals; try a small dose first to check for reaction.

Artemisia vulgaris—MUGWORT

AERIAL PARTS

Actions: Gentle nervine; useful for menopausal tensions and for mild depressions and stress.

How to use: Take up to 2 ml (40 drops) of tincture tree times a day or drink a weak infusion.

Combinations: Combine with wood betony, skullcap, or vervain for menopausal tension with emotional

stress; combine tinctures up to a total of 5 ml per dose.

Precautions: Avoid in pregnancy and when breast-feeding.

COPING WITH STRESS

Stress is part of everyday life helping us to remain alert and active; it triggers production of adrenaline, the "flight or fight" hormone; failure to respond physically leads to a "negative stress response" with excess physical tension.

KEY SYMPTOMS:
• Dry mouth, easy tears; palpitations or panic attacks.
• Constant tiredness, difficulty sleeping or concentrating,
• Inability to relax, headaches, muscular aches and pains, stomach upsets.

REMEDIES:

Eleutherococcus senticosus—SIBERIAN GINSENG

ROOT

Actions: Helps the body to cope more efficiently with stress and improves stamina; useful as a preventative before exams, a busy time at work or long-haul air travel to combat jet lag.

How to use: Take up to 600 mg a day for 10–14 days before the stresses are due to peak. This can be a useful stress preventative before exams.

Combinations: Use as a simple of combine with reishi mushroom in capsules.

Matricaria chamomilla—GERMAN CHAMOMILE

FLOWERS

Actions: Calming and mildly sedative to encourage relaxation and also act as a tonic for the digestive system stress-related upsets.

How to use: Use in infusions.

Combinations: Combine with lemon balm or wood betony in infusions; add a few jasmine flowers to the mix if available.

EXHAUSTION & TIREDNESS

Often dismissed as a symptom but may be related to destructive emotions, over-work or chronic illness.

KEY SYMPTOMS:
- Difficulty getting out of bed each morning.
- Lacking the energy to complete tasks.
- Difficulty concentrating.

Important: Constant or excessive tiredness may be a sign of undiagnosed illness; seek professional help if symptoms have no apparent cause.

REMEDIES:

Panax ginseng—KOREAN GINSENG
ROOT
Actions: Energy tonic, traditionally used in China for older people and ideal to help the body adjust to changing seasons.

How to use: Best taken in periods of up to four weeks, 600 mg in capsules or tablets or up to 10 ml of tincture daily.

Combinations: Use as a simple or combine with *huang qi*, ginkgo or *ashwaghanda* and a little ginger or galangal.

Precautions: Avoid long-term or excessive use in pregnancy; may add to macho aggression in young very *yang* men.

Salvia officinalis Purpurescens Group or *Salvia officinalis*—PURPLE or GREEN SAGE
AERIAL PARTS
Actions: Restorative, hormonal and antioxidant; stimulates the nervous and digestive systems.

How to use: Take in infusion, tinctures or powdered in capsules (up to 1 g daily).

Combinations: Use with rosemary, gotu kola, wood betony, hibiscus or thyme in infusions.

Precautions: Avoid high doses in pregnancy and completely in epilepsy.

CHRONIC FATIGUE SYNDROME

Variously called post-viral syndrome or myalgic encephalomyelitis (ME), the problem has been variously linked to viral infection, immune weakness and psychological disturbances.

KEY SYMPTOMS:
- Muscle fatigue and weakness after even minor exercise.
- Headaches, muscular pains, breathing problems.
- Weariness and difficulty concentrating.

REMEDIES:

Astragalus membranaceous—HUANG QI
ROOT
Actions: Stimulating for both the immune system and energy levels; traditionally used in China for younger people who are often affected by ME.

How to use: Use in tinctures, decoction or powdered in capsules (up to 600 mg daily).

Combinations: With ginseng and echinacea; support with evening primrose oil, zinc, and vitamin C supplements and gotu kola, milk thistle, and cardamom in infusions.

Withania somnifera—ASHWAGHANDA
ROOT
Actions: A nutritive and rejuvenating tonic to act on both physical and mental energies.

How to use: In tinctures, decoctions or use 250 mg to 1 g of powder per dose in capsules or with a little water; take up to 5 g daily in warm milk sweetened with a little sugar.

Combinations: Add a little long pepper to enhance action; combine with ginseng and licorice in decoctions. Support with liver stimulants and 25 ml daily of cleavers juice to cleanse the lymphatic system. Eat plenty of shiitake mushrooms to help the immune system.

Echinacea spp.—Echinacea
ROOT OR LEAVES
Actions: Antiviral and antifungal to combat associated infection and possible candidiasis.

How to use: In tinctures or capsules (two 200 mg, three times daily); in decoction or infusion depending on part used.

Combinations: Combine with cleavers, milk thistle and galangal tinctures; use in infusions with gotu kola and in decoctions with *huang qi* or ginseng. Support with evening primrose, zinc and vitamin C supplements as before.

Precautions: High doses may rarely cause dizziness and nausea.

Seasonal Affective Disorder (SAD)

Depression and emotional problems associated with short daylight hours and dark winter days. Often helped by special artificial daylight lighting systems.

Key Symptoms:
- Clear seasonal association with depression.
- Insomnia, weariness, occasional sugar cravings.

Remedies:

Hypericum perforatum—ST. JOHN'S WORT
Aerial Parts
Actions: Proven anti-depressive increasingly used as an alternative to orthodox drugs.

How to use: In tinctures, teas or capsules.

Combinations: Use with wood betony, basil or lemon balm infusions or tinctures.

Precautions: Reports suggest long-term or excessive use may be associated with cataracts.

Rosmarinus officinalis—ROSEMARY
Aerial Parts or Essential Oil
Actions: Stimulating for the nervous system, antioxidant and tonifying for the digestion.

How to use: Take the fresh or dried leaves in infusions or tinctures; use 5–10 drops of oil in bath-water.

Combinations: Mix with basil, sage and thyme for a stimulating and uplifting tea; add with 2–3 drops of rose geranium oil to baths.

Shock

Emotional shock is associated with sudden fears; physical shock may follow traumatic accidents.

Key Symptoms:
- Cold sweat, palpitations, breathlessness, shivering, confusion.

Remedies:

Capsicum frutescens—CAYENNE
Fruit
Actions: Stimulates blood circulation and tissues throughout the body; warming, restorative and normalising.

How to use: Take up to 5 drops of tincture in a little water or directly to the tongue.

Combinations: Use the drops of tincture in a cup of sage or chamomile infusion. Drink plenty of fluids.

Alpinia spp.—GALANGAL
Root
Actions: Warming and stimulating; especially effective for calming palpitations, irregular heartbeat and feelings of panic.

How to use: Take up to 5 drops of tincture directly to the tongue; use in a decoction

Combinations: Use the drops of tincture in a cup of skullcap infusion; drink plenty of fluids.

Gynecological Problems

A holistic approach to health care is seldom more relevant than when coping with the commonplace disorders of a woman's reproductive cycle: premenstrual syndrome, menstrual pain, infertility, vaginal itching, painful intercourse, heavy menstrual bleeding, menopausal problems, and so on. Emotions and spiritual disharmonies can be even more significant than physical disorders, but the verdict of "no abnormalities detected" after a battery of invasive tests can simply result in repeat prescriptions for tranquilizers, hormone replacement therapy, or even recommendations for a hysterectomy.

Traditional Chinese medicine closely associates the female reproductive system with the liver. Important energy channels link the organs and the liver is considered to "store the blood" giving obvious links with monthly menstrual bleeding in this medical model. The Chinese also regard the liver as controlling the flow of *qi* or energy around the body. Common PMS symptoms can be explained in terms of liver disharmony: irritability – the liver is linked with the emotion of anger; abdominal bloating and menstrual pain – stagnation of qi in the lower abdomen; digestive upsets and sweet cravings – excess liver energy "invading the spleen" and causing deficiency and weakness; and so on. Treatment for PMS can often, therefore, center on herbs designed to stimulate and move liver energy – and this approach can also often clear up the sort of irritable bowel symptoms that many women find worsen during the premenstrual phase.

Modern Western herbal treatments, too, can adopt a multidimensional holistic approach: for example, hormone regulators like chaste-tree can be combined with uterine tonics such as motherwort or black cohosh to ease menstrual disorders.

In Chinese medicine, menopausal symptoms are explained in terms of a "run-down" in kidney energy. The kidney is considered to store the body's "vital essence" or *jing*. This can be considered the body's life force – a combination of creative and reproductive energies. The sort of symptoms we associate with the menopause are thus explained by the TCM practitioner, in terms of kidney energy deficiency. Chinese medicine associates the kidney with body fluids, the ears and hearing, and the lower back. Typical symptoms of weakening kidney energy can include night sweats, dizziness and tinnitus, back pain, and thirst. In the classic five element model, the kidney (water element) also controls the heart (fire element) so weak kidney energy leads to "flaring of heart fire" with hot flushes, insomnia, palpitations, etc. Chinese treatments for menopausal symptoms therefore generally focus on kidney tonics or calming heart herbs.

In Ayurveda, sexual energy is seen as an aspect of the creative an spiritual forces and should be respected as such. Ayurveda also sees the reproductive organs as linked to the *chakras* – the body's energy centers. The root *chakra*, for example, is closely linked with the uterus and is associated with our sense of belonging, or "groundedness," and women who are unhappy with their role in life may suffer from reproductive disorders as a physical aspect of this disharmony. A hysterectomy can also unsettle the root *chakra* leaving some women unable to concentrate, settle or relax. They seem to have a restless, rootless quality that can be very difficult to ease.

Case Studies

Premenstrual syndrome

Patient: Lucy, a 29-year-old marketing manager, suffering from increasingly severe premenstrual syndrome. Her work kept her on a permanent "high" and she found it difficult to relax and unwind. She also felt under pressure from her live-in boyfriend to fulfill a domestic role while her mother persisted in dropping hints about grandchildren.

History and presenting complaint: Lucy's symptoms included abdominal bloating, tender, swollen breasts, and mood swings with extremes of irritability, anger, and depression that were growing in severity. Symptoms lasted for at least 12 days before each period. Her periods were also irregular, painful, and becoming increasingly heavy.

Treatment: Regular relaxation was a priority forcing Lucy to completely unwind from the stresses of the day. Herbal medicine focused on clearing liver *qi* stagnation and included *chai hu, bai shao, dang gui, bai zhi, fu ling,* peppermint, ginger and licorice.

Outcome: Within six weeks Lucy's PMS was dramatically reduced with little fluid retention and much less irritability. Over the following two months her irregular menstrual cycle also returned to normal, menstrual cramps were significantly reduced, and the monthly bouts of breast tenderness gradually disappeared. She brought her boyfriend along for one consultation so that he could learn a little more of her *qi* problems and she also had a good "heart-to-heart" talk with her mother putting the grandchildren issue firmly into the background. Two years later Lucy came back for further herbal treatment – this time as a happily married expectant mother suffering from morning sickness and with her future part-time career plans already mapped out.

PREMENSTRUAL SYNDROME

Can be associated with hormonal imbalance or stagnant energy (*qi*) levels.

KEY SYMPTOMS:

- Irritability of anger.
- Depression and emotional upsets.
- Abdominal bloating.
- Breast swelling and tenderness.
- Food cravings (especially for sweets).
- Constipation and/or diarrhea.

REMEDIES:

Vitex agnus-castus—CHASTE-TREE

BERRIES

Actions: Acts on the pituitary gland to stimulate and normalize hormonal function.

How to use: Take 10 drops of tincture in water each morning in the second half of the cycle.

Combinations: Use as a simple, but can be combined with other PMS strategies, such as evening primrose oil & vitamin B supplements.

Precautions: High doses can cause a sensation of ants creeping over the skin (formication).

Alchemilla vulgaris—LADY'S MANTLE

LEAVES

Action: Regulates menstrual cycle with gentle hormonal action; astringent.

How to use: Up to 5 ml of tincture three times daily or standard infusion with other herbs.

Combinations: Add 10–20 drops of pasque flower, black cohosh, mugwort or *dang gui* to tinctures or add white deadnettle and wood betony to infusions.

Precautions: Avoid in pregnancy.

Paeonia lactiflora—BAI SHAO YAO

ROOT

Actions: Balances liver function and soothes liver energy (*qi*); nourishes blood and *yin*.

How to use: Best used in combinations of tinctures; for decoction use up to 40 g of mixed herbs in 500 ml water taken in three equal doses during the day.

Combinations: For decoction use 10 g *bai shao yao* with 5 g each of *bai zhu, dang gui, chai hu,* licorice, and *fu ling* with 1 g of fresh ginger. Add 5 g *chen pi* if there is breast tenderness.

Precautions: Avoid if symptoms include diarrhea.

Oenothera biennis—EVENING PRIMROSE

SEED OIL

Actions: Contains gamma-linolenic acid for prosta-glandin production; eases breast tenderness.

How to use: Take 250–500 mg in capsules daily.

Combinations: Use as a simple but can be combined with other PMS strategies such as vitamin B supplements and infusions of lady's mantle.

MENSTRUAL PAIN (DYSMENORRHOEA)

May be due to blood stagnation before bleeding starts or to uterine cramping once the flow begins.

KEY SYMPTOMS:

- Lower abdominal pain either before or at the start of a period.
- Pain spreading to thighs or legs.
- Abdominal bloating.
- Flow may be scanty with excess clots.

REMEDIES:

Pulsatilla vulgaris—PASQUE FLOWER

AERIAL PARTS

Actions: Nervine and anodyne good for all pains involving reproductive organs.

How to use: Take up to 20 drops of tincture three times a day for symptomatic relief or 5 g to 500 ml of water in infusions.

Combinations: Add 10–15 g of St. John's wort to infusions.

Precautions: Use only the dried plant as the fresh is irritant.

Viburnum prunifolium—BLACK HAW

ROOT BARK

Actions: Antispasmodic specific for uterine muscle. Symptomatic remedy for cramping pain.

How to use: Take 20 ml of tincture in water; repeat once or twice during the day if need be.

Combinations: Use as a simple or add 10–20 drops of Jamaican dogwood per dose.

Precautions: Use in the recommended dose for a maximum of two consecutive days.

Angelica polyphorma var. *sinensis*—DANG GUI

ROOT

Actions: Regulates menstrual function, nourishes the blood, liver *qi* stimulant.

How to use: Best used in combinations; decoction of 30 g in 500 ml water taken in three doses.

Combinations: Combine with 5–10 g of *chai hu*, mugwort, *bai shao yao*, or *chuan xiong* and 1 g of fresh ginger in a decoction. Available in many patent remedy forms in health food or Chinese herb shops.

Precautions: Avoid large doses during pregnancy.

Caulophyllum thalictroides—BLUE COHOSH

RHIZOME

Actions: Antispasmodic with steroidal component that stimulates the uterus; best for pain due to blood stagnation.

How to use: Use standard decoction or tinctures; best combined with other herbs.

Combinations: Add 10–20 drops of skullcap, motherwort, yarrow, false unicorn root, *mu dan pi*, or *chi shao yao* tinctures per dose.

Precautions: Avoid in early pregnancy.

HEAVY PERIODS (MENORRHAGIA)

Always seek professional advice for sudden or unusual changes in menstrual flow. Often the condition appears to have no pathological cause and herbs can help. Heavy periods can increase the risk of iron-deficient anemia.

KEY SYMPTOMS:

- Flooding.
- Excessive clots.
- Prolonged bleeding—more than seven days.
- Shortened menstrual cycles.

REMEDIES:

Calendula officinalis—POT MARIGOLD

FLOWER PETALS

Actions: Astringent with wide ranging menstrual action for regulating the cycle and other functions.

How to use: Standard infusion or tincture.

Combinations: Add up to 1 ml of shepherd's purse, lady's mantle, or American cranesbill tinctures per dose as additional astringents. Total dose of tincture should not exceed 5 ml.

Capsella bursa-pastoris—SHEPHERD'S PURSE

AERIAL PARTS

Actions: Astringent and anti-haemorrhagic herb specific for urogenital bleeding. Eases the root *chakra*.

How to use: Standard infusion or tincture.

Combinations: Add 5 drops of goldenseal tincture per dose or use with white deadnettle in infusions.

Artemisia vulgaris var. *indicus*—AI YE

AERIAL PARTS

Actions: Styptic and warming herb for the meridians; useful if bleeding is prolonged.

How to use: Use 15 g to 500 ml of water for infusions or up to 2.5 ml (50 drops) of tincture three times a day.

Combinations: Add shepherd's purse, self-heal, or *bhringaraj* to tincture or infusion; or combine infusion with a decoction of *dang gui*.

Precautions: Do not use in pregnancy without professional advice.

Lamium album—WHITE DEADNETTLE

FLOWERING TOPS

Actions: Astringent and antispasmodic; regulates uterine blood flow and acts on reproductive organs.

How to use: Standard infusion or tincture.

Combinations: Combine with American cranesbill or lady's mantle.

MENOPAUSAL SYNDROME

Associated with hormonal changes and, in Chinese medicine with kidney energy (*qi*) weakness.

KEY SYMPTOMS:

- Irregular menstruation.
- Hot flushes and night sweats.
- Mood swings and depression.
- Vaginal dryness (eyes may be dry also).
- Palpitations and/or hypertension.
- Forgetfulness.

REMEDIES:

Vitex agnus-castus—CHASTE-TREE

BERRIES

Actions: Acts on the pituitary gland to stimulate and normalize hormonal function.

How to use: 10 drops of tincture in water each morning; or use two 200 mg capsules.

Combinations: Use as a simple or combine in capsules with goldenseal powder to relieve hot flushes. Drink sage tea to relieve night sweats.

Precautions: High doses can cause a sensation of ants creeping over the skin.

Chamaelirium luteum—FALSE UNICORN ROOT

RHIZOME

Actions: Stimulates ovarian hormones and can be helpful for early menopause after hysterectomy or to "kick-start" the system after years of oral contraceptive pills.

How to use: Take 5–10 drops of tincture 4–6 times daily.

Combinations: Use as a simple or combine with 2 ml of lady's mantle, black cohosh, or wild yam tincture per dose. Ease any vaginal dryness with pot marigold cream with 1–2 drops of rose oil added.

Leonurus cardiaca—MOTHERWORT

LEAVES

Actions: Nervine heart tonic, and uterine stimulant. Good for palpitations and anxiety.

How to use: Take a standard infusion or tincture

Combinations: Combine with other sedating nervines like lavender or vervain or with sage and mugwort to ease night sweats.

Polygonum multiflorum—HE SHOU WU

TUBER

Actions: Kidney *qi* tonic and nourishes the blood. Useful for early menopause.

How to use: Best used in combinations in decoction (50 g of the combination to 750 ml water) or in tonic wines.

Combinations: Combine with *nu zhen zhi, gou qi zi, shu di huang* and cinnamon in decoction.

Precautions: Avoid if symptoms include diarrhea or if there is any liver disease. Do not use in pregnancy, when breastfeeding or if suffering from estrogen-sensitive cancers.

VAGINAL THRUSH

Often related to general systemic weakness allowing opportunist yeasts to proliferate in the vagina.

KEY SYMPTOMS:
- Milky discharge.
- Characteristic white plaques on inner surface of vagina.
- Itching.

REMEDIES:

Melaleuca alternifolia—TEA TREE

ESSENTIAL OIL

Actions: Effective antifungal that does not irritate the vaginal membranes.

How to use: Use in creams; dilute 5 ml in 25 ml of water and soak a little of the mixture into a tampon inserted for 4 hours; or 2 ml to 40 g cocoa butter for 12 pessaries.

Combinations: Use as a simple or instead of water dilute the oil with pot marigold infusion for use on a tampon or add 10 drops thyme oil to the pessary mix.

Calendula officinalis—POT MARIGOLD

FLOWER PETALS

Actions: Antifungal, astringent and healing.

How to use: Use the infusion as douche; marigold creams or the infused oil as a lotion.

Combinations: Add 5 drops of echinacea tincture to the douche or eat a garlic clove daily to combat underlying fungal infections.

VAGINAL ITCHING (PRURITUS VULVAE)

Irritation which may be associated with menopausal syndrome, psychological factors or infection.

KEY SYMPTOMS:
- Itching (without other symptoms of thrush).
- Dryness.
- Possibly pain on intercourse.

REMEDIES:

Rosa x *damascena*—DAMASK ROSE

ESSENTIAL OIL

Actions: Cooling, soothing, astringent and anti-inflammatory with an uplifting effect to drive away melancholy.

How to use: Use rosewater as a lotion or add 2 drops of rose oil to creams.

Combinations: Make a cream with 5 ml pasque flower tincture, 10 ml lady's mantle tincture and 15 ml rosewater to 70 g of emusifying ointment.

Precautions: Do not take essential oils internally without professional guidance. Rose oil is expensive and often adulterated; use only good quality genuine rose oil.

Verbena officinalis—VERVAIN

AERIAL PARTS

Actions: Gentle nervine stimulating for liver and uterus; antidepressant and energising.

How to use: Take a standard infusion or up to 5 ml of tincture three times day.

Combinations: Combine with lavender, oats or lady's mantle tinctures: useful for pruritis of nervous origin.

Precautions: Avoid in pregnancy.

HYSTERECTOMY

Post-operative help can be given with herbs to relieve symptoms of premature menopause or disordered root *chakra*.

KEY SYMPTOMS:
- Menopausal syndrome.
- Difficulty in concentrating, forgetfulness.
- Irritability, short-temper, constant feeling of excitability and movement.
- A lack of calm contentment.

REMEDIES:

Ligustrum lucidem—NU ZHEN ZI

BERRIES
Actions: Stimulates kidney energy and also alleviates symptoms of early menopause.

How to use: Take as a standard tincture or in combination with other herbs in decoctions.

Combinations: Add tonic herbs such as *wu wei zi* or *ling zhi* (reishi mushroom) to decoctions; add 1–2 ml of rose or wood betony tinctures for additional support.

Ocimum basilicum—BASIL

LEAVES AND ESSENTIAL OIL
Actions: Antidepressant; tonic for the root chakra; stimulates the adrenal cortex and kidney *yang.*

How to use: Eat 2–3 fresh leaves with salads; take a standard tincture or use dilute oil as a massage.

Combinations: Add 2 drops of rose oil to 20 drops basil oil in 10 ml of carrier oil for massage; add 10–20 drops of pasque flower to tincture per dose.

Precautions: Do not take essential oils internally unless under professional guidance.

Stachys officinalis—WOOD BETONY

AERIAL PARTS
Actions: Sedative, stimulant for cerebral circulation and root chakra; eases fears and worry.

How to use: Standard infusion or tincture.

Combinations: Add equal amounts of Lavender, vervain or basil to infusions or tinctures (no more than 30 g of the combination in infusions or 5 ml of tincture per dose); add 10–20 drops of chaste tree tincture to the morning dose.

PREGNANCY & CHILDBIRTH

For generations of women, herbal remedies were the only option when it came to easing the ills of pregnancy and the trials of childbirth. Although nowadays we are far more cautious about using herbs during pregnancy they still have an important role to play.

During pregnancy herbs can be safely used as an alternative to orthodox drugs, which may be harmful: butternut is a suitably gentle laxative in constipation, while nettle tea, watercress, or burdock can help if there is anemia, and powdered slippery elm or marshmallow root will ease heartburn. Women who suffer from regular bouts of cystitis can safely use buchu, couchgrass, cornsilk, or echinacea instead of antibiotics.

Morning sickness is often best treated with a variety of remedies: ginger for a few days, followed by chamomile or peppermint, black horehound, or fennel. When women feel sick much of the time, any regular remedy stands the risk of contributing to the general feelings of nausea – no matter how antiemetic it happens to be. A selection of tinctures in dropper bottles that can be used as the sufferer feels fit is often the best solution.

Herbal teas can also be helpful throughout labor – betony, raspberry leaf, or chamomile spiked with a rose petals and cinnamon are especially useful and pleasant to take. In the weeks before the birth herbs can also be used to prepare the uterus for its coming exertions with tonic herbs or dilute jasmine oil massaged into the abdomen in the last three weeks. After the birth, basil and motherwort tea can help clear the placenta and all new mothers should also take homoeopathic Arnica 6X tablets every 15–30 minutes for a few hours to help repair stressed tissues

Cross references
Anemia, p. 184; Constipation, p. 186; Cramp, p. 159; Indigestion, p. 189; Varicose Veins, p. 182.

CASE HISTORY

BLEEDING IN PREGNANCY

Patient: Julie, 32, happily married with two daughters, ages 2 and 4, and just embarking on her third pregnancy.

History and presenting complaint: Julie had suffered from continuous bleeding throughout her first two pregnancies and spent much of the nine months confined to bed at her mother's house. With two lively under-fives, she was worried that the third pregnancy would go the same way leading to severe disruption for the entire family. This time slight spotting started during the sixth week of her pregnancy. In traditional Chinese medicine many uterine bleeding disorders can be attributed to a weakness in the *chong* (vital) and *ren* (responsibility) acupuncture channels. The *ren* channel is regarded as being responsible to all the *yin* channels in the body and is also called the "conception vessel" as it starts in the uterus. The *chong* channel communicates with all the other channels and also starts in the uterus. These channels are closely linked with childbirth and any coldness and deficiency here can lead to bleeding during or after pregnancy.

Treatment: An herbal remedy containing *dang gui*, *shu di huang*, *ai ye*, *bai shao yao*, licorice, and *chuan xiong* was used to warm and nourish the deficient chong and ren channels.

Outcome: Within two weeks the uterine bleeding had stopped completely, and Julie continued with a normal pregnancy without the need for protracted bed rest and without further bleeding and produced a healthy third daughter at term.

PROBLEMS WITH INFERTILITY

While modern fertilization techniques can be very successful, they are often invasive and require dedication from both partners. Herbs can help improve general health and readiness for conception – but they are not a magic formula for success, nor can they solve the mechanical causes of infertility such blocked fallopian tubes. Professional herbal treatment can help if endometriosis, chronic cystitis, ovarian cysts or candidiasis are interfering with conception.

REMEDIES:

Chamaelirium luteum—FALSE UNICORN ROOT

RHIZOME
Actions: Potent uterine and hormone tonic, helpful for weaknesses in the female reproductive system

including inflammations affecting the Fallopian tubes.

How to use: Take a decoction, 1 teaspoon per cup simmered for 20 minutes or up to 5 ml of tincture per dose.

Combinations: Combine with black cohosh or add Siberian ginseng or valerian if stress is a factor.

Precautions: Excess may cause nausea and vomiting.

Angelica polyphorma var. *sinensis*—DANG GUI

ROOT

Actions: Nourishing tonic for the reproductive system; helps to strengthen and normalize the menstrual cycle.

How to use: Take in tincture, decoction or use 600 mg powdered root in capsules daily.

Combinations: Use as a simple; take 10 drops of chaste tree tincture daily to help regulate hormones if required.

Precautions: Do not take in pregnancy so limit treatment to the 10 days from the start of each period if actively trying to conceive.

Alchemilla xanthoclora—LADY'S MANTLE

AERIAL PARTS

Actions: Acts to regulate the menstrual cycle and normalize function.

How to use: Take in infusions or tinctures.

Combinations: Use with red clover flowers, stinging nettles, and marigold petals (2 teaspoons of the mix per cup) as a general tonic for the female reproductive system. Add a pinch of peppermint to improve the flavor if need be.

Precautions: Best used to tonify the system before attempting to conceive; should be avoided in pregnancy so limit treatment to the 10 days from the start of each period only if sexually active.

MORNING SICKNESS

Nausea and vomiting theoretically on rising in the morning but often lasting all day. Severe cases (*hyperemesis gravidarum*) may require hospital treatment because of the risk of liver disease and loss of body fluids.

KEY SYMPTOMS:

- Vomiting often on rising although may persist throughout the day.
- Symptoms generally confined to the first three months of pregnancy.

REMEDIES:

Zingiber officinale—GINGER

ROOT

Actions: Highly antiemetic and has been successfully used in hospital trials involving *hyperemesis gravidarum* patients.

How to use: Use up to 1 g of powdered herb in capsules per dose; or 10 drops of tincture as required.

Combinations: Best as a simple but alternate with lemon balm, fennel, basil, chamomile or peppermint as need be.

Precautions: Do not exceed stated dose; use with care in early pregnancy.

Matricaria chamomilla—GERMAN CHAMOMILE

FLOWERS

Actions: Reduces feelings of nausea and calms the stomach; suitably relaxing nervine in stressful situations.

How to use: Drink 1 cup of a standard infusion before rising or take 5–10 drops doses of tincture as required.

Combinations: Best as a simple – but can alternate with lemon balm, fennel, basil, ginger or peppermint as need be.

Precautions: Do not exceed stated dose.

AERIAL PARTS

Actions: Antiemetic and sedative also useful for nervous dyspepsia.

How to use: Use up to 2 ml of tincture up to three times daily or sip a weak infusion.

Combinations: Best as a simple – but can alternate with lemon balm, fennel, chamomile, basil, ginger, or peppermint as need be.

PREPARING FOR THE BIRTH

Herbs have long been used as "*partum praeparators*" to help the body prepare for childbirth and tonify the uterine muscles.

REMEDIES:

Rubus idaeus—RASPBERRY

LEAVES

Actions: Tonifies the uterus.

How to use: Drink one cup of standard infusion daily in the final eight weeks of pregnancy.

Combinations: As a simple during pregnancy; add rose petals and wood betony to the infusion during labor.

Mitchella repens—SQUAW VINE

AERIAL PARTS

Actions: Uterine tonic and stimulant; also astringent and restorative for the nervous system.

How to use: Drink one cup of a standard infusion or 10 ml tincture daily last eight weeks or pregnancy.

Combinations: As a simple of combine with raspberry leaves. Can also be used as a cream for sore nipples during breastfeeding.

DURING LABOR

Herbal support during labor generally depends on the help of a sympathetic midwife or doctor. During the first stage, before orthodox medicine takes over, herbal infusions can help to calm the nerves, stimulate the womb and encourage the establishment of regular contractions.

REMEDIES:

Stachys officinalis—WOOD BETONY

AERIAL PARTS

Actions: Stimulates the uterus to encourage contractions while its sedating effect helps to calm the mother.

How to use: Take regular sips of an infusion throughout the first stage of labor.

Combinations: Use with rose petals, motherwort, squaw vine, and raspberry leaves.

Precautions: Avoid during pregnancy except during labor.

Jasminium officinale—JASMINE

ESSENTIAL OIL & FLOWERS

Actions: Tonifying and stimulating for the uterus to encourage contractions and parturition; mildly anaesthetic and sedating to calm the mother.

How to use: Use 5 drops in 5 ml of almond oil as abdominal massage during labor. Use the flowers in an infusion to soak a hot compress to apply to the lower abdomen. Replace with another hot compress as it cools.

Combinations: Use with 5 drops of lavender essential oil or add 2 drops of clove or nutmeg oil; adding 1 drop of sage oil may also help but can overstimulate so use with care. Add marigold, mugwort, or wood betony to the compress infusion.

Precautions: Jasmine oil is expensive and often adulterated, only buy from reliable sources.

Caulophyllum thalictroides—BLUE COHOSH

RHIZOME

Actions: Oxytocic (encourages uterine contractions) to hasten labor and childbirth; stimulates the womb and helps combat any exhaustion.

How to use: Use up to 1 g of powder per dose stirred into warm milk or take drops of tincture diluted in a little water on the tongue.

Combinations: Use with black cohosh or mugwort in tinctures or use betony tea sweetened with a little honey instead of milk.

Cautions: Avoid in the first six months of pregnancy.

Rosa x *damascena*—DAMASK ROSE

ESSENTIAL OIL & PETALS

Actions: Calming for the nerves and spiritually up-lifting; stimulates and tonifies the uterus.

How to use: Use petals in infusions or to soak a compress; add 1 drop of oil to 5 ml of almond oil as an abdominal massage and use the oil in a diffuser to scent the birthing room.

Combinations: Use with motherwort and wood betony in infusions.

Precautions: Rose oil is expensive and often adulterated, buy only from reliable sources; do not use rose petals from garden hybrids.

PERINEAL TEARS

Perineal tears occur frequently in childbirth and can be painful and slow to heal. These herbs can also help perineal bruising and soreness.

KEY SYMPTOMS:
- Tears in the perineum during birth, which may require stitches.
- Pain on intercourse can be a lingering symptom.

REMEDIES:

Hypericum perforatum—ST. JOHN'S WORT

FLOWERING TIPS

Actions: Anti-inflammatory, healing, and astringent.

How to use: Use the infused oil or add a strong infusion to a hip bath.

Combinations: Add lavender and pot marigold essential oils to the infused oil or add the dried herbs to infusions for baths.

Ranunculus ficaria—PILEWORT

ROOT OR LEAVES

Actions: Very astringent.

How to use: Apply pilewort cream to affected areas.

Combinations: Combine the infusion with distilled witch-hazel in lotions.

Precautions: Do not take internally or use on open wounds.

Symphytum officinale—COMFREY

LEAVES OR ROOT

Actions: Healing—encourages cell growth and can help limit scar tissue.

How to use: Apply cream, infused oil or ointment to affected areas or use an infusion in hip baths.

Combinations: Add 2 ml of lavender essential oil to 10 ml of the infused comfrey oil base.

Precautions: Do not use on open wounds.

SORE NIPPLES

Sore nipples may be due to the baby's inability to latch on to the breast correctly. The whole areola (dark area around the nipple) needs to be sucked, not just the nipple. Yeast infections can also cause irritation.

KEY SYMPTOMS:
- Sore, cracked nipples.

REMEDIES:

Calendula officinalis—POT MARIGOLD

FLOWER PETALS

Actions: Antiseptic, anti-inflammatory, and soothing for dry skin and yeast infections.

How to use: Use cream on sore nipples, applying after every feeding.

Combinations: Use as a simple or combine with squaw vine as a cream.

Matricaria chamomilla—GERMAN
CHAMOMILE

ESSENTIAL OIL & FLOWERS

Actions: Anti-inflammatory and antimicrobial to combat possible infections and soreness.

How to use: Use one drop of oil in a little breast milk or wheatgerm oil to massage the nipple after feedings; use flowers in creams or a compress soaked in infusion; a used chamomile tea bag makes a suitable poultice.

Combinations: Use as a simple or combine with marigold in creams and compresses.

MASTITIS & ENGORGEMENT

Engorgement is most common in the first five days after the birth when the milk may be in excess of baby's needs. Mastitis (breast inflammation) is usually caused by bacterial infection through damaged nipples or a blockage in the milk duct.

KEY SYMPTOMS:
- Pain and inflammation.
- Lumpy tender breasts.

REMEDIES:

Brassica olearacea—CABBAGE

LEAF

Actions: Anti-inflammatory and healing; useful to relieve both engorgement and mastitis.

How to use: Place a slightly softened fresh leaf between breast and bra.

Combinations: Use as a simple. A poultice of fresh common plantain leaves is a good alternative to cabbage. An infusion of red clover, chamomile, and marigold flowers (1 teaspoon of the mix per cup) taken 3–4 times a day will also help.

Salvia officinalis Purpurescens Group or *Salvia officinalis*—PURPLE or GREEN SAGE

LEAVES

Actions: Hormonal and drying for body secretions helping to reduce milk flow.

How to use: Drink half a cup of sage infusion once or twice a day; at weaning increase to one cup three times daily to dry up milk completely.

Combinations: In engorgement, express surplus with a hand pump; using a warm compress soaked in lavender or chamomile infusion will help encourage milk flow.

Precautions: Do not take in excess if continuing breastfeeding.

INSUFFICIENT MILK

A poor milk supply can be related to inadequate nutrition, lack of rest, or stress – although some women are just naturally short of milk and find breast–feeding a problem in successive pregnancies. Large babies can also prove very demanding and it may be necessary to supplement feedings from an early stage.

REMEDIES:

Galega officinalis—GOAT'S RUE

AERIAL PARTS

Actions: Increases milk flow and encourages development of the breasts.

How to use: Use 15 g dried herb to 500 ml water as an infusion or take or up to 2 ml of tincture three times a day.

Combinations: Can combine with other galactagogues, such as fennel, dill, vervain, fenugreek, milk thistle, stinging nettles, and borage.

Precautions: Strong tasting herbs may flavor the breast milk.

Anethum graveolens—DILL

SEEDS

Actions: Stimulates milk flow and is carminative to help combat colic and wind in the baby as well.

How to use: Take three cups of infusion daily; vary the mix with additional herbs to avoid becoming bored with the flavor.

Combinations: Use with any of the herbs listed with goat's rue above. Add borage or vervain for mild depression. Take 10 drops of chaste-tree or saw palmetto tincture to stimulate hormones and tonify the mammary glands.

Precautions: Strong tasting herbs may flavor the breast milk.

INVOLUTION & AFTERPAINS

The uterus gradually contracts back to its pre-pregnancy shape following the birth, which may lead to uncomfortable afterpains in the first few days. Complete involution can take two months. The process is helped by breastfeeding, which releases the hormone oxytocin into the bloodstream to improve lactation, so afterpains are common at feeding times.

KEY SYMPTOMS:
- Cramping pains often at feeding times.

REMEDIES:

Viburnum prunifolium—BLACK HAW

ROOT BARK

Actions: Specific antispasmodic for the uterus helping to ease painful contractions; also sedative and calming for the nervous system.

How to use: Use in decoctions or tincture (up to 10 ml per dose).

Combinations: Use with wild yam in decoctions or add the tincture to raspberry leaf or squaw vine infusions with a pinch of grated ginger.

Actaea racemosa—BLACK COHOSH

ROOT AND RHIZOME

Actions: Antispasmodic and relaxing for the uterus; mild analgesic with an aspirin-like action.

How to use: Take 10 drops of tincture in a little water, as required up to 5 ml per day (100 drops) total.

Combinations: Use with blue cohosh; add to raspberry leaf or squaw vine infusions.

Precautions: Excess can cause nausea and vomiting.

Caulophyllum thalictoides—BLUE COHOSH

RHIZOME

Actions: Oxytocic (encourages uterine contractions) to stimulate the womb. Also helpful to speed labor and help combat exhaustion in childbirth.

How to use: Use drops of tincture diluted with a little water on the tongue as required, or up to 1 g of powder per dose stirred into warm milk.

Combinations: Use with black cohosh or mugwort in tinctures, or use wood betony tea sweetened with a little honey instead of milk.

Precautions: Avoid in the first six months of pregnancy.

MALE REPRODUCTIVE PROBLEMS

Men are often more reluctant than women to seek help for any health problems – and that can be doubly so when it comes to disorders involving the reproductive system. Prostate and testicular cancers often go undiagnosed because of this reluctance and regular health checks for both these disorders are essential: testicular cancer is common among younger men and all men over age 50 should get a regular prostate check.

The prostate gland contributes to the seminal fluid and opens into the ureter, just below the bladder. Its benign enlargement, so common in older men, is believed to be caused by the conversion of the male hormone testosterone into dihydrotestosterone. Saw palmetto, long used for prostate problems, is now known to prevent this conversion so can actually combat the likely underlying causes of enlargement.

Physical inactivity also sometimes seems a trigger for prostate problems especially in the newly-retired who may find it difficult to adjust to a non-work routine: creative energies and vigor seem to stagnate and decline as a result. The gland's growth restricts urine flow and leads to characteristic hesitancy and dribbling, while retention of urine can result in low grade urinary infection with lethargy and tiredness. This in turn contributes to the physical inactivity and may be associated with weight gain, sluggishness, and stagnation. Keeping active – both physically and mentally – is important to maintain energies and vigor.

In traditional Chinese medicine, reproductive energies (also associated with creativity) reside in the kidneys. This energy supply is limited and non-renewable. Ayurveda, too, makes the same connection between sexual and creative energies while both theories argue that this vital energy can be damaged by excessive sexual activity, or "marrying too early" as conservative Chinese texts tend to phrase it. Sexual exhaustion, they argue, leads to debility, fatigue, loss of libido, and impotence.

Modern Western society tends to place great emphasis on the importance of the male sex drive, which can be another reason why those suffering from related problems are reluctant to seek treatment. In our culture, impotence is more often associated with stress, nervous tension, and overwork, or occasionally physical problems needing surgery.

In contrast, Eastern medicine will advise sexual abstinence as a treatment for impotence using tonic herbs for the kidney to restore energies: *ashwagandha, shatavari, bala, shu di huang, shan yao,* and *jin yin zi* are among the many herbs used to treat male reproductive problems by strengthening kidney energies. The well-known aphrodisiac tonics of Ayurveda (pp. 239–240) are not only used to strengthen sexual energies, but are also a tool for refreshing creative and spiritual energies.

Cross references
See also: Urethritis, p. 198, Lumbago, p. 157.

CASE HISTORY

BENIGN PROSTATE ENLARGEMENT
Patient: George, 58, recently divorced and now with a younger partner, feeling very stressed at work and hoping to take early retirement.

History and complaint: George complained of a general lack of energy, tiredness, and prostate problems. Increased frequency of urination, especially at night, coupled with hesitancy had led to a prostate check with his doctor who had confirmed mild benign prostate enlargement and had suggested that surgery might be necessary, while offering antibiotics to combat any infection.

Treatment: George was given a tincture containing saw palmetto, Siberian ginseng, and hydrangea to combat the prostate enlargement and any urinary infection as well as relieve problems of stress. *Ashwagandha* tablets were given as a supplement with buchu and couchgrass tea used to combat infection.

Outcome: Within six weeks symptoms were significantly reduced. Medication has continued long-term reducing the dosage to a low maintenance level as symptoms diminished. Surgery has been averted.

IMPOTENCE/LOSS OF LIBIDO

Stress, over-work, alcohol, and excess caffeine can all contribute to low libido. In other cases the explanation may be physical; painful piles are a common cause.

KEY SYMPTOMS:
- Little interest in sexual activity.
- Difficulty achieving or sustaining an erection.
- Premature ejaculation.

Note: Professional help is often necessary in chronic cases.

REMEDIES:

Turnera diffusa var. *aphrodisiaca*—DAMIANA

AERIAL PARTS

Actions: Aphrodisiac and antidepressant; uplifting for the nervous system and stimulates sexual performance.

How to use: Use in infusions, tablets or tinctures.

Combinations: Add a clove to each cup of infusion or add saw palmetto, ashwagandha, or Korean ginseng to tinctures; traditionally combined in tablets with cola and saw palmetto. Take vervain tea if premature ejaculation is a problem.

Withania somnifera—ASHWAGANDHA (WINTER CHERRY)

ROOT

Actions: Stimulating aphrodisiac and rejuvenative tonic to benefit the whole system and enhance sexual performance.

How to use: Take in milk decoction or capsules, up to 1 g per dose or use powder in warm milk sweetened with a little sugar.

Combinations: With ginseng or saw palmetto; add a pinch of long pepper to decoctions. Massage before love making can also help – use 1 drop of rose oil and 5 drops of sandalwood in 5 ml of almond oil as body massage for both partners. Heat the same oils in a diffuser in the bedroom.

INFERTILITY

Recent studies suggest that junk food and contaminants in the form of pesticides or polluted water contribute to a low sperm count.

KEY SYMPTOMS:
- Problems with conception.
- Low sperm count.

Note: Sperm may be damaged by high temperatures; loose trousers rather than tight jeans can help to keep them cool.

Polygonum multiflorum—HE SHOU WU

ROOT

Actions: Kidney tonic to stimulate reproductive energies.

How to use: Use in decoctions, tinctures, tonic wine or capsules.

Combinations: Add one clove to each cup of decoction; use in tonic wine with ginseng or *ashwagandha*.

Precautions: Avoid in diarrhea associated with spleen weakness or phlegm or if there is any liver disease. Do not take for prolonged periods.

Centella asiatica—GOTU KOLA

AERIAL PARTS

Actions: Rejuvenating and stimulating tonic to increase energies.

How to use: In infusions, tinctures or capsules.

Combinations: With damiana in infusions; add skullcap, vervain, or chamomile if stress is contributing to the problem.

PROSTATE PROBLEMS

Prostatitis is an inflammation often associated with infection in the prostate gland; benign prostate enlargement is very common in men over 50.

KEY SYMPTOMS:
- Frequent urination, urgency at night.
- Pain in the crotch and lower back.
- Dribbling and difficulty with urination.
- Retention of urine may be acute.

Note: Any prostate enlargement requires professional evaluation to check for possible malignancy.

REMEDIES:

Serenoa serrulata—SAW PALMETTO

BERRIES

Actions: Diuretic and urinary antiseptic with specific hormonal action on the male reproductive system reducing benign prostate hypertrophy; reputed aphrodisiac.

How to use: Use 10 g of berries to 500 ml water for a decoction or take up to 2 ml of tincture three times a day.

Combinations: Use as simple or combine with hydrangea or horsetail to increase action on the prostate.

Lamium album—WHITE DEADNETTLE

FLOWERING TOPS

Action: Astringent and soothing with a specific action on the reproductive system reducing benign prostate hypertrophy.

How to use: Standard infusion or up to 15 ml of tincture daily.

Combinations: Use as a simple of with cornsilk hydrangea or, couchgrass as a healing diuretic and to enhance the action on the prostate. Useful as a tea after prostate surgery to speed recovery and reduce risk of infection.

Hydrangea arborescens—HYDRANGEA

ROOT AND RHIZOME

Actions: Diuretic and soothing, especially helpful in prostatitis or where prostate enlargement leads to urine retention and infection.

How to use: Use in decoction of tinctures.

Combinations: With bearberry, yarrow or buchu in prostatitis; with saw palmetto and pasque flower in benign prostate enlargement.

Urtica dioica—STINGING NETTLE

AERIAL PARTS & ROOT

Actions: Extracts from root and leaves have been shown in studies to combat prostate enlargement and reduce symptoms.

How to use: Use in infusion, decoctions, tinctures, or capsules.

Combinations: With white deadnettle, horsetail, or marshmallow leaf; take echinacea tablets if there is associated infection.

PROBLEMS OF THE ELDERLY

For those people who regard the body as a machine, the problems of old age are associated with mechanical decay – joints suffer from wear and tear leading to osteoarthritis; the digestive system rebels against a life-time of low fibre foods and laxatives, leading to constipation and diverticulitis; and mental acuity is blunted. In Chinese medicine, the problems of old age are more likely to be associated with a run-down in vital energy: declining kidney essence – a key factor in menopausal syndrome – can account for the incontinence, tinnitus and deafness that affect so many older people. Strengthening tonic herbs, such as *he shou wu, nu zhen zi*, or *bhringaraj*, can often help with these problems.

The Chinese also use *qi* (energy) weakness, to explain some of the constipation problems of the elderly—a specific herb for this is *huo ma ren*, the seeds of *Cannabis sativa* or marijuana. (In the West, these are generally supplied pre-boiled to prevent illicit cultivation.) Depending on precise symptoms these may be prescribed in combination with herbs like apricot seeds (*xing ren*), bitter orange, *bai shao yao*, rhubarb root, or *dang gui*. Herbal tonics can also counter symptoms of mental confusion: in China ginseng has always been popular among those wealthy enough to afford it, while in Ayurvedic medicine *chyavan prash* (see p. 225), a mixture of around 20 herbs, sometimes with silver or gold foil added, has played a similar role. Such *qi* tonics may not prevent dementia, but they can certainly improve energy levels and increase alertness.

Herbs can also help in distressing conditions like Parkinson's disease. Deadly nightshade, a highly toxic remedy unsuitable for home use, was the main treatment to reduce some of the symptoms of Parkinsonism until recently. As well as reducing salivation, this antispasmodic herb helps to control tremors and is the original source of atropine, which is still prescribed by conventional practitioners for the disease. The related plants henbane and thorn apple can also be effective but are not for home use. Some argue that the whole plants are considerably more effective for controlling Parkinsonism than synthetic atropine or other artificially derived drugs. Important: the metabolism of the elderly is often slow, and doses for old people may need to be lower than for adults in their prime.

CASE HISTORY

HARDENING OF THE ARTERIES AND CONFUSION

Patient: William was 88, bedridden and confused, requiring constant attention from his wife, then age 72, and home care attendants.

History and complaint: William's wife, an enthusiastic supporter of complementary medicine, sought treatment for her husband after doctors had diagnosed hardening of the cerebral arteries and suggested there was nothing to be done beyond terminal care.

Treatment: William was given a tincture containing ginkgo, wood betony, linden, *shi di huang*, and a little ginger. The normal adult dose was reduced by half to compensate for his age and frailty.

Outcome: William slowly improved a little, became more lucid, and started reading again; after four months he was able to leave his room and go downstairs for the first time in nearly two years. Medication was continued at a reduced dose and with the addition of various herbs, such as *dang shen*, *gotu kola*, and *ashwagandha*. William celebrated his ninetieth birthday with a happy family party and died peacefully in his sleep nearly six months later.

Cross references

See also: Arthritis, p. 155; Constipation, p. 186; Prostate Problems, p. 221; Tonic Herbs, pp. 238–252.

HARDENING OF THE ARTERIES (ATHEROSCLEROSIS)

Fatty deposits in the arteries lead to restricted blood supply and increase the risk of heart attacks and strokes; in the elderly, hardening of the cerebral arteries can also increase confusion and concentration problems.

KEY SYMPTOMS:

- Depending on arteries affected, there may be cold feet and hands, pallor, mental confusion, breathlessness, or heart disorders.
- Eye disorders, pain in the legs on walking (intermittent claudication).

REMEDIES:

Ginkgo biloba—GINKGO

LEAVES

Actions: Significantly improves and tonifies circulation, especially cerebral circulation; inhibits platelet activating factor which tends to make the blood thick and sticky.

How to use: Take in tablets, tinctures, or infusions of fresh leaves; numerous commercial extracts are available,

Combinations: Use with garlic in capsules or hawthorn and linden in teas and tinctures.

Viscum album—MISTLETOE

TWIGS

Actions: Strengthens capillary walls, reduces inflammation and encourages repair; also cardiac depressant slowing heart rate.

How to use: Take 10–20 drops of tincture three times a day.

Combinations: Combine with lesser periwinkle or ginkgo tinctures up to a 5 ml dose. Drink with buckwheat or linden infusion to help repair arteriole walls.

Precautions: Do not use the berries, which are toxic.

Vinca minor—LESSER PERIWINKLE

Actions: Contains vincamine, which improves cerebral blood flow in arteriosclerosis and can be helpful after a stroke. Tonic for the cerebral arterioles.

How to use: Standard infusion and tincture.

Combinations: Combine tincture with recommended mistletoe dose (see above) or use with linden and wood betony in infusions.

URINARY INCONTINENCE

Involuntary urination which may be associated with weakened pelvic floor muscles, obstruction to the bladder outflow or lack of kidney *qi*. Double incontinence is generally related to other chronic conditions and requires professional support.

KEY SYMPTOMS:
• Urgent and frequent urination.
• Bed-wetting.
• Lack of bladder control with leakage often following coughing or laughter.

REMEDIES:

Equisetum arvense—HORSETAIL

AERIAL PARTS
Action: Healing and tonifying for the urogenital system and urinary mucosa.

How to use: Take 10 ml of juice twice a day or decoct 2 g in 200 ml water for 2 hours or take in 10 ml doses up to three times daily.

Combinations: Use as a simple or add or with 2–5 ml of St. John's wort or 10–20 drops of sweet sumach tincture daily.

Astraglus membranaceous—HUANG QI

RHIZOME
Actions: Replenishes vital energy and helps to regulate water metabolism.

How to use: Take a decoction with other herbs, or 600 mg powdered herb in capsules or 2–3 ml of tincture daily.

Combinations: Combine with *dang gui, chuan xiong,* and *chi shao yao* in a decoction.

Precautions: Avoid herb if the condition involves excess heat or *yin* deficiency.

Cupressus sempervirens—CYPRESS

ESSENTIAL OIL
Action: Astringent and relaxing oil, good for all types of excess fluid production.

How to use: Add 50 drops to 25 ml of almond oil and massage a little into the lower abdomen twice a day.

Combinations: Use a simple or add 10–25 drops of niaouli to the diluted cypress oil and massage using the mixture.

Precautions: Do not take essential oils internally.

OSTEOPOROSIS

"Brittle bone" syndrome most commonly associated with calcium and other mineral loss in post-menopausal women leading to softening and weakening of bones. Regular exercise, limited alcohol intake, fish oil and calcium supplements are important preventatives.

KEY SYMPTOMS:
• Increased risk of fractures.
• Damage to the backbone leads to stooping and loss of height.
• Tendency often runs in families.

REMEDIES:

Angelica polyphorma var. *sinensis*—DANG GUI
ROOT
Actions: Nourishes blood and body tissues to stimulate the system and ensure healthy metabolism.

How to use: Take in decoction or tincture; use up to 600 mg daily in capsules or powder.

Combinations: Use with herbs like false unicorn root in decoctions to help stimulate hormones or with true unicorn root or sage in tinctures or powders for a similar hormonal effect.

Precautions: Avoid in pregnancy.

Urtica dioica—STINGING NETTLES

AERIAL PARTS

Actions: Important mineral source to provide essential nutrients and circulatory stimulant to help tissue nourishment.

How to use: Use in infusion or tincture.

Combinations: With sage in infusions or tinctures or add 10 ml of horsetail juice per dose to either tinctures or infusion.

FORGETFULNESS & CONFUSION

This is common in old age and can be helped by tonic herbs to strengthen kidney *qi*, *yin*, or *yang* energies as appropriate (see pp. 242–247).

REMEDIES:

Salvia officinalis Purpurescens group or *Salvia officinalis*—PURPLE or GREEN SAGE

LEAVES

Action: Traditionally held to improve the memory and longevity; tonifies *qi*.

How to use: Take a 1–2 cups of infusion or 10 ml of tincture daily.

Combinations: Use as a simple or combine with rosemary, thyme, or gotu kola.

Precautions: Contains thujone which can trigger epileptic fits in sufferers.

Centella asiatica—GOTU KOLA

AERIAL PARTS

Action: Used in Ayurvedic medicine to promote mental calm and clarity.

How to use: Take a cup of infusion or a tincture of 5–10 ml doses, 1–2 times daily.

Combinations: Take as a simple or combine with bhringaraj in infusion or tincture.

Emblica officinalis—AMALAKI

FRUIT

Action: Yin tonic widely used in Ayurveda for senility.

How to use: Eat fresh or dried (Indian gooseberry) or stewed fruit.

Combinations: Generally taken in *chyavan prash* (an herb jelly sold in Indian markets and restaurants) or with *ashwagandha* or *shatavari*.

ENDOCRINE & GLANDULAR PROBLEMS

The body has a large number of glands that produce important chemicals and secretions to ensure that the system runs smoothly. The "endocrine" or "ductless gland" system includes the pituitary, thyroid, parathyroid, and adrenal glands, ovaries, testes, placenta, and parts of the pancreas. These glands are responsible for producing a variety of hormones, which are then secreted into the bloodstream. Any dysfunction soon upsets body chemistry and can lead to a range of symptoms. Problems with endocrine glands can include various menstrual disorders associated with hormones produced by the pituitary glands and ovaries as well as obvious thyroid disorders and diabetes which is linked to the islets of Langerhans in the pancreas.

There are also "exocrine" or "duct" glands which produce secretions via a duct onto a surface of the body: this group includes the glands which secrete saliva or sweat and sometimes these too can cause health problems. The parotid glands, for example, are one of three pairs of glands which produce saliva and inflammation here leads for parotitis, common with mumps. Mumps can also affect the endocrine glands – notably the ovaries and testes. Problems affecting sweat glands are common in skin disorders: infection leading to boils while the sebaceous glands, which produce oils or sebum to lubricate the gland, can lead to sebaceous cysts filled with yellowish, cheesy sebum which can grow to considerable size and often need surgical removal.

In addition to these glands, we often speak of "lymph glands," which are part of the lymphatic system that transports various fluids around the body. This is really a misnomer as these are nodes or small swellings act as filters for the lymph, preventing foreign particles from entering the bloodstream and also producing lymphocytes, which are a type of white blood cell important in the immune system. These "glands" often swell when there is an infection and the lymphocytes battle with invading micro organisms. Glandular fever involves the lymphatic system, and the characteristic "swollen glands" are much enlarged lymph nodes.

Herbs are useful for problems affecting all these various "glands" – influencing body chemistry to normalize production of particular hormones and enzymes as well as combating infections and inflammations. Traditional medicine understood little of these hidden endocrine glands or the lymphatic system. Chinese and Ayurvedic treatment have no real concept of "hormones" or body chemistry, although there are many herbs used to treat "hard swellings" that would commonly have been associated with lymphatic problems and are often cleansing and antimicrobial remedies.

Cross references

See also: Tonsillitis, p. 174; Mumps, p. 234; Menstrual Irregularities, pp. 209–211; Boils, p. 164; Weak Immune System, p. 164.

CASE HISTORY

LATE-ONSET DIABETES

Patient: Henry, 72, a retired accountant, overweight and not inclined to exercise with a fondness for sweet foods and good wine. His wife was a long-time convert to herbalism although Henry had little enthusiasm for any type of medication.

History and presenting complaint: Henry had been feeling rather lethargic and out of sorts for some time when a routine blood test by his GP indicated late-onset diabetes. He had been given a diet sheet, ordered to lose weight, and was told to monitor urine sugar levels for one month after which time the GP would decide if medication was needed. After two weeks, the tests were regularly showing raised fasting glucose levels of up to 111 mmol/l.

Treatment: Henry was reluctant to take anything which looked like medicine so the emphasis was on herbs as food supplements. Two fenugreek capsules were prescribed after each meal with regular use of foods that both have a hypoglycemic effect and increase insulin production – garlic, onions coriander, barley, peas, cranberries, bilberries, cashew nuts, cinnamon, and cloves – all of which Henry fortunately liked. An herbal tea of goat's rue with the occasional addition of bilberry leaf and disguised with a little peppermint was also used.

Outcome: Within a few days Henry was regularly recording 5.5 or 14 mmol/l in his fasting urine tests and within two weeks the morning reading was consistently 0–5.5 mmol/l so that Henry's GP decided not to prescribe hypoglycemic drugs. As blood sugar levels have fallen the lethargy and confusion have also been eased and strict dietary control has kept Henry's weight to healthier levels. His condition has continued to be closely monitored at the local diabetic clinic and the daily urine tests have remained satisfactory.

LATE-ONSET DIABETES

Caused by lack of insulin leading to high levels of blood sugar. It is often associated with obesity and poor diet and is generally non-insulin dependent.

KEY SYMPTOMS:
- Excessive thirst and urination.
- Mental confusion.
- Weight loss.
- Lethargy.

REMEDIES:

Trigonella foenum-graecum—FENUGREEK

SEEDS

Action: Hypoglycemic; in trials it has reduced urine sugar levels by 50%.

How to use: Take up to 1 g powdered herb or in capsules after meals or make a decoction; can be used in cooking.

Combinations: Eat a high fiber diet with plenty of garlic; add powdered cloves or cinnamon to capsules if desired.

Precautions: Blood or urine sugar levels should be regularly monitored. Maintain dietary control.

Galega officinalis—GOAT'S RUE

AERIAL PARTS

Actions: Enlarges the islets of Langerhans in the pancreas which are responsible for insulin production.

How to use: Take an infusion or tincture before meals.

Combinations: Use as a simple or combine with stinging nettles or bilberry leaf; add 2–4 ml sweet sumach tincture per dose. Eat a high fiber diet with plenty of garlic.

Precautions: Blood or urine sugar levels should be regularly monitored. Maintain dietary control.

Vaccinium myrtillus—BILBERRY

LEAVES

Actions: Hypoglycemic; increases insulin production.

How to use: Drink an infusion before meals.

Combinations: Add goat's rue or stinging nettles to infusions. Eat a high fibre diet with plenty of garlic.

Precautions: Leaves contain hydro-quinone and should not be used continuously. Blood or urine sugar levels should be regularly monitored. Maintain dietary control.

THYROID PROBLEMS

Over-activity of the thyroid gland leads to thyrotoxicosis and the body; under-activity causes myxedema.

KEY SYMPTOMS:
- Constipation, weight gain, apathy and general lethargy in myxedema.
- Weight loss, diarrhea, sweating, and hyperactivity in thyrotoxicosis.

Note: Thyroid problems should always be referred to a health care professional.

REMEDIES:

Fucus vesiculosis—BLADDERWRACK

THALLUS

Actions: A good source of iodine which is essential for normal function of the thyroid gland; metabolic stimulant to combat sluggishness in myxedema.

How to use: Take in tablets or capsules, up to 2 g daily; use in tinctures or infusions.

Combinations: Use with parsley, damiana and oats in tinctures and infusions; add ginseng or ginkgo to powders and capsules. Add vervain or St. John's wort if depression is a problem in myxedema.

Precautions: Avoid in overactive thyroid.

Lycopus virginicus—BUGLEWEED

AERIAL PARTS

Actions: Largely used to relieve the symptoms of an overactive thyroid – especially rapid heartbeat and palpitations. It can be helpful for low blood sugar levels.

How to use: Use in infusions and tinctures

Combinations: With motherwort, parsley and lemon balm in infusions to calm the system and reduce palpitations and other symptoms.

Precautions: Avoid in pregnancy and under-active thyroid.

Leonurus cardiaca—MOTHERWORT

AERIAL PARTS

Actions: Calming and normalising or the heart in overactive thyroid problems.

How to use: Use in infusions and tinctures.

Combinations: Use with half as much pasque flower and blue flag in tinctures or with an equal amount of lemon balm in infusions.

GLANDULAR FEVER

Thought to be caused by the Epstein-Barr virus, glandular fever (infectious mononucleosis) is common in young adults. It has a long incubation period and symptoms may persist for several weeks leaving sufferers feeling drained and debilitated.

KEY SYMPTOMS:

* Enlarged and tender lymph nodes in neck, armpits and groin.
* Loss of appetite and general lethargy.
* Headache, fever, sore throat.

Note: Herbal remedies should be used to support any orthodox treatment; always consult you health care professional in cases of glandular fever.

Galium aparine—CLEAVERS

AERIAL PARTS

Actions: Especially cleansing for the entire lymphatic system.

How to use: Best taken as juiced fresh herb, process enough fresh cleavers in a food-mixer to make 2 tablespoons juice when strained; alternatively use tinctures, infusion, or *capsules.*

Combinations: Add the fresh juice to a cup of echinacea and blue flag decoction with a pinch of pow-

dered dried cayenne and the juice of half a lemon, take every 3–4 hours. Take garlic supplements to combat possible infections and drink additional red clover and marigold infusions.

Inula helenium—ELECAMPANE

ROOT

Actions: Tonic and restorative, antimicrobial and expectorant to help clear any associated infections.

How to use: Use as a restorative to combat any lingering debility in decoctions, tincture, or syrup.

Combinations: With wood betony infusion; add a couple of drops of wormwood or calumba tincture per cup to stimulate appetite. Take up to 600 mg Korean ginseng for up to 1 month after lymphatic swellings subside.

HYPOGLYCEMIA (LOW BLOOD SUGAR)

Low blood sugar is caused by insulin overproduction often associated with erratic eating habits or over-consumption of refined sugars.

KEY SYMPTOMS:

* Hunger, dizziness, headaches, fatigue, irritability.
* Memory lapses, visual disturbances, panic attacks, and twitching limbs in more severe cases.
* Symptoms usually eased by eating sweet foods.

REMEDIES:

Artemisia absinthum—WORMWOOD

AERIAL PARTS

Actions: Bitter digestive tonic to stimulate digestive enzymes and normalize glucose metabolism.

How to use: Take 2–3 drops of tincture directly to the tongue at the first sign of symptoms.

Combinations: Add the wormwood tincture to a cup of chamomile, white horehound, or wood betony if preferred; drink these same herbal infusions instead of caffeine drinks and chew licorice root instead of eating sugar-based sweets.

Precautions: Avoid in pregnancy, breastfeeding and epilepsy.

CHILDREN'S COMPLAINTS

GENTLE HERBS can be ideal for many children's ailments: soothing and relaxing remedies like chamomile or linden flowers can ease over-excitement and encourage sleep. In fevers, cooling herbs such as elderflower, yarrow, or catmint can be freely given while purple coneflower is an ideal antibiotic. For coughs try hyssop, licorice, or white horehound in syrups, while for persistent catarrh try replacing milk products with soya-based preparations and using herbs like ground ivy and eyebright in capsules or as tincture. Soya is a good source of calcium so eliminating dairy products from a child's diet is unlikely to cause any deficiencies. Hyperactivity can also be related to food allergy: avoid colorants (E102 and E110 in particular). Constipation in children needs gentle aperients rather than stimulating laxatives – try psyllium seeds disguised in breakfast cereal or butternut rather than rhubarb root or senna. Unfortunately, many herbs do taste quite unpleasant and persuading small children to swallow them can be a problem. Babies may be persuaded to take weak soothing chamomile or linden flowers infusions from a bottle while breastfeeding mothers can take the remedy which is then passed into milk, especially useful with colic remedies like dill or fennel. Toddlers will generally accept powders or tinctures mixed with half a teaspoon of honey while capsules are ideal as soon as the child is old enough to swallow them. Dilute tinctures given in drop doses on the tongue can be acceptable or flavor with peppermint, licorice or raspberry vinegar as appropriate. Reduced alcohol tinctures can also be useful for long-term use in young children (see p. 148).

Children's Doses

Children's doses need to be reduced depending on age or size. All doses given in the tables in this section are full adult doses, unless otherwise specified, so need to be reduced depending on the child. The following proportions are for average children – adapt as need be for those that are above or below average sizes.

Age	Dose
0–1 year	5% of adult dose
1–2 years	10% of adult dose
3–4 years	20% of adult dose
5–6 years	30% of adult dose
7–8 years	40% of adult dose
9–10 years	50% of adult dose
11–12 years	60% of adult dose
13–14 years	80% of adult dose
15-plus	100% of adult dose

DIAPER RASH

The painful raw area around the anus and buttocks of diaper rash may be due to irritant stools or wet diapers. It can be related to yeast infections, especially if the mother is breastfeeding while on antibiotics.

KEY SYMPTOMS:
- Sore, red, painful inflammation around the anus and buttocks in diaper rash.

REMEDIES:

Calendula officinalis—POT MARIGOLD

FLOWER PETALS

Actions: Anti-inflammatory, antimicrobial, soothing, and astringent to encourage healing and combat possible infections.

How to use: Use the infused oil as a lotion for the affected area after each diaper change.

Combinations: Add 1–2 drops of tea tree or thyme oil to 10 ml of infused oil if there is any infection.

Plantago major—PLANTAIN

LEAVES

Action: Locally healing and soothing.

How to use: Apply ointment or infused oil frequently as required; put fresh, crushed washed leaves in the diaper at each change.

Combinations: Add 1–2 drops of tea tree oil to infused oil if fungal infection develops.

Symphytum officinale—COMFREY

LEAVES OR ROOT

Actions: Encourages cell growth of connective tissues; demulcent and soothing.

How to use: Apply ointment or infused oil frequently as required; use a paste of powdered root as a poultice on affected areas.

Combinations: Use arrowroot powder instead of baby talc when changing the diaper.

Precautions: Can cause rapid healing so ensure affected area is clean.

CRADLE CAP

Cradle cap is a scaly dermatitis affecting the scalp often due to overactive sweat glands it is not serious or contagious.

KEY SYMPTOMS:

- Scaly crust over the scalp in cradle cap.

REMEDIES:

Viola tricolor—HEARTSEASE

AERIAL PARTS

Actions: Soothing anti-inflammatory useful for a wide range of skin disorders.

How to use: Use standard infusion as a wash to bathe affected areas; alternatively apply cream. (Soften hard crusts with vegetable left on the scalp overnight if need be.)

Combinations: Add lemon balm or ground ivy to the wash or cream.

Arctium lappa—BURDOCK

ROOT

Actions: Cleansing and tonifying for the sweat and oil glands of the scalp in cradle cap.

How to use: Use 5 drops of tincture in a bottle of warm water for small babies under 10 kg; 10 add drops for larger ones (over 10 kg).

Combinations: Can combine with heartsease.

COLIC

Colic is caused by spasmodic contractions of the intestines associated with gas and tension. It often follows rushed or tense feeding times.

KEY SYMPTOMS:

- Pain – causing small babies to scream loudly.
- Abdomen may feel tense and bloated.
- Wind and flatulence.

REMEDIES:

Foeniculum vulgare—FENNEL

SEEDS

Action: Carminative and reduces griping pains.

How to use: Give babies 5–10 drops of tincture in a bottle of water or add to feedings. Breastfeeding mothers should drink a cup of standard infusion before feedings.

Combinations: Dill can be used in the same way as an alternative.

Matricaria chamomilla—GERMAN
CHAMOMILE

FLOWERS & ROOT

Action: Sedative, carminative and antispasmodic.
Good for excitement and nervous tummies.

How to use: Use homoeopathic Chamomilla 3X
(made from the root) – for babies 5–10 drops up to
three times daily or 1–5 crushed pillules.

Combinations: Use as a simple; breastfeeding mothers
can drink chamomile tea (made from the flowers) to relax them and, if breastfeeding, also soothe
baby's colic.

Nepeta cataria—CATMINT

AERIAL PARTS

Action: Carminative, antispasmodic, and can
encourage sleep in restless babies.

How to use: Add 5–10 drops of tincture to a bottle
of warm water or a feeding; or give a weak infusion
(20% of a standard brew) by bottle.

Combinations: Use as a simple.

TEETHING

Teething pains can affect babies from the age of 4 or
5 months.

Chamaemelum nobile—ROMAN CHAMOMILE

ESSENTIAL OIL & ROOT

Action: Sedative, carminative and antispasmodic.

How to use: Use homoeopathic Chamomilla 3X
(made from the roots) – for babies 5–10 drops up
to three times daily or 1–5 crushed pillules or put 1
drop of essential oil of Roman chamomile on a wet
swab and apply to the gum.

Combinations: Use as a simple or add 1 drop of clove
oil to the swab. Give a weak linden infusion by
bottle.

Precautions: Do not exceed the stated dose of essential oil.

GASTRIC UPSETS

Bilious attacks in children can be a type of migraine
so persistent problems could be related to food
intolerance. Diarrhea can be due to similar factors as
in adults (see p. 187).

KEY SYMPTOMS:

- Sudden diarrhea and vomiting.
- Complaints of "tummy ache."

REMEDIES:

Agrimonia eupatoria—AGRIMONY

AERIAL PARTS

Actions: Astringent and healing for gastric mucosa;
stimulates bile flow, helpful in food allergies; ideal
for childhood diarrhea.

How to use: Standard infusions and tincture (see dosage chart). Breastfeeding mothers should also drink
an infusion to deliver the remedy in her breast milk.

Combinations: Can combine with chamomile, catmint or lemon balm for nervous tummies; marshmallow for inflammations.

Precautions: Avoid in constipation.

Geranium maculatum—AMERICAN
CRANESBILL

LEAF OR ROOT

Actions: Astringent and tonifying for diarrhea and
gastritis.

How to use: Standard infusions and tincture (see dosage chart).

Combinations: Can combine with agrimony, meadowsweet, marshmallow or chamomile to enhance
the action.

SLEEPLESSNESS

Sleepless babies increase tension in the entire
household. Check the room temperature and if the
problem is associated with insecurity, use a lot of
love.

Chamaemelum nobile—ROMAN CHAMOMILE

ESSENTIAL OIL & FLOWERS

Actions: Sedative, carminative, and antispasmodic. Ideal for over-excitement.

How to use: Add 100–500 ml of standard infusion or 2–3 drops of essential oil to bath-water.

Combinations: Use as a simple; breastfeeding mothers can drink chamomile tea to relax both them and their babies.

Precautions: Do not exceed stated dose of essential oil.

Eschscholzia Californica—CALIFORNIA POPPY

AERIAL PARTS

Actions: Sedative, mild hypnotic, and antispasmodic: good for over-excitement.

How to use: Use standard infusion or tincture (see dosage chart) about 30 minutes before bedtime.

Combinations: Add a little honey to make it more palatable for children; can add chamomile or a little skullcap to increase soothing and sedating action.

THREADWORMS

Parasitic worms are common in children and can be due to poor hygiene. Cases are generally mild but the eggs can survive for two weeks so treatment needs to be continued for several weeks.

KEY SYMPTOMS:
- Anal itching caused by eggs.
- Worms may be visible in stools or anus.

REMEDIES:

Brassica olearacea—CABBAGE

LEAVES

Actions: Traditional remedy for intestinal worms; antibacterial and healing.

How to use: Give a glass of cabbage juice each morning for 3 days. Repeat for the next two weeks.

Combinations: Can combine with carrot juice. An alternative traditional cure is to feed the child nothing but grated carrot for two days.

Allium ursinum—RAMSOMS (WILD GARLIC)

AERIAL PARTS & BULB

Actions: Similar to garlic – potent antiseptic.

How to use: Drink a standard infusion (see dosage chart) of the whole herb or 10 ml of juice once a day for three days. Use the infusion as an enema once a week. Repeat for the next two weeks.

Combinations: As a simple or use garlic instead for older children.

NITS & HEAD LICE

Nits are static and are the eggs of head lice; they are generally found at the back of the head and nape of the neck. Lice move and are more visible.

KEY SYMPTOMS:
- Lice easily in the hair and nits seen on examination.
- Itching scalp.

REMEDIES:

Melaleuca alternifolia—TEA TREE

ESSENTIAL OIL

Actions: Effective antiseptic – also antibacterial and antifungal.

How to use: Put a few drops of oil on a fine comb and comb the hair thoroughly; add 5–10 drops to shampoo or hair rinse daily.

Combinations: Use as a simple, repeat daily until the infestation clears; can be combined with well diluted lemon oil (no more than 5 drops in 25 ml of carrier oil as it can irritate).

Azadirachta indica—NEEM

BARK

Actions: Antimicrobial and antiparasitic; a strong and effective herbal insecticide.

How to use: Use a strong decoction as a final rinse after washing hair or infuse the bark in a bottle of soap-based shampoo for two weeks and use that to wash hair.

Combinations: Use as a simple or combine the decoction with an equal amount of almond oil and use to massage the scalp at night.

Precautions: Use with caution on very young children.

HYPERACTIVITY

Excessive overactivity in children can be related to food intolerance or over-exuberant liver *qi* and liver fire.

KEY SYMPTOMS:

- Excessive and abnormal activity.
- Problems concentrating, clumsiness, frustration.
- Abnormally frequent temper tantrums.
- Sleeping problems, constant thirst.

REMEDIES:

Prunella vulgaris—XIA KU CAO

FLOWER SPIKES

Actions: Used in Chinese medicine for calming liver fire associated with over-excitability.

How to use: Standard infusion or tincture (see dosage chart).

Combinations: Combine with calming nervines such as chamomile, passion flower, St. John's wort, or wood betony. Add a small amount of vervain or *bai shao yao* to soothe the liver.

Thymus vulgaris—THYME

ESSENTIAL OIL & AERIAL PARTS

Actions: Recent studies have suggested that inability to concentrate may be associated with lipid imbalance and trials using evening primrose and fish oils with thyme oil have had significant results.

How to use: Use in prepared capsules or add 5 drops of thyme oil to 10 ml of evening primrose oil as a

massage for lower back or abdomen. Use the dried herbs in infusions or syrups.

Combinations: Use borage seed oil instead of evening primrose internally; combine the dried herb with *xia ku cao* and vervain; add agrimony for food allergies.

Precautions: Only use thyme oil internally under professional supervision or in licensed remedies.

BEDWETTING

Can be a congenital disorder or due to insecurity, emotional upsets or urinary tract infections.

KEY SYMPTOMS:

- Persistent urination in bed by children over 3 years of age.
- Check for problems with a tight foreskin in boys.

REMEDIES:

Rhus aromatic—SWEET SUMACH

ROOT BARK

Actions: Astringent and tonic for the urinary system; traditionally used for bedwetting in childhood although scientific evidence for efficacy is scant.

How to use: Give 10–15 drops of standard tincture up to three times daily (see dosage chart).

Combinations: Can combine with cornsilk or horsetail if urinary infection is suspected; combine with St. John's wort or wood betony for related nervous problems.

Arctostaphylos uva-ursi—BEARBERRY

LEAVES

Actions: Astringent and urinary antiseptic to soothe and combat and irritation and infections.

How to use: In infusions, tinctures or capsules for older children who can swallow them (see dosage chart).

Combinations: Use with American cranesbill, cornsilk and passion flower or skullcap in infusions; add valerian to tinctures.

TRAVEL SICKNESS

Nausea and vomiting related to motion, as in car journeys and sea sickness, is common in childhood.

REMEDIES:

Zingiber officinale—GINGER

ROOT

Actions: Antiemetic and carminative.

How to use: Use 1–2 200 mg capsules before travelling.

Combinations: Best as a simple; ginger sweets and cookies can be useful for younger children or give crystallised ginger to chew during the journey.

Mentha x piperita—PEPPERMINT

AERIAL PARTS & ESSENTIAL OIL

Actions: Antiemetic and antispasmodic.

How to use: Use drop doses of diluted tincture while travelling.

Combinations: Older children can be given peppermint sweets.

Precautions: Do not use peppermint oil with babies or toddlers.

MUMPS

Mumps is a viral disease that usually in children the salivary glands. In adults the infection may also involve the testes or ovaries and can lead to infertility. The pancreas can also be involved.

KEY SYMPTOMS:
- Difficulty swallowing.
- Enlarged salivary glands can easily be felt in the throat.
- Mild fever, irritability.

Note: In children, the condition is usually mild but adult sufferers should always seek professional help. A notifiable disease in some countries.

REMEDIES:

Salvia officinalis Purpurescens Group or *Salvia officinalis*—PURPLE or GREEN SAGE

AERIAL PARTS

Actions: Antiseptic and astringent to soothe throat discomfort.

How to use: Use the infusion as a gargle repeating every 30–60 minutes if possible while symptoms are severe.

Combinations: Use with thyme or rosemary in gargles, add a pinch of powdered cayenne to each dose; take with chamomile, lemon balm and betony in soothing infusions.

Calendula officinalis—POT MARIGOLD

FLOWER PETALS

Actions: Astringent, anti-inflammatory and antiseptic to combat infection and irritation.

How to use: In infusions (see dosage chart).

Combinations: Use with lemon balm, echinacea leaves, and yarrow in infusions: add 10 drops of poke root tincture or 10 ml of cleavers juice to each dose. Older children can take additional echinacea in tablets or capsules.

MEASLES (PAROTITIS)

A highly contagious viral disease with an incubation period of 1–2 weeks, often occurs in spring and autumn.

KEY SYMPTOMS:
- Typical symptoms of a heavy cold with harsh dry cough and nasal congestion.
- A blotchy, orange-red rash usually starts behind the ears and extends to the whole body.
- Blood-shot, light-sensitive eyes often followed by blepharitis.

Note: A notifiable disease in many countries, it usually occurs in local epidemics. Complications include pneumonia and middle-ear infections; seek professional help.

REMEDIES:

Echinacea spp.—ECHINACEA

ROOT

Action: Important antibacterial and antiviral, also strengthens resistance to infections; for all septic or infectious conditions.

How to use: Give two 200–250 mg capsules of powdered root three times a day or use 10 ml tinctures (see dosage chart).

Combinations: Effective as a simple or add elderflower, yarrow, or catmint tinctures in feverish conditions. Add 2–5 drops of fresh ginger tincture if nausea is a problem.

Precautions: High doses may occasionally cause nausea and vomiting.

Hyssopus officinalis—HYSSOP

AERIAL PARTS

Action: Relaxing expectorant particularly suitable for children's coughs and respiratory infections.

How to use: Give up to 10 ml of tincture daily or a standard infusion (see dosage chart).

Combinations: Use with marshmallow leaf or ribwort plantain or add white horehound to soothe the mucous membranes in dry irritable coughs.

Euphrasia officinalis—EYEBRIGHT

AERIAL PARTS

Actions: Antiseptic and anti-inflammatory to soothe inflamed eyes and eyelids.

How to use: Use a well-strained infusion of eyebright (1 teaspoon to 1 cup of boiling water, allow it to cool) in eye baths to soothe irritation.

Combinations: Use with pot marigold or self-heal in eye baths; sponge feverish children with a marigold or basil infusion as well.

CHICKEN POX (VARICELLA)

In children, chicken pox is usually a mild, if highly contagious, infection.

KEY SYMPTOMS:

- Rashes that soon turn into white spots, which then blister and form irritating scabs.
- Mild fever, spore throat, nasal congestion.

Note: Scratching or damaging the scabs can lead to scars. In adults the same virus produces shingles, affecting specific nerves, which can be severe and lead to lingering nerve pain.

REMEDIES:

Lonicera japonica—JIN YIN HUA

FLOWER BUDS

Actions: Cooling for feverish conditions, antibacterial, and anti-inflammatory.

How to use: Give a standard infusion or tincture (see dosage chart).

Combinations: Add elderflower, peppermint/catmint (depending on age) or a little *lian qiao* to infusions or tinctures.

Scutellaria lateriflora—SKULLCAP

AERIAL PARTS

Actions: Sedating and calming for children irritated by fever and itching scabs.

How to use: In infusions (see dosage chart).

Combinations: Use with chamomile, yarrow, lemon balm, elderflower, or boneset to combat feverish symptoms and catarrh. Give additional echinacea capsules or drops of tincture.

Hamamelis virginianum—WITCH HAZEL

BARK

Actions: Astringent and cooling to soothe irritation.

How to use: Use the diluted tincture or a cooled decoction in compresses to sponge the child's body.

Combinations: Use with rosewater or borage juice (restricted herb in some geographies) or use chickweed cream to ease the irritation of rashes.

German Measels (Rubella)

An infectious viral disease with an incubation period up to three weeks.

Key Symptoms:
- Mild fever, headache, drowsiness.
- Nasal congestion, sore throat, swollen glands in the neck and behind the ears.
- Irritant pink rash starting from the face and spreading down the body.

Note: Can cause birth defects if women are affected in early pregnancy; a notifiable disease in some countries.

Remedies:

Thymus serpyllum—WILD THYME

Aerial Parts

Actions: Astringent and antiseptic to ease symptoms.

How to use: In infusions (see dosage chart).

Combinations: Use with chamomile, elder flowers and sage in teas; soothe irritant rash as suggested under chicken pox above and take additional echinacea to combat infection.

Melissa officinalis—LEMON BALM

Aerial Parts

Actions: Sedating and calming for irritated and tense children; some antiviral activity reported.

How to use: Use in infusions to drink (see dosage chart) or to soak a compress and sponge the child externally.

Combinations: With hyssop, chamomile, elder flowers or pot marigold in infusions; add a little spearmint to improve the flavor if required. Add 10 ml of cleavers juice or 10 drops of poke root tincture to each cup to combat swollen glands.

Whooping Cough

Whooping cough often starts slowly with a mild cough and cold with sticky mucus, but a distressing convulsive cough soon follows.

Key Symptoms:
- Cough gradually develops over a week until it becomes convulsive.
- Characteristic whoop when coughing after 14 days, often followed by vomiting.
- Breathlessness.

Note: Before the age of three whooping cough can be dangerous: professional help should be sought in all cases.

Remedies:

Tussilago farfara—COLTSFOOT

Flowers

Actions: Antitussive and antispasmodic to ease convulsive coughing; expectorant to help clear sticky mucus and congestion.

How to use: In infusions, tinctures or syrups (see dosage chart).

Combinations: With thyme and white horehound in infusions and syrups; massage the child's chest with 5 drops of hyssop, basil or cypress oil in 5 ml of almond oil to help ease congestion. Use echinacea or add 10 drops of wild indigo tincture per dose to combat infection.

Precautions: Coltsfoot contains pyrrolizidine alkaloids and is restricted in some geographies.

Lactuca virosa—WILD LETTUCE

Aerial Parts

Actions: Sedating to soothe and relax exhausted children.

How to use: Use in infusions or tinctures.

Combinations: Use with wild thyme, mullein, elecampane, white horehound or licorice in combined infusion/decoctions, syrups or tinctures to combat and soothe convulsive coughing.

Precautions: Large doses may cause drowsiness and confusion.

CROUP

A bacterial or viral infection leading to inflammation and obstruction of the larynx which usually affects children aged between about 6 months and two years.

KEY SYMPTOMS:
- Difficulty breathing – noisy, gulping breaths.
- Usually worse at night when feverishness and anxiety increases.

Note: Seek professional help if the condition does not ease within 48 hours.

REMEDIES:

Eucalyptus globulus—EUCALYPTUS

ESSENTIAL OIL
Actions: Strongly antimicrobial, antispasmodic and expectorant to ease congestion, infection and breathing problems.

How to use: Use 5 drops in a steam inhalation or add to 5 ml of almond oil and use as a chest rub. Maintain a damp, humid atmosphere in the child's room – use a wet towel over the radiator or run the hot water in the sink.

Combinations: Add lavender, hyssop or thyme oil to rubs and inhalants.

Precautions: Do not take essential oils internally.

Marrubium vulgare—WHITE HOREHOUND

AERIAL PARTS
Actions: Combats bronchial spasms and helps to clear mucus and phlegm; restorative and bitter to stimulate the digestion.

How to use: In infusions or syrups (see dosage chart).

Combinations: Add a pinch of ginger or cayenne to each dose or combine with catmint, echinacea leaves, and thyme in infusions or syrups. Support with chest rubs and additional echinacea or garlic supplements to combat infection.

AYURVEDIC TONICS

In Ayurveda, tonic herbs can be nutritive to strengthen the body, aphrodisiac to reinvigorate the sexual organs and inner energies, or rejuvenative to help creativity and awareness. Nutritive tonics (*bruhana karma*) tend to be sweet in taste and are usually strengthening for *kapha* – the humor associated with earth and water, and important for weight gain – and will decrease *vata* (air) and *pitta* (fire). Aphrodisiac remedies are known as *vajikarana* from "*vaji*" a stallion, as they supply the energy and vitality of a horse – also renowned in Indian tradition for its sexual activity. This focus on reproductive energy also strengthens all the body's tissues (*dhatus*). By increasing sexual energy, the vajikarana not only help to create new life in conception but also help to renew our own lives. The rejuvenative remedies (*rasayana karma*) are among the most important in Ayurveda. These can be compared with the Taoist longevity tonics (see p. 242) to help prevent decay and aging, while enhancing mental clarity and spiritual awareness, which is so important in India's "science of life." Some herbs contain all three properties.

BRUHANA KARMA

Bruhana karma tonics are generally heavy, oily, or mucilaginous. They strengthen muscles and fats, build tissues, increase body fluids, and are restorative in debility, convalescence, emaciation, or physical weakness. As mucilaginous remedies they are often demulcent and soothing for mucous membranes so can be especially helpful in stomach or respiratory disorders. They also tend to be calming and sedating as they decrease air and fire elements and emphasize earth and water. Because they are heavy, these tonics can also be hard to digest, especially in conditions where *agni* (digestive fire) is weak, so warming, carminative herbs – such as ginger, galangal, or cinnamon are sometimes added. In Ayurveda, the action of these *bruhana karma* is enhanced by taking them in milk, *ghee* (clarified butter), or with added sugar or honey.

Emblica officinalis—AMALAKI

Amalaki is both a nutritive remedy and a *rasayana* for *pitta* conditions. The fruits are a very rich source of vitamin C (up to 3 g per fruit) and it also stimulates the appetite. *Amalaki* is the basis for *chyavan prash* – an herbal jelly used in India as a general tonic.

Parts used: Fruit.

Actions: Nutritive tonic, rejuvenative, aphrodisiac, laxative, astringent, styptic.

How to use: Use 250-1000 mg of powder per dose or in a decoction.

Combinations: Used with herbs like *gokshura*, *ashwagandha*, *shatavari*, and cinnamon in *chyavan prash*.

Precautions: Avoid in diarrhea or dysentery.

Sesamum indicum—TILA/SESAME

Sesame seeds, known as *tila* in India, are rich in calcium to help strengthen tissues and are also rejuvenative for *vata* conditions. The seeds are regarded as *sattvic*, to renew spiritual energies, and are a popular food among yogis.

Parts used: Seeds.

Actions: Nutritive and rejuvenative tonic, demulcent, laxative, antioxidant, anti-anemia.

How to use: Use up to 2 g of the powder per dose or a decoction of seeds; sesame oil is used externally with lime water for burns and sores or with a little camphor as a massage for migraines and vertigo.

Combinations: The seeds can be made into a confection with *shatavari*, ginger, and raw sugar and eaten daily.

Sida cordifolia—BALA

Bala is a type of wild mallow, and the name in Sanskrit means "giving strength." It is a good heart tonic and one of the herbs which are nutritive, rejuvenating, and an aphrodisiac. It is mainly used for *vata* disorders, often in sesame oil.

Parts used: Root.

Actions: Rejuvenative, nutritive, and aphrodisiac tonic, demulcent, diuretic, analgesic, wound herb, stimulant.

How to use: Use in milk decoction with sugar or take up to 1 g of powder per dose; with sesame oil it is used for nerve pains and muscle cramps.

Combinations: Used with ginger or black pepper for fevers or with basil, elecampane, mullein, and cinnamon as a lung tonic after influenza or in chronic respiratory problems.

Other nutritive tonics featured elsewhere in the book:

dang gui
di huang
flax seeds
Korean ginseng
licorice
lotus seeds
marshmallow

saw palmetto
shatavari
slippery elm
Solomon's seal
vidari-kanda
wild yam

VAJIKARANA

The aphrodisiac tonics focus on reproductive tissues, helping both sexual vitality and strengthening or regenerating inner organs. Although these herbs are sometimes used as aphrodisiacs they are more important as tissue energy tonics to nurture the reproductive organs – especially important in infertility – and to help encourage the creative energies associated with reproduction and strengthen the whole body. *Vajikaranas* are divided into tonics and stimulants: tonics improve the tissues and stimulants improve functionality.

Ipomoea digitata—VIDARI-KANDA

A member of the morning glory family, and relative of the sweet potato (*I. batatas*) *vidari-kanda*, is a versatile tonic that is sometimes called Indian ginseng. Related species are used in India for a wide range of ailments – from snakebites to leprosy.

Parts used: Root, leaves.

Actions: Nutritive, aphrodisiac and rejuvenating tonic, stimulates milk flow, hormonal action.

How to use: Use 5 g of powder in a milk decoction with ghee and honey as a daily tonic for debility and weakness in the reproductive organs.

Tribulis terrestris—GOKSHURA

Gokshura is an important remedy for urinary tract problems including stones, cystitis and infections. It also strengthens kidney function so it is a good tonic for the reproductive system. It is *sattvic* (promotes clarity and mental awareness) and has a calming effect on the nervous system.

Parts used: Fruit.

Actions: Rejuvenative and aphrodisiac tonic, diuretic, analgesic, clears urinary stones

How to use: Use in a milk decoction to enhance its aphrodisiac action; 250-100 mg of powder per dose; included in medicated oils for scalp massage as a treatment for baldness.

Combinations: Used with *ashwagandha* as a rejuvenating mixture or with dry ginger as an analgesic for nerve pains.

Polygonatum odoratum—MEDA/SOLOMON'S SEAL

Solomon's seal is rare in the wild and most cultivated specimens are a cross between *P. odoratum* and *P. multiflorum*. In India, *meda or mahameda*, is an important ingredient in *ashtavarga* (see p. 128) and is another of the flexible, all-around tonics.

Parts used: Rhizome.

Actions: Nutritive, aphrodisiac and rejuvenative tonic, demulcent, expectorant, stops bleeding.

How to use: Use in milk decoction or take up to 3 g of powder twice a day with warm milk and ghee.

Combinations: Meda is one of eight members of the lily family which go into *ashtavarga* use as a fertility tonic, taken during breastfeeding and for chronic wasting disease.

Other *vajikarana* tonics featured elsewhere in the book:

asafoetida	hibiscus
ashwagandha	Korean ginseng
cloves	long pepper
damiana	lotus seeds
dang gui	rose
di huang	saffron
fenugreek	*shatavari*
garlic	*vidari-kanda*
he shou wu	wild yam

RASAYANA KARMA

Rasayana means substances that enter (*ayana*) the vital essence (*rasa*) – herbal remedies that penetrate and revitalize spiritual energies and enhance well-being. *Rasayanas* are sometimes called longevity tonics, but that has to be seen against the Indian tradition of immortality as a continued existence in a universal whole rather than the survival of the individual. *Rasayana* tonics are also described as rejuvenating remedies to renew mind, body and spirit and combat aging and decay. Like the nutritive tonics, many are sweet to taste but they are also pungent, hot spicy remedies that are particularly appropriate for *kapha* conditions. In Ayurvedic theory plants possess a substance called *soma*, which is an almost magical nectar to renew the whole being, and *rasayanas* are believed to provide plenty of this vital energy-giving substance to increase understanding and awareness.

Centella asiatica—GOTU KOLA

Indian pennywort or *gotu kola* is known as *brahmi* in Sanskrit as it increases knowledge of *Brahman*, the supreme reality. It is one of the most important *rasayanas* in Ayurvedic medicine, helping to revitalize the brain and nervous system, combat aging and senility, and improve the memory. It is a specific tonic for *pitta* while clearing excess *vata* and *kapha*, so is calming, *sattvic*, and an important aid for spiritual renewal.

Parts used: Aerial parts.

Actions: Rejuvenative tonic, cooling in fevers, immune stimulant, cleansing, bitter digestive stimulant, laxative, sedative.

How to use: Use up to 1 g powder per dose or in infusions (½ teaspoon per cup); a paste made of the powder is used externally for eczema and skin sores.

Combinations: Use with basil as a cooling remedy in fevers and food poisoning; with rosemary or wood betony in teas when studying, or with *ashwagandha*, licorice and sandalwood for nervous irritability and mental weakness.

Precautions: Avoid in pregnancy and epilepsy.

Crocus sativus—SAFFRON

Traditionally used in India as a blood tonic, stimulant and aphrodisiac, saffron is very restorative and in Ayurveda is used to strengthen feelings of devotion and compassion. It is especially good for the female reproductive system and is also one of the best anti-*pitta* herbs. The herb is known as *nagakeshara* in Sanskrit; safflower (*Carthamus tinctorius*) is often used as a low-cost substitute although it is not as effective. Saffron helps to enhance other tonic herbs so is often added to other remedies.

Parts used: Flower stigma.

Actions: Aphrodisiac and rejuvenative tonic, promotes menstruation, carminative, antispasmodic, stimulating.

How to use: Although expensive, a little goes a long way. Use it in cooking or simmer a pinch in milk as a decoction.

Combinations: Use with *shatavari* or *dang gui* as a tonic for the female reproductive organs and function especially for menopause.

Eclipta prostata—BHRINGARAJ

Bhringaraj is important in both Ayurvedic and Chinese medicine (*han lian cao*) as a kidney tonic. Its Indian name actually means "ruler of the hair" and as in Chinese theory, healthy head hair is said to indicate healthy kidneys. It combats aging and helps rejuvenate bones, teeth, sight, hearing, and memory. It calms the mind and encourages restful sleep. It is also rejuvenative for predominantly *pitta* people and a good liver tonic.

Parts used: Aerial parts.

Actions: Astringent, antibacterial, a *yin* tonic that nourishes the kidneys and liver and stops bleeding; take for kidney weakness or heavy menstrual or postpartum bleeding.

How to use: Take an infusion or up to 10 ml of tincture a day.

Combinations: Use with *gotu kola* as a general tonic; *bhringaraj* oil is sold in India as a hair tonic to combat graying and balding. In Chinese medicine it is combined with a variety of other herbs, including *di huang*, for various blood disorders.

Other *rasayana* tonics featured elsewhere in the book:

aloe vera	Korean ginseng
amalaki	long pepper
ashwagandha	myrrh
bala	oatstraw
bibhitaki	saw palmetto
dang gui	sesame
di huang	*shatavari*
elecampane	Solomon's seal
garlic	spikenard
guggul	*vamsha rochana*
haritaki	*vidari-kanda*
he shou wu	wild yam

CHINESE TONICS

Use of tonic herbs in China goes back to the early Taoists. They believed that the ideal way of life to achieve prosperity, longevity, and immortality was to encourage "virtue." Virtue meant conforming to nature and living in harmony with all things. Herbal tonics were part of this "cultivation of the Way," helping to integrate physical and spiritual growth and encourage determination to follow the path of virtue. Today many of these herbs are described as "longevity tonics" – although a better description is perhaps "virtue tonics."

Note: There are four major groups of tonics: energy or qi tonics, blood tonics, yang tonics, and tonics. A correct diagnosis is important because the use of inappropriate tonic remedies, such as a *yang* tonic when *yang* energies are already in excess, can make the condition worse. Seek professional help for severe or persistent problems.

QI TONICS

In China, illness is often defined in terms of energy deficiency and is treated with *qi* tonics. *Qi* – usually understood in the West as our inner energy level – actually comes in a wide variety of types. *Qi* is a mixture of energies derived from the food we eat and the air we breathe, plus an element inherited from our parents that is with us from birth. These ingredients then combine and are transformed to make the different sorts of *qi* that circulate in the body.

Zizyphus jujube—DA ZAO

Da Zao literally means "big date" and the fruits are one of the important "harmonizers" of Chinese medicine, often added – like licorice (*gan cao*) – to prescriptions to help modify and blend any conflicts in the action of the different ingredients. *Da zao* are sometimes called *hong zao* or red dates.

Parts used: Fruit.

Actions: Energy tonic for spleen and stomach; nourishes blood, nutritive, sedative, calms the spirit; moderates toxic herbs.

How to use: Take 3-10 dates per dose in decoctions or eat fresh.

Combinations: With ginseng or *dang gui* as appropriate.

Astragalus membranaceous—HUANG QI

Huang qi is an important *qi* tonic traditionally used for younger people while ginseng was considered better for those over forty. The two herbs are also frequently used together as a general tonic. *Huang qi* is included in Shen Nong's list of "superior" remedies and research in recent years has confirmed its importance as an immune tonic

Parts used: Root.

Actions: Antispasmodic, diuretic, stimulates bile flow, antibacterial, lowers blood sugar, nervous stimulant, lowers blood pressure, immune stimulant; tonic for *qi* and blood; used to stabilize *wei qi* (defense energy), accelerate wound healing and regulates water metabolism.

How to use: Decoction or tincture.

Combinations: Use with ginseng for fatigue and general debility, with *bai zhu* for stomach weakness, with *dang gui* for deficient blood associated with prolonged bleeding; with *fu ling* and cinnamon twigs for edema in the peripheries.

Atractylodes macrocephala—BAI ZHU

Bai zhu is one of the main *qi* tonics for spleen or stomach *qi* deficiency syndromes. The herb has been used in China since the Tang Dynasty (650 A.D.). It is included in the famous "four noble ingredients decoction" (*Si Jun Zi Tang*) – an important energy-giving brew – with ginseng, *fu ling*, and licorice.

Parts used: Rhizome.

Actions: Energy tonic for spleen and stomach; diuretic and carminative; helps to regulate *qi* and strengthen the lower limbs.

How to use: Take a decoction or tincture.

Combinations: Can be combined with *ban xia* and *chen pi* for stomach weakness or with cinnamon and *fu ling* for lung problems.

Important energy tonics featured elsewhere in this book include:

cordyceps	Korean ginseng
da zao	licorice
dang shen	reishi mushroom
elecampane	rosemary
fu ling	*shan yao*
he shou wu	

BLOOD TONICS

In Chinese medicine, blood and body fluids are classed as *yin* and are often nourished by herbs that are *yin* in character. Blood deficiency can be due to anemia, although Chinese medicine also cites liver disharmony, heart weakness or psychological factors as causes. In the East, blood tonics are widely used by women to encourage healthy reproductive functionality, to regulate the menstrual cycle, and as a general tonic after childbirth.

SYMPTOMS OF BLOOD DEFICIENCY

- Dizziness, vertigo; poor eyesight.
- Lethargy, palpitations.
- Dry skin, thirst.
- Menstrual irregularities.
- Pale tongue; pallid face and lips.

Lycium chinense—GOU QI ZI

Both fruits and root bark (*di gu pi*) are used in Chinese medicine – the root bark is listed among Shen Nong's "superior woods" as a remedy for "evil *qi*" although today the fruits are a more common remedy.

Parts used: Berries.

Actions: Good *yin* tonic for the kidneys, nourishes blood, cooling, stops bleeding, lowers blood sugar.

How to use: Take decoction or tincture; eat dried berries as currants or use in cooking and tonic wines.

Combinations: Can be combined with *ju hua* for high blood pressure associated with liver disharmony; use with *he shou wu*, *shu di huang*, and *chen pi* for kidney exhaustion linked to overwork or old age; with *wu wei zi* for general debility.

Rehmannia glutinosa—DI HUANG

Shu di huang is the prepared form of the herb made by stir-frying the sliced tubers with wine. It is a major blood tonic. The raw herb, *sheng di huang*, is colder and it is sometimes cooked (without wine) to produce *gan di huang*. Both of these forms are more helpful for *yin* and body fluids as well as used to clear heat.

Parts used: Root – either raw or cooked.

Actions: Demulcent, laxative, stops bleeding, also a *yin* tonic specific to nourish kidney *yin*; *sheng di huang* is used as a nourishing and cooling *yin* remedy, while *shu di huang* is better to nourish blood.

How to use: Take up to 10 ml tincture three times a day or up to 15 g per dose in a decoction.

Combinations: Use *shu di huang* with *shan zhu yu*, *shan yao*, *mu dan pi* and *gou qi zi* for menopausal problems; *sheng di huang* combines with *qing hao* and *mu dan pi* for *yin* deficiency.

Polygonum multiflorum—HE SHOU WU

He shou wu (also known in the West as *fo ti* from its Cantonese name) is an important blood tonic that also helps kidney and liver energy. The root is the main herb, although fleeceflower stems (*ye jiao teng*) are also used as a heart and liver tonic to calm the nerves and improve blood circulation. It is especially useful for menopause.

Parts used: Root.

Actions: Antibacterial, heart tonic, hormonal action, raises blood sugar, laxative, liver stimulant, reduces blood cholesterol; used to replenish liver and kidney *jing* and nourish blood; also to detoxify "fire poisons" and clear external wind.

How to use: Take as decoction, tincture or use in tonic wines.

Combinations: Use with ginseng and *dang gui* for chronic debility; with *xuan shen* and *lian qiao* to relieve abscesses and swelling due to "fire poisons."

Precautions: Avoid in diarrhea associated with spleen weakness or phlegm or if there is any liver disease. Do not use in pregnancy, when breastfeeding or if suffering from estrogen-sensitive cancers.

Important blood tonics featured elsewhere in this book include:

amalaki	*nu zhen zi*
bai shao yao	reishi mushroom
chuan xiong	*san qi*
dang gui	*sang shen*
echinacea	*shatavari*
mai men dong	stinging nettle

YANG TONICS

Yang tonics are mainly used for deficient *yang* syndromes that commonly afflict the kidney, spleen, and heart. Many remedies (such as sea horses and gecko) reflect the less acceptable side of Chinese medicine although there are also some suitable herbs.

SYMPTOMS OF *YANG* DEFICIENCY
- Frequent colds or infections, fatigue.
- Fluid retention; coldness, and pallor.
- Pale, puffy tongue; slow, tired pulse.
- Withdrawal, introspection.

Psoralea corylifolia—BU GU ZHI

The name *bu gu zhi* literally means "tonify bone resin," and the berries of this plant have been used as a *yang* tonic since at least 450 A.D. The herb is particularly good for both kidney and spleen *yang*, and modern research has also shown it to be effective as an external remedy for alopecia, psoriasis and vitiligo.

Parts used: Fruit.

Actions: Strengthens kidney *yang*, diuretic, astringent, antibacterial, stops uterine bleeding.

How to use: Take a decoction.

Combinations: Combine with wu *zhu yu*, *wu wei zi*, nutmeg, and ginger for early morning diarrhea associated with kidney weakness.

Precautions: Can cause photosensitivity of the skin.

Eucommia ulmoides—DU ZHONG

Du zhong was one of the herbs listed in Shen Nong's herbal; the tree is the only surviving member of its genus and was first collected by Western plant hunters in the 1880s. Extracts have been used in recent years to treat high blood pressure, with a decoction of the stir-fried herb proving particularly effective.

Parts used: Bark.

Actions: Diuretic, hypotensive, reduces cholesterol levels, sedative, uterine relaxant, tonifies liver and kidney *qi*, smooths the flow of *qi* and blood to strengthen bones and muscles; helps prevent miscarriage.

How to use: Take in decoction, tincture or up to 500 mg daily powdered in capsules.

Combinations: With *bu gu zhi* for deficient kidney *yang* deficiency or with *gui zhi* for problems associated with cold and damp.

Precautions: Avoid in deficient *yin*.

Epimedium grandiflorum—YIN YANG HUO

Yin yang huo translates rather incongruously as "licentious goat wort," and modern research has confirmed its aphrodisiac action: it will increase sperm production and stimulate the sensory nerves to increase sexual desire. It focuses on kidney energy and also on the liver to help normalize menstrual activity.

Parts used: Aerial parts.

Actions: Aphrodisiac, antibiotic, reduces blood pressure, diuretic (in low doses), tonifies the kidneys and strengthens *yang*; expels wind, cold and dampness; controls liver *yang*.

How to use: Take in tinctures or infusions.

Combinations: With *wu wei zi* and *gou qi zi* for weak kidney *yang* associated with impotence and infertility.

Important *yang* tonics featured elsewhere in this book include:

cinnamon	ginger
cordyceps	walnut
fenugreek	*wu wei zi*

YIN TONICS

Yin tonics are suitable for deficient *yin* syndromes that are most common in the lungs, stomach, liver and kidneys. These remedies also help to promote body fluids – moistening tissues and having a laxative effect. They are also used to help clear phlegm by making it less sticky and heavy. Modern research has shown that many popular yin tonics also tend to reduce high blood pressure and cholesterol levels.

SYMPTOMS OF *YIN* DEFICIENCY
* Feverishness and night sweats; thirst and dry mouth.
* Debility following a long illness.
* Red, shiny tongue; fast pulse.

Codonopsis pilosula—DANG SHEN

Dang shen is often used as a less expensive alternative to Korean ginseng and is traditionally taken by nursing mothers. It is a popular ingredient of "Change of Season Soup" (which also contains *huang qi*, *shan yao* and *gou qi zi*) used whenever there are major shifts in the weather to help the body adapt.

Parts used: Root.

Actions: Demulcent and expectorant acting on lung and spleen; widely used as a substitute for ginseng, it is rather milder and more *yin* in character, it is particularly good for nourishing stomach *yin*.

How to use: Take a decoction or tincture or drink as a tonic wine.

Combinations: Use with *fu ling*, *bai zhu* and licorice.

Dendrobium officinale—SHI HU

Shi hu – also known as *suk gok* from its Korean name – is a member of the lily family used in Chinese medicine since the days of Shen Nong. It mainly affects stomach, lung and kidney *yin*. Modern studies have shown that it lowers body temperature and is a mild analgesic.

Parts used: Stems.

Actions: *Yin* tonic is particularly good for the kidney; also strengthens lung and stomach and increases body fluids; cooling; used to nourish *jing* and for dry coughs and fevers; reputedly increases sexual vigor.

How to use: Take a tincture or decoction made with 60 g of herb in 750 ml of water.

Combinations: Traditionally Taoists used *shi hu* with liquorice as a general tonic; with *sheng di huang* and *xuan shen* for low-grade fevers and heat problems.

Schizandra chinensis—WU WEI ZI

Although the taste of *wu wei zi* is generally described as "sour" the name actually means "five taste seeds" and it is regarded as combining all five of the classic Chinese tastes. The herb is listed in the *Shen Nong Ben Cao Jing* and has long been regarded as an aphrodisiac.

Parts used: Fruit.

Actions: Astringent, sedative and aphrodisiac; effective kidney and skin tonic; take for insomnia and anxiety; an all-round tonic that acts on all organs; good for allergic skin conditions and traditionally taken by women as a beauty aid.

How to use: Take an infusion or tincture; or take 200-250 mg powdered herb in capsules three times day.

Combinations: Often used with *dan shen* and *mai men dong*; with dry ginger in lung deficiency.

Important *yin* tonics featured elsewhere in this book include:

bai shao yao	*huang qin*
bhringaraj	*san qi*
chen pi	*sang shen*
da zao	*sheng di huang*
da zhong	Solomon's seal
fu ling	*tian men dong*

WESTERN TONICS

Although tonic herbs are less common in modern Western herbal medicine, European tradition still boasts many plants regarded as potent energy and spiritual remedies. Much of this tradition is now lost in the mists of folklore but the magical associations of many herbs are still apparent in surviving shamanic rituals. Numerous psychotropic herbs have been used in all cultures to raise mental awareness and alter emotional states. In North America, the native medicine man smoked tobacco or took peyote (*Lophophora williamsii*) before seeking the spiritual cause of the patient's illness. In Europe, medieval witches favored henbane, deadly nightshade or mandrake to alter emotional states, while the Siberian shaman used the fly agaric toadstool (*Amanita muscaria*). Today, South American shaman use extracts of a vine (*Banisteriopsis caapi*) known in

Columbia as *yage* and in Peru and Ecuador as *ayahuasca* to achieve a trance-like state to aid spirit travelling and healing. Other herbs have a less dramatic effect, and old herbals are full of references to plants that "make the heart merry and glad" or "take away melancholy," while others, like guarana (see p. 135), were used to combat fatigue on long journeys.

ENERGY TONICS

The uplifting effect of a cup of tea or coffee is appreciated by all – yet we would rarely put these herbs in the same category as ginseng or guarana. Caffeine-based herbs provide only a superficial energy tonic; others have a more deep-seated effect. Rosemary (p. 99) contains a chemical called borneol, which acts as a powerful stimulant to the nervous system to overcome fatigue. This same compound is also found in other common culinary herbs such as sage (p. 102) and thyme (p. 115), both of which can be used in stimulating and energy-giving teas.

Eleutherococcus senticosus—SIBERIAN GINSENG

Varieties of *Eleutherococcus* have been used in traditional Chinese medicine for some 2,000 years, although it was only "rediscovered" in the West in the 1950s. The herb was then used extensively by Soviet athletes to increase stamina and enhance performance. It helps the body to cope with increased stress levels and improves concentration and mental activity. It is usually regarded as gentler in action than Korean ginseng and may be a preferred choice for women.

Parts used: Root.

Actions: Helps to combat stress, antiviral, aphrodisiac, immune and circulatory stimulant, regulates blood pressure, lowers blood sugar levels, tonic stimulant for adrenal hormones.

How to use: Take 10 drops of tincture, three times a day or up to 1 g in tablets or capsules daily; it is better to take Siberian ginseng before a particularly stressful period – such as in the weeks before exams or an arduous business trip – rather than in the heat of a crisis.

Combinations: Usually taken as a simple or can be combined with saw palmetto or oats.

Cola nitida—KOLA NUTS

Cola contains up to 2.5% caffeine with traces of theobromine, making it a rather more effective stimulant than coffee (which contains up to around 0.3% caffeine). Like other caffeine sources, cola essentially provides a short-term energy boost rather than acting as a more deep-seated energy tonic. It was used in the original Coca-Cola recipe – the "coca" being provided by cocaine leaves. Tablets containing 5 g of cola, called "Forced March," were regularly issued to troops in the early years of the twentieth century to provide an energy boost.

Parts used: Seeds.

Actions: Diuretic, stimulant, antidepressant, astringent, tonic, nerve stimulant.

How to use: Use powdered in capsules up to 3 g per dose or in decoctions (up to ½ teaspoon per cup).

Combinations: Use with damiana and saw palmetto for sexual problems, with skullcap for depression and nervous debility.

Serenoa serrulata—SAW PALMETTO

Saw palmetto berries originate in the southeastern states of the U.S. and were a popular food among Native Americans and early settlers. They were highly valued for their tonic effect as a strengthening remedy in debility and convalescence. Researchers have demonstrated that saw palmetto prevents the conversion of the male hormone testosterone into dihydrotestosterone, which is believed to be responsible for benign prostate enlargement. The herb also encourages breakdown of any DHT that has formed, thus both preventing and helping to relieve the problem.

Parts used: Fruit.

Actions: Urinary antiseptic, combats benign prostate enlargement, tonic nutrient, diuretic, sedative, antispasmodic, stimulant.

How to use: Take 150 mg in tablets twice a day; use ½ teaspoon per cup in decoctions.

Combinations: Often used with cola and damiana as a tonic for elderly men, used with Siberian ginseng as a general energy tonic; used with horsetail and white deadnettle in prostatitis.

Useful energy tonics featured elsewhere in this book:

American ginseng	guarana
cardamom	rosemary
damiana	sage
elecampane	thyme

NERVE TONICS

In the West nervous disorders and stress are blamed for many physical ills ,while a great many herbs are labeled as nerve tonics, nervines, sedatives, or "thymoleptics" (basically an antidepressant). For generations, herbs have been used to "lift the spirits" or "gladden the heart," although in earlier centuries these terms often implied treatment for humoral imbalance rather than nervous or psychological weaknesses.

Elettaria cardamomum—CARDAMOM

Cardamom is an effective digestive stimulant used to relieve indigestion and abdominal discomfort. It also acts as an energy tonic and stimulant for the nervous system – traditionally thought to stimulate the mind and heart and "bring joy." It is good for productive coughs and also eases feelings of nausea. It has been used in Europe since ancient Greek times and was described by William Cole in the seventeenth century as "chief of all seeds."

Parts used: Seed, essential oil.

Actions: Carminative, stimulating, soothing for the digestive system, appetite stimulant, expectorant, promotes sweating, anti-spasmodic.

How to use: Use the crushed seeds in infusions or tinctures; use 2-5 drops of essential oil in 5 ml of carrier oil as massage, add to bath water or take 1 drop on a sugar lump.

Combinations: Use in massage with rosemary or thyme; combine in infusions with *gotu kola* for debility and digestive weakness; use with fennel and lemon balm for nervous digestive upsets.

Turnera diffusa var. *aphrodisiaca*—DAMIANA

Damiana is a popular stimulant and aphrodisiac used to combat fatigue and give energy. It is an aromatic shrub largely found in Central and South America and acts as a tonic for the nervous system. It can be helpful in convalescence and general debility, both as a tonic and to encourage the appetite. Damiana can also be helpful for menstrual problems, loss of libido, impotence, and prostate disorders.

Parts used: Leaves.

Actions: Aphrodisiac, antidepressant, diuretic, digestive tonic, nervous stimulant, stimulant for the reproductive organs.

How to use: Use in infusions, tinctures or take up to 1 g in capsules or tablets daily.

Combinations: Combine with saw palmetto and kola for male sexual problems, with oats and vervain for depression, with raspberry leaf and St. John's wort for menstrual discomfort and irregularity.

Calamintha nepeta—CALAMINT

Today, calamint is generally grown as a garden ornamental rather than a medicinal herb, not least because, like pennyroyal (*Mentha pulegium*), it contains pulegone, a potent uterine stimulant. Earlier herbalists were more enthusiastic, regarding the herb as an effective remedy for a "sorrowful spirit" – or as John Gerard put it, "the seed of calamint relieves infirmities of the heart, taking away melancholy and making a man merry and glad."

Parts used: Whole plant, seeds.

Actions: Nerve tonic, stimulant, diaphoretic, carminative, uterine stimulant.

How to use: Use in infusions or decoctions (seed).

Combinations: Use with St. John's wort for insomnia, with lemon balm for depression and nervous tension, with fennel seeds for digestive problems.

Precautions: Do not use in pregnancy.

Important nerve tonics featured elsewhere in this book:

black cohosh	skullcap
cola	St John's wort
damiana	valerian
gotu kola	vervain
oats	wood betony

MIND TONICS

Today, Western herbs tend to be labeled as "sedative" rather than "spiritual" or "emotional" remedies – although many certainly have these properties. Wood betony, for example, acts on the liver and can ease emotions like frustration and anger, while borage can help us take a more optimistic view of life and realize that it is in our power to make essential changes. In the 1930s, Dr. Edward Bach "discovered" the Bach Flower Remedies, which affect specific moods. Australian "Bush Essences" and American "Quintessentials" also act on the emotions.

Hibiscus rosa-sinensis—HIBISCUS

Hibiscus flowers form the basis of *karkade*, a chilled tea traditionally served as a restorative to travelers in Egypt arriving after a long journey, and they are also a popular ingredient in many modern Western herbal teas. In India, the plant is sacred to Ganesh, the god of wisdom, who destroys obstacles and helps realize goals. Hibiscus is a good herb for helping such determination.

Parts used: Flowers.

Actions: Stops bleeding (including excessive menstrual bleeding), eases menstrual cramps and pain associated with urinary tract inflammations, uterine stimulant, promotes menstruation, demulcent, antispasmodic, cooling in fevers.

How to use: Use in infusions or tinctures; *karkade* is made by macerating the petals in cold water, then bringing the mix to a boil and straining immediately; sweeten, chill and serve; tea bags are readily available from health food shops.

Combinations: Use with rose petals for improving determination and resolution; use with raspberry leaf for menstrual problems.

Precautions: Avoid in pregnancy.

Satureja montana—WINTER SAVORY

Winter savory is usually classified as a culinary herb ideal for flavoring soups and stews. Like other culinary plants it is an effective digestive remedy, but it shares with basil the ability to lift the spirits and stimulate the mind. It can help to clear melancholy and depression and improve concentration and mental activity.

Parts used: Aerial parts.

Actions: Diaphoretic, carminative, stimulant, promotes menstruation, antispasmodic, astringent, antibacterial, stimulates pituitary gland.

How to use: In infusions and tinctures; the essential oil is used internally in parts of Europe but should not be used externally as it can irritate the skin.

Combinations: Use with basil in infusions and teas as a mental pick-me-up; use the oil in infusers to scent rooms.

Precautions: Avoid in pregnancy.

Pulsatilla vulgaris—PASQUE FLOWER

Pasque flower is generally regarded in modern herbal medicine as a soothing and analgesic remedy for the reproductive organs. It is an important sedative and can be used by patients trying to reduce dependence on benzodiazepine tranquillizers. It is calming and restorative for the emotions and has been used effectively for obsessive syndromes in mental illness and in schizophrenia. In homeopathy, pulsatilla is often prescribed for over-dependence and indecisiveness.

Parts used: Aerial parts of dried plant.

Actions: Nerve relaxant (especially for women), mild sedative, antibacterial, mild analgesic, antispasmodic.

How to use: Use 10-50 drops of 1:10 tincture per dose, three times a day; take 250 mg in capsules per dose; use prepared homeopathic remedies.

Combinations: With passion flower for insomnia and hyperactivity; with black cohosh and motherwort for menopausal problems, with skullcap and wood betony for emotional upsets.

Precautions: Do not use the fresh plant, which is an irritant.

Important herbs to affect mind and spirit featured elsewhere in this book:

basil	saffron
borage	sage
gotu kola	sandalwood
jasmine	skullcap
lemon balm	spikenard
mugwort	vervain
reishi mushroom	wood betony
rose	

OTHER MEDICINAL HERBS

AMERICAN CRANESBILL: *Geranium maculatum*
Parts used: Root, leaves.
Actions: Astringent, styptic, tonic.

ARBOR VITAE: *Thuja occidentalis*
Parts used: Leaf tips.
Actions: Anthelmintic, astringent, antimicrobial, anti-inflammatory, muscle stimulant, antiseptic.

ARNICA: *Arnica montana*
Parts used: Flowers.
Actions: Wound healer, immunostimulant.
Caution: Do not use on broken skin; use homeopathic *Arnica* internally only.

BAN XIA: *Pinellia ternata*
Parts used: Tuber.
Actions: Antitussive, expectorant, antiemetic, anti-catarrhal.

BARBERRY: *Berberis vulgaris*
Parts used: Bark, root, berries.
Actions: Cooling, anti-inflammatory, antiseptic, bitter digestive stimulant.

BAYBERRY: *Myrica cerifera*
Parts used: Bark.
Actions: Stimulant, astringent, diaphoretic.

BEARBERRY: *Arctostaphylos uva-ursi*
Parts used: Leaves.
Actions: Urinary antiseptic, astringent.
Caution: High doses may cause nausea.

BENZOIN: *Styrax benzoin*
Parts used: Essential oil, gum.
Actions: Expectorant, astringent, antispasmodic.

BIRCH: *Betula pendula*
Parts used: Sap, bark, leaves.
Actions: Bitter, astringent, antirheumatic.

BISTORT: *Polygonum bistorta*
Parts used: Root.
Actions: Astringent, stops diarrhea and bleeding, anti-catarrhal.

BITTER CANDYTUFT: *Iberis amara*
Parts used: Aerial parts.
Actions: Antispasmodic, relaxant, tonifies the digestive tract, carminative, traditionally used for gout and rheumatism.

BLACK HOREHOUND: *Ballota nigra*
Parts used: Aerial parts.
Actions: Antiemetic, stimulant, antispasmodic.

BLUE COHOSH: *Caulophyllum thalictroides*
Parts used: Rhizome.
Actions: Tonic, antispasmodic, anti-inflammatory, uterine stimulant, diuretic, antirheumatic.
Cautions: Avoid in early pregnancy.

BLUE FLAG: *Iris versicolor*
Parts used: Rhizome.
Actions: Anti-inflammatory, diuretic, stimulant, cathartic.

BOGBEAN: *Menyanthes trifoliata*
Parts used: Leaves.
Actions: Antirheumatic, bitter, tonic.

BOLDO: *Peumus boldo*
Parts used: Leaves.
Actions: Liver stimulant, diuretic.

BONESET: *Eupatorium perfoliatum*
Parts used: Aerial parts.
Actions: Diaphoretic, peripheral vasodilator, laxative, antispasmodic, antiviral, expectorant, cholagogue.
Cautions: High doses may cause vomiting.

BROOM: *Cytisus scoparius*
Parts used: Flowering tops.
Actions: Diuretic, laxative, hypertensive, uterine stimulant.

Caution: Avoid in high blood pressure and pregnancy; prolonged use may lead to liver damage.

BUCHU: *Agathosma betulina*
Parts used: Leaves.
Actions: Diuretic, tonic, urinary antiseptic, diaphoretic.

BUCKWHEAT: *Fagopyrum esculentum*
Parts used: Leaves.
Actions: Hypotensive, vasodilator, repairs blood vessel walls.

BUGLEWEED: *Lycopus virginicus*
Parts used: Aerial parts.
Actions: Sedative, astringent, tonic, vasoconstricor, antitussive, hyperglycaemic, styptic.
Caution: Avoid in pregnancy.

CALIFORNIA POPPY: *Eschscholzia californica*
Parts used: Aerial parts.
Actions: Analgesic, hypnotic, sedative.

CALUMBA: *Jateorhiza palmata*
Parts used: Root.
Actions: Bitter digestive tonic, carminative, hypotensive.

CASCARA SAGRADA: *Rhamnus purshiana*
Parts used: Bark.
Actions: Purgative, digestive tonic.

CATMINT: *Nepeta cataria*
Parts used: Aerial parts.
Actions: Carminative, antispasmodic, diaphoretic, sedative, cooling, digestive stimulant.

CENTAURY: *Centaurium erythraea*
Parts used: Aerial parts.
Actions: Bitter, liver stimulant.

CHAI HU: *Bupleurum chinense*
Parts used: Root.

Actions: Energy tonic, liver stimulant, cooling, antibacterial, anti-inflammatory, analgesic, cholagogue, reduces cholesterol levels.

CHASTE-TREE: *Vitex agnus-castus*
Parts used: Berries.
Actions: Stimulates pituitary gland and hormone production.
Caution: High doses may cause formication.

CHICORY: *Cichorium intybus*
Parts used: Root.
Actions: Diuretic, laxative, tonic.

CLOVES: *Syzygium aromaticum*
Parst used: Flower buds, essential oil.
Actions: Stimulant, carminative, antiemetic, antiseptic, anodyne, antispasmodic.

CORNFLOWER: *Centaurea cyanus*
Parts used: Flowers.
Actions: Tonic, stimulant, anti-inflammatory.

CORNSILK: *Zea mays*
Parts used: Stamens.
Actions: Diuretic, healing for urinary mucosa, tonic, demulcent.

CYPRESS: *Cupresses sempervirens*
Parts used: Essential oil.
Actions: Antiseptic, antispasmodic, sedative, diuretic.

DILL: *Anethum graveolens*
Parts used: Seeds.
Actions: Carminative.

DU HUO: *Angelica pubescens*
Parts used: Root.
Actions: Antirheumatic, analgesic, anti-inflammatory.

EVENING PRIMROSE: *Oenothera biennis*
Parts used: Seed oil.
Actions: Important source of gamma-linolenic acid needed for prostaglandin production.

EYEBRIGHT: *Euphrasia officinalis*
Parts used: Whole herb.
Actions: Anti-catarrhal, antiseptic, anti-inflammatory.

FALSE UNICORN ROOT: *Chamaelirium luteum*
Parts used: Rhizome.
Actions: Diuretic, uterine tonic, emetic.

FRINGE TREE: *Chionanthus virginicus*
Parts used: Root bark.
Actions: Cholagogue, liver stimulant, tonic, diuretic.

GERANIUM: *Pelargonium odorantissimum*
Parts used: Essential oil.
Actions: Antidepressant, analgesic, diuretic, sedative, tonic.

GLOBE ARTICHOKE: *Cynara scolymus*
Parts used: Aerial parts.
Actions: Liver tonic and restorative, cholagogue.

GOAT'S RUE: *Galega officinalis*
Parts used: Aerial parts.
Actions: Hypoglycemic, insulin stimulant, galactagogue, diuretic.

GOLDEN ROD: *Solidago virgaurea*
Parts used: Aerial parts.
Actions: Anti-inflammatory, anti-catarrhal, healing, urinary antiseptic, sedative, hypotensive, diaphoretic.

GREATER CELANDINE: *Chelidonium majus*
Parts used: Aerial parts.
Actions: Diuretic, cleansing, liver stimulant, anti-inflammatory.
Caution: Avoid in pregnancy.

GROUND IVY: *Glechoma hederacea*
Parts used: Leaves.
Actions: Astringent, anti-catarrhal.

GUMPLANT: *Grindelia camporum*
Parts used: Aerial parts.

Actions: Antispasmodic, expectorant, cardiac depressant.
Caution: Avoid in low blood pressure, may irritate the kidneys.

HERB ROBERT: *Geranium robertianum*
Parts used: Leaves.
Actions: Astringent, styptic.

HOLY THISTLE: *Cnicus benedictus*
Parts used: Aerial parts.
Actions: Bitter digestive stimulant, expectorant, antiseptic, wound herb.

HORSE CHESTNUT: *Aesculus hippocastanum*
Parts used: Bark, seeds.
Actions: Anti-inflammatory, astringent.
Caution: Large amounts of seed coating can be toxic.

HUAI JIAO: *Sophora japonica*
Parts used: Fruit.
Actions: Hemostatic, laxative.
Caution: Avoid in pregnancy.

HUAI NIU XI: *Achyranthes bidentata*
Parts used: Root.
Actions: Circulatory stimulant, liver tonic, analgesic.

HUANG LIAN: *Coptis chinensis*
Parts used: Root.
Actions: Cholagogue, antibacterial, analgesic, sedative, anti-inflammatory.

HUO MA REN: *Cannabis sativa*
Parts used: Seeds.
Actions: Stimulating laxative.

HYDRANGEA: *Hydrangea arborescens*
Parts used: Rhizome, root.
Actions: Diuretic, laxative, kidney stimulant.

INDIAN TOBACCO: *Lobelia inflata*
Parts used: Aerial parts.
Actions: Relaxant, expectorant, diaphoretic, emetic, antispasmodic, anti-asthmatic.

Caution: Restricted in some geographies; use only as directed by a professional practitioner.

IRISH MOSS: *Chondrus crispus*
Parts used: Whole plant (thallus).
Actions: Demulcent, expectorant, antiemetic, nutritive.

JAMAICAN DOGWOOD: *Piscidia erythrina*
Parts used: Root bark.
Actions: Sedative, anodyne.
Caution: Do not exceed stated dose.

JIE GENG: *Platycodon grandiflorum*
Parts used: Root.
Actions: Expectorant, antifungal, antibacterial, hypoglycemic.

KING'S CLOVER: *Melilotus officinale*
Parts used: Flowering aerial parts.
Actions: Demulcent, diuretic, antispasmodic, anti-coagulant.
Caution: Do not use with blood-thinning drugs such as warfarin or if there is a blood-clotting problem.

LEMON: *Citrus x limon*
Parts used: Essential oil, fruit.
Actions: Anti-inflammatory, anti-histaminic, diuretic, venous tonic.
Caution: Only use organic oil and ensure it is well-diluted to avoid potential skin irritation.

LESSER PERIWINKLE: *Vinca minor*
Parts used: Leaves, root.
Actions: Astringent, circulatory stimulant, improves cerebral blood flow.

LIAN QIAO: *Forsythia suspensa*
Parts used: Fruit.
Actions: Anti-inflammatory, antibacterial, antipyretic.
Caution: Avoid in diarrhea or *yin* deficiency.

LIGNUM VITAE: *Guaiacum officinalis*
Parts used: Heartwood.
Actions: Antirheumatic, anti-inflammatory, circulatory stimulant.

LILY-OF-THE-VALLEY: *Convallaria majolis*
Parts used: Leaves.
Actions: Heart tonic, diuretic, purgative, emetic.
Caution: Restricted herb in some geographies; use only under professional guidance.

LINDEN: *Tilia x europaea*
Parts used: Flowers.
Actions: Sedating nervine, diaphoretic, vasodilator, healing for blood vessel walls, hypotensive.

LOVAGE: *Levisticum officinale*
Parts used: Roots, seeds.
Actions: Warming digestive tonic, carminative, diaphoretic, expectorant, anti-catarrhal.

MAI MEN DONG: *Ophiopogon japonicus*
Parts used: Tuber.
Actions: Promotes secretion of body fluids, tonic, sedative, antitussive, hypoglycemic, antibacterial.

MARSH CUDWEED: *Gnaphthalium uliginosum*
Parts used: Aerial parts.
Actions: Astringent, anti-catarrhal, anti-inflammatory, tonifying to mucosa.

MISTLETOE: *Viscum album*
Parts used: Young leafy twigs.
Actions: Slows heart rate, hypotensive, antitumor.
Caution: Do not use berries, which are toxic and restricted in some geographies; avoid in pregnancy.

MOUSE-EAR HAWKWEED: *Hieracium pilosella*
Parts used: Aerial parts.
Actions: Antispasmodic, expectorant, anti-catarrhal, diuretic, wound herb.

NU ZHEN ZI: *Ligustrum lucidem*
Parts used: Berries.
Actions: Tonic, diuretic, immunostimulant.

OAK: *Quercus robur*
Parts used: Bark.
Actions: Strong astringent.

PARSLEY PIERT: *Aphanes arvensis*
Parts used: Aerial parts.
Actions: Diuretic, demulcent.

PELLITORY-OF-THE-WALL: *Parietaria diffusa*
Parts used: Aerial parts.
Actions: Diuretic, demulcent, soothing for urinary mucosa.

PILEWORT: *Ranunculus ficaria*
Parts used: Roots, leaves.
Actions: Astringent, used for hemorrhoids.
Caution: Do not take internally.

PRICKLY ASH: *Zanthoxylum americanum*
Parts used: Bark.
Actions: Circulatory stimulant, diaphoretic, carminative, tonic.

QUASSIA: *Picrasma excelsa*
Parts used: Wood.
Actions: Anthelmintic, bitter.

RAMSOMS/WILD GARLIC: *Allium ursinum*
Parts used: Aerial parts, bulbs.
Actions: Antimicrobial, hypoglycemic, lowers serum cholesterol levels.

SAFFLOWER: *Carthamnus tinctorius*
Parts used: Flowers.
Actions: Laxative, diuretic, anti-inflammatory.

SHAN ZHU YU: *Cornus officinalis*
Parts used: Fruit.
Actions: Tonic, diuretic, hypotensive, antimicrobial.

Slippery elm: *Ulmus fulva*
Parts used: Bark.
Actions: Demulcent, nutritive, astringent.

Soap bark: *Quillaja saponaria*
Parts used: Inner bark.
Actions: Expectorant, detergent, anti-inflammatory.
Caution: Do not take internally.

Southernwood: *Artemisia abrotanum*
Parts used: Aerial parts.
Actions: Anthelmintic, antiseptic, bitter, uterine stimulant.
Caution: Avoid in pregnancy.

Squaw vine: *Mitchella repens*
Parts used: Aerial parts.
Actions: Uterine stimulant, tonic, restorative, astringent, diuretic.

Sweet sumach: *Rhus aromatica*
Parts used: Root bark.
Actions: Astringent, tonic, anti-diabetic, diuretic.

Tormentil: *Potentilla erecta*
Parts used: Root.
Actions: Astringent – especially for gut wall.

True unicorn root: *Aletris farinosa*
Parts used: Rhizome. roots.
Actions: Estrogenic, tonic, digestive stimulant, sedative.

Wall germander: *Teucrium chamaedrys*
Parts used: Aerial parts.
Actions: Bitter digestive stimulant, anti-catarrhal, antimicrobial, anti-inflammatory.
Caution: Research suggests that long-term use may cause liver damage; do not exceed the stated dose.

White bryony: *Bryonia alba*
Parts used: Root.
Actions: Antirheumatic, cathartic.

White deadnettle: *Lamium album*
Parts used: Flowering tops.
Actions: Astringent, antispasmodic, tonic for reproductive system.

White horehound: *Marrubium vulgare*
Parts used: Aerial parts.
Actions: Stimulating expectorant, antispasmodic, bitter digestive remedy, soothing tonic for the mucosa.

Wild indigo: *Baptisia tinctoria*
Parts used: Root, leaves.
Actions: Antiseptic, antibacterial, antipyretic, laxative.
Caution: Do not exceed stated dose; excess may cause vomiting.

Wild lettuce: *Lactuca virosa*
Parts used: Leaves, sap.
Actions: Sedative, hypoglycemic, hypnotic, anaphrodisiac.
Caution: May cause drowsiness, do not drive or operate machinery; excess may cause stupor and confusion and reduce sex drive.

Wood sage: *Teucrium scorodonia*
Parts used: Aerial parts.
Actions: Astringent, diaphoretic, antirheumatic, carminative, wound herb, cholagogue.

Woundwort: *Stachys palustris*
Parts used: Aerial parts.
Actions: Antiseptic, antispasmodic, wound herb.

Wu zhu yu: *Evodia rutæcarpa*
Parts used: Fruit.
Actions: Analgesic, antibacterial, warming, stimulant.

Xiang fu: *Cyperus rotundus*
Parts used: Tuber.
Actions: Carminative, analgesic, uterine antispasmodic, encourages *qi* flow.

Yellow dock: *Rumex crispus*
Parts used: Root.
Actions: Strong laxative, cholagogue, cleansing.

Yellow jasmine: *Gelsemium sempervirens*
Parts used: Root.
Actions: Analgesic, sedative, hypotensive, eases neuralgia.
Caution: Restricted in some geographies; overdose may cause nausea and double vision.

Ze xie: *Alisma plantago*
Parts used: Rhizome.
Actions: Diuretic, hypotensive, antibacterial, liver cleanser.

Zhi zi: *Gardenia jasminoides*
Parts used: Fruit.
Actions: Antipyretic, sedative, hypotensive, antibacterial, cholagogue.

CONSULTING AN HERBALIST

While many people use herbs as safe and effective home remedies for minor ailments, persistent or more serious problems need professional help. Finding a practitioner with whom you feel empathy and can trust can be just as important in treatment as taking the right herbs. Some herbalists follow a semi-orthodox path prescribing remedies to ease symptoms, while others will focus on holistic treatments and urge major lifestyle changes. Some will use only Western herbs, others a combination of Chinese or Ayurvedic remedies. Some will talk mainly of pathological conditions, others will suggest *qi* stagnation, allergies, or focus on emotional stress.

If possible, choose your practitioner by personal recommendation from like-minded friends to ensure a good relationship with someone who understands your problem and whom you can also understand. Alternatively, ask the national regulatory body for a list of members and speak to likely practitioners before making an appointment: ask about their experience of treating ailments similar to yours and their general therapeutic approach. A wide range of ailments are commonly treated: both the sort of problems one may normally take to a GP – infections, aches and pains, menstrual disorders, high blood pressure, urinary dysfunction, or digestive problems – as well as those chronic conditions for which herbalism is often seen as a "last resort," such as rheumatoid arthritis, ME, or emphysema.

WHO ARE THE HERBALISTS?

National practices and regulations vary around the world. In the UK, the national Institute of Medical Herbalists was founded in 1864, and is the oldest professional body of medical herbalists in the world. Students must complete several years' training, which today includes a degree course in herbal medicine at an accredited institution plus 500 hours of supervised clinical training, before being accepted into membership. Members use the initials MNIMH or FNIMH after their names, which gives the patient some guarantee that they are consulting a suitably trained practitioner. In the U.S., the American Herbalists Guild was started by well-known herbalist Michael Tierra in 1989. As with the NIMH, there are strict criteria for membership, which includes four years of academic training and 400 hours of clinical experience. Practitioners generally use RH(AHG) (registered herbalist AHG)" after their names. The AHG website provides details of the many colleges in the U.S. that offer herb courses and their graduates' qualifications, so finding out about the nature of your chosen practitioner's training can be straightforward.

Other national practices can vary considerably: in France, herbal practitioners, or *phytothérapeute*, are almost always trained doctors who have studied plant medicine at the post-graduate level; in Germany, alternative practitioners qualify as "heilpraktiker" and have comparable status to orthodox GPs while in many Eastern European medical schools "*materia medica*," the study of herbal remedies, remains an important part of the student curriculum. In Australia, trained herbalists become full members of the National Herbalists Association and use the initials NHAA after their names. They are officially classed as Health Care Professionals by the Commonwealth Government.

In China, traditional herbal medicine is taught in dedicated colleges and is available to patients at special hospitals as an alternative to Western medicine, while in Japan, herbal remedies are available on their equivalent of the National Health Service. In other countries, including some US states, it is illegal for anyone to prescribe herbal remedies or set themselves up as a herbal practitioner, although self-medication with herbs is permitted. In others, just about anyone, well-trained or not, can set up in business as a medical herbalist and dispense all manner of inappropriate "cures."

What Does an Herbalist Do?

During a consultation, an herbalist will use patient listening and probing questions to uncover all the relevant symptoms along with time-honored diagnostic techniques: feeling pulses, looking at tongues, testing urine and blood pressure with clinical examinations dependent on palpation, auscultation, and percussion. A first consultation will generally take at least an hour and subsequent ones 20 minutes or so. As well as reviewing the current illness, the herbalist will ask about medical history – previous health problems that may be contributing to the current imbalance, family tendencies and allergies, diet, lifestyle, stresses, and worries.

Existing orthodox medication also needs to be checked. Herbalists would certainly not recommend dropping vital drugs, but any incompatibility of these with herbal remedies obviously needs to be considered when prescribing plant medicines. Similarly, many patients turn to herbs because they are anxious to phase-out their drugs, for whatever reason, and a safe program of replacing them with gentler herbal remedies needs to be devised – preferably with the support and co-operation of the patient's GP.

Many herbalists still dispense their own remedies so at the end of the consultation the patient may leave with an assortment of appropriate tinctures, ointments, or capsules – or perhaps a bag of dried herbs to brew at home. Whatever the remedy, it will have been specially selected to help the health problems of the individual patient rather than be just a standard selection of ready-made products.

Herbalists like to see patients fairly soon after the first consultation to check on progress – perhaps after two or three weeks – with regular meetings every four to six weeks for three months or more in chronic cases. Herbal medication is likely to be altered slightly after each consultation to reflect changes in the condition. Just as all patients are different, so too are all herbalists; healing is a two-way process, and the patient must take responsibility for their own health and actively participate in any cure.

GLOSSARY

Adrenal cortex: Part of the adrenal gland, which produces corticosteroid hormones.

Alkaloid: Active plant constituent containing one or more nitrogen atoms usually in a heterocyclic ring structure.

Alterative: Cleansing – stimulating efficient removal of waste products.

Analgesic: Relieves pain.

Anodyne: Allays pain.

Anthelmintic: Destroys and helps expel intestinal worms.

Antibiotic: Destroys or inhibits the growth of micro-organisms.

Anticoagulant: Hinders blood clotting.

Antiemetic: Helps to prevent vomiting and suppress nausea.

Anti-hydrotic: Limits the production of water-based fluids including sweat.

Antipyretic: Cooling; reduces fevers.

Antispasmodic: Reduces muscle spasm and tension

Antitussive: Inhibits the cough reflex helping to stop coughing

Aperient: Mild laxative.

Arthralgia: Pain in a joint.

Astringent: Precipitates proteins from the surface of cells or mucous membranes, producing a protective coating: binding and contracting effect.

Ayurvedic: Traditional system of Indian medicine that translates as "science of life."

Bitter: Stimulates secretion of digestive juices and encourages appetite.

Black bile: One of the four Galenical humors associated with the earth element and considered cold and dry.

Blood: Apart from the familiar substance, "blood" was one of the four Galenical humors associated with the air element and considered hot and damp.

Blood stagnation: Concept in traditional Chinese medicine where the blood circulation is retarded or where blood vessels become blocked for any reason. Considered to interfere with the normal flow of *qi* (q.v.) through the body.

Bulk laxative: Increases the volume of feces producing larger, softer stools.

Cardioactive: Affecting heart function.

Carminative: Relieves flatulence, digestive colic, and gastric discomfort.

Cathartic: Drastic purgative.

Channel: See meridian.

Cholagogue: Stimulates bile flow from the gallbladder and bile ducts into the duodenum.

Choleretic: Encourages free flow of bile by increasing cholesterol excretion.

Choleric: Galenical state related to yellow bile.

Circulatory stimulant: Increases blood flow.

Cold conditions: Traditional concept associated with chills, poor circulation, thirst for hot drinks, feeling cold, fatigue, sharp pain, frequent urination, or *yang* deficiency.

Colic: Spasmodic pain affecting smooth muscle – e.g. guts, gallbladder, urinary tract, etc.

Coumarin: Active plant constituent, generally smelling of new mown hay, that encourages blood clotting.

Cream: Oil/fat/water-based plant extract that is miscible with skin.

Decoction: Water-based plant extract produced by boiling herbs in water.

Demulcent: Softens and soothes damaged or inflamed surfaces, such as the gastric mucosa.

Diaphoretic: Encourages sweating.

Diuretic: Encourages urine flow.

Doctrine of Signatures: Theory that the appearance of a plant indicates its inherent medicinal properties.

Eclectic: System of herbal medicine developed in the U.S. in the nineteenth century.

Emetic: Causes vomiting.

Emmenagogue: Encourages menstrual flow.

Emollient: Softens and soothes the skin.

Essential oil: Volatile oil extracted from plants usually by steam distillation and containing a mixture of active constituents. Generally highly aromatic.

Expectorant: Encourages the loosening and removal of phlegm from the respiratory tracts.

Febrifuge: Reduces fever.

Galactagogue: Encourages lactation (milk production).

Galenical: Traditional system of Western medicine based on the four humors theory of Ancient Greece.

Glycoside: Active plant constituent containing one or more sugar molecules.

Haematuria: Blood in the urine.

Hemostatic: Stops or slows bleeding.

Hot conditions: Traditional concept associated with fevers, increased metabolic rate, thirst for cold drinks, increased heat sensitivity, irritability. burning pains, thick catarrh, or *yin* deficiency.

Humor: Theoretical body fluid important in Galenical and Ayurvedic medicine.

Hyperglycemic: Raises blood sugar levels.

Hypertensive: Raises blood pressure.

Hypoglycemic: Lowers blood sugar levels.

Hypotensive: Lowers blood pressure.

Immunostimulant: Enhances and increases the body's immune (defense) mechanism.

Infusion: Water-based plant extract produced by pouring boiling (or almost boiling) water on the herb.

Jung: The "vital essence" of traditional Chinese medicine responsible for creative and reproductive energies and stored in the kidneys.

Kapha: Ayurvedic humor – associated with dampness or phlegm.

Laxative: Encourages bowel motions.

Melancholic: Galenical state related to black bile.

Meridian: In Chinese medicine, a conduit that can be compared with an imaginary line or channel linking points on the surface of the body with internal organs in which *qi* flows. Traditional Chinese Medicine defines fourteen main channels and eight extra channels. The surface points are used in acupuncture.

Mucilage: Complex sugar molecules that are soft and slippery and protect mucous membranes and inflamed tissues.

Narcotic: Causes stupor and numbness.

Nervine: Affects the nervous system – may be stimulating, sedating or relaxing.

Neuralgia: Pain along a nerve.

Ointment: Oil/fat-based plant extract that is immiscible with skin.

Peripheral circulation: Blood supply to limbs, skin and muscles (includes heart muscle).

Phlegm: In modern Western medicine similar to catarrh or sputum; Galenical humor associated with the water element and considered cold and damp; *Kapha* (q.v.); associated with spleen deficiency in traditional Chinese medicine.

Phlegmatic: Galenical state related to phlegm.

Physiomedicalism: System of herbal medicine developed in the U.S. in the nineteenth century.

Pitta: Ayurvedic humor, associated with fire or bile.

Prostaglandins: Hormone-like substances with a wide range of functions including chemical messengers, causing uterine contractions.

Purgative: Drastic laxative.

Qi (ch'i): The body's vital energy.

Rubefacient: Irritates the skin causing redness by increasing blood flow to the surface.

Sanguine: Galenical state related to blood.

Saponins: Active plant constituents, similar to soap, producing a lather in water; can irritate the digestive tract; expectorants; some chemically resemble steroidal hormones.

Sedative: Soothing and calming.

Simple: A single herb used as a remedy on its own.

Steroids: Group of chemicals with a characteristic multi-ring molecular structure. naturally occurring steroids include the sex hormones and adrenaline.

Styptic: Stops external bleeding

Tannin: Active plant constituents which combine with proteins. Originally derived from plants used for tanning leather. Astringents (q.v.).

Terpene: Complex active plant constituents with a carbon ring structure, generally highly aromatic and included in essential oils.

Tincture: Alcohol-water-based plant extract.

Tonic: Restoring, nourishing and supporting for the system.

Tonify: Strengthen and restore.

Topical: local administration of a herbal remedy e.g. to the skin or eye; effect herb has in local treatment.

Vasoconstrictor: Stimulates blood vessels reducing their diameter.

Vasodilator: Relaxes blood vessels increasing their diameter.

Vata: Ayurvedic humor, associated with wind or air

Vulnerary: Heals wounds.

Wei qi: Chinese concept of defence energy comparable with the immune system.

Yang: Aspect of being equated with male energy – dry, hot, ascending, exterior.

Yellow bile: Galenical humor associated with the fire element and considered hot and dry; Kapha (q.v.); associated with spleen deficiency in traditional Chinese medicine.

Yin: Aspect of being equated with female energy – damp, cold, descending, interior.

INDEX

A

Abscesses, 164

Acacia. See Australian wattle

Acetylsalicylic acid, 12

Aches, 154–159

Achillea millefolium. See Yarrow

Achyranthes bidentata. See Huai niu xi

Acne, 175, 176–177

Aconitine, 12

Actaea racemosa. See Black cohosh

Actium lappa. See Burdock

Adrenal stimulant, 34, 58, 83

Aerial parts, 140–141

Aesculus hippocastanum. See Horse chestnut

After pains, 219

Agaric, 132

Agathosma betulina. See Buchu

Agni, 4

Agrimonia. See Agrimony

Agrimony, 20, 50, 172, 173, 187, 192, 196, 231

AIDS, 133

Ai ye, 211, 214

Alchemilla vulgaris. See Lady's mantle

Alchemilla xanthoclora. See Lady's mantle

Aletris farinosa. See True unicorn root

Alisma plantago. See Ze xie

Alkaloids, 12

Allergic conditions, 194–196

Allium sativa. See Garlic

Aloe, 4, 23, 151, 178

Aloe vera. See Aloe

Alopecia, 178–179

Alpine lovage, 71

Alpinia. See Galangal

Alpinia galangal. See Galangal

Alterative, 29, 116

Althaea officinalis. See Marshmallow

Amalaki, 225, 238

Amanita muscaria. See Fly agaric

American cranesbill, 187, 189, 211, 231, 233, 253

Ammi visnaga. See Khella

Amni visnaga. See Khella

Analgesic, 19, 60, 63, 66, 69, 71, 78, 79, 84, 86, 88, 90, 94, 99, 101, 133

Anaphrodisiac, 61

Anemia, 23, 184

Anemopaegma arvense. See Catuaba

Anethum graveolens. See Dill

Angelica, 27, 154, 156, 169, 190

Angelica polyphorma var. sinensis. See Dang gui

Angelica pubescens. See Du huo

Angina pectoris, 24, 26, 183–184

Anise, 22

Anodyne, 121

Anthelmintic, 23, 30, 49, 67, 106, 112, 114, 132

Antibacterial, 31, 35, 39, 40, 41, 45, 47, 57, 65, 69, 71, 73, 76, 77, 81, 84, 89, 93, 94, 97–98, 104, 105, 106, 128

Antibiotic, 22, 29, 46, 102, 115, 213

Anti-catarrhal, 42, 62, 64, 88, 91, 103, 118, 131

Antidepressant, 32, 34, 66, 77, 83, 97–98, 99, 107

Antiemetic, 75, 78, 80, 83, 120, 127

Antifungal, 23, 24, 28, 36, 40, 42, 57, 65, 71, 76, 81

Anti-hydrotic, 47, 101

Anti-inflammatory, 19, 21, 27, 29, 33, 34, 35, 36, 44, 45, 48, 51, 52, 54, 56, 58, 59, 60, 63, 64, 67, 72, 73, 75, 80, 84, 88, 92, 94, 101, 103, 104, 112, 117, 122, 124, 125, 126, 130, 131

Antimicrobial, 44, 87, 108, 125, 131, 132

Antioxidant, 102, 107, 129

Antiparasitic, 20, 22, 65, 88

Antipyretic, 58, 93, 101, 104, 105. *See also* Febrifuge

Antirheumatic, 27, 28, 29, 30, 32, 34, 35, 50, 51, 60, 68, 72, 74, 79, 88, 99, 101, 110, 113, 125, 136

Antiscorbutic, 50, 108, 119

Antiseptic, 29, 36, 39, 40, 42, 44, 49, 66, 72, 74, 76, 83, 89, 90, 97–98, 99, 101, 102, 114, 115, 120, 127, 128, 132

Antispasmodic, 19, 26, 27, 40, 41, 45, 47, 49, 50, 66, 67, 69, 71, 73, 75, 78, 80, 81, 84, 86, 87, 90, 91, 92, 97–98, 99, 102, 105, 115, 116, 117, 121, 123, 124, 127

Antitumor, 31, 37, 125, 126, 132, 133, 136

Antitussive, 19, 31, 72, 94, 115

Antiviral, 20, 47, 64, 76, 77, 97–98, 107, 133

Anxiety, 133, 201–202

Aperient, 29

Aphanes arvensis. See Parsley piert

Aphrodisiac, 66, 82, 97–98, 135, 136

Aphthous stomatitis, 172

Apium graveolens. See Celery

Appetite stimulant, 56, 80, 192

Apples, 74

Arbor vitae, 177, 253

Arctium lappa. See Burdock

Arctostaphylos uva-ursi. See Bearberry

Arnica, 155, 179, 253
Arnica cream, 150
Arnica tablets, 150
Arrow, 163
Artemisia absinthum. See
   Wormwood
Artemisia abrotanum. See
   Southernwood
Artemisia vulgaris. See Ai ye;
   Mugwort
Arthritis, 58, 129, 130, 134, 136,
   154, 155
Artichoke, 189, 190, 254
Asclepias tuberosa. See Pleurisy root
Ashwagandha, 4, 126, 206, 221,
   225
Asparagus, 31
Asthma, 132, 134, 169
Astragalus membranaceus. See
   Huang qi
Astringent, 18, 20, 21, 36, 37, 38,
   42, 43, 48, 53, 55, 57, 59, 62,
   63, 66, 67, 79, 82, 92, 93, 94,
   96, 97–98, 99, 100, 101, 102,
   109, 110, 111, 114, 115, 119,
   120, 122, 124, 132
Atherosclerosis, 223–224
Atropine, 12
Australian wattle, 130
Avena sativa. See Oats
Avicenna, 2–3
Avocado, 136–137
Ayahuasca, 10, 247–248
Ayurveda, 3–5, 14–15
Ayurvedic herbs, 128–130
Ayurvedic tonics, 238–242
Azadirachta indica. See Neem

B
Bach Flower Remedies, 150, 154,
   160, 200, 205, 250
Backache, 129, 157
Bad breath, 193
Bai shao yao, 154, 190, 209, 214.

See also White peony
Bai zhu, 164, 186, 209, 243
Bala, 239
Bamboo, 87, 166
Banisteriopsis caapi. See Ayahuasca
Ban xia, 186, 243, 253
Baptisia tinctoria. See Wild indigo
Barberry, 188, 191, 253
Bark, 141
Basil, 4, 83, 201, 203, 207, 213,
   215, 216, 251
Bayberry, 168, 253
Bearberry, 4, 197, 198, 233, 253
Bedwetting, 233
Beech, Wooster, 11
Benzoin, 253
Berberis vulgaris. See Barberry
Bergamot, 41
Betula pendula. See Birch
Bhringaraj, 241
Bibhitaki, 173
Bilberry, 120, 227
Bile stimulant, 62, 123, 129
Birch, 253
Bistort, 172, 253
Bitter candytuft, 190, 253
Black cohosh, 11, 19, 156–157,
   158, 209, 211, 217, 219
Black haw, 210, 219
Black horehound, 191, 213, 216,
   253
Black root, 11
Bladderwrack, 54, 227
Bleeding, 59, 82, 87, 214
Blepharitis, 171–172
Bloating, 191
Blood, 180–185
Blood pressure, 180–182. *See also*
   Hypotensive
Blood tonics, 243–245
Blue cohosh, 11, 210, 216–217,
   219, 253
Blue flag, 177, 228, 253. *See also*
   Iris versicolor

Bogbean, 154, 155, 156, 253
Boils, 164
Boldo, 189, 253
Boletus edulis. See Ceps
Boneset, 10, 50, 163, 253
Borage, 34, 203, 233, 235
Borago officinalis. See Borage
Brassica oleracea. See Cabbage
Breast engorgement, 218
Bronchitis, 128, 133, 134, 168–
   169
Broom, 182, 253
Bruhana karma, 238–239
Bryonia alba. See White bryony
Buchu, 25, 157, 197, 198, 213, 253
Buckwheat, 185, 223, 253
Bugleweed, 227–228, 253
Bu gu zhi, 245
Bulbs, 141
Bupleurum chinense. See Chai hu
Burdock, 3, 29, 156, 176, 179, 230
Bush herbs, 130–132
Butternut, 67, 186

C
Cabbage, 35, 176–177, 196, 232
Calamint, 250
Calendula officinalis. See Pot
   marigold
California poppy, 204, 232, 253
Calocybe gambosa. See St. George's
   mushroom
Calumba, 192, 253
Camellia sinensis. See Tea
Camphor, 128–129
Candidiasis, 133
Cannabis sativa. See Hemp; Huo
   ma ren
Cantharellus cibarius. See
   Chanterelles
Capsella bursa-pastoris. See
   Shepherd's purse
Capsicum frutescens. See Cayenne
Capsules, 146–147

Cardamom, 4, 166, 191, 249
Cardiac stimulant, 104
Cardiac tonic, 43, 70, 99, 124
Cardioprotective, 114, 129
Carminative, 24, 27, 28, 39, 40, 41, 52, 64, 68, 69, 70, 71, 78, 80, 81, 83, 89, 99, 102, 121, 127
Carthamnus tinctorius. See Safflower
Cascara sagrada, 253
Catarrh, 167. *See also* Anti-catarrhal
Caterpillar fungus, 133–134
Catmint, 163, 164, 231, 235, 237, 253
Cat's claw. *See* Peruvian cat's claw
Catuaba, 135
Caulophyllum thalictroides. See Blue cohosh
Cayenne, 4, 39, 158–159, 183, 207
Celandine, 177. *See also* Greater celandine; Lesser celandine
Celery, 4, 28, 155, 156, 157, 198
Cell proliferator, 111
Centaurea cyanus. See Cornflower
Centaury, 189, 253
Centella asiatica. See Gotu kola
Ceps, 134
Chai hu, 190, 209, 253–254
Chakras, 4
Chamaelirium luteum. See False unicorn root
Chamomile, 186, 189, 190, 191, 192, 195, 196, 201, 204, 207, 215, 218, 228, 231, 235. *See also* German chamomile
Chandana. See Sandalwood
Chanterelles, 134
Chaste-tree, 209, 211, 215, 254
Chelidonium majus. See Greater celandine
Cherry, winter. *See* Ashwagandha
Chest rub, 131
Chicken pox, 235
Chickweed, 110, 175

Chickweed cream, 150
Chicory, 189, 254
Chilblains, 129
Childbirth, 213–219
Children, 229–237
Chinese decoctions, 149
Chinese medicine, 5–8, 14, 174–175, 185, 208
Chinese tonics, 242–247
Chionanthus virginica. See Fringe tree bark
Chocolate, 134
Cholagogue, 23, 36, 45, 50, 67, 69, 78, 99, 102, 105, 113
Choleretic, 97–98
Choleric, 3
Cholesterol, 22, 23, 32, 37, 58, 85, 129, 136, 184–185
Chondrus crispus. See Irish moss
Christmas rose, 3
Chronic fatigue syndrome, 206–207
Chuan xiaong, 190, 214
Cichorium intybus. See Chicory
Cinchona pubescens. See Jesuit's bark
Cinnamomum camphora. See Camphor
Cinnamomum cassia. See Gui zhi; Rou gui
Cinnamomum zeylanicum. See Cinnamon
Cinnamon, 4, 40, 163–164, 166, 226
Circulation, 180–185. *See also* Cardiac stimulant; Hypertensive; Hypotensive
Circulatory stimulant, 27, 38, 39, 42, 52, 57, 69, 84, 89, 95, 99, 102, 103, 104, 109, 119, 127
Citrus. See Orange, bitter
Citrus aurantium. See Neroli; Zhi ke; Zhi shi
Cleavers, 55, 174, 176, 177, 178,

179, 207, 228
Clove, 4, 191, 226, 231, 254
Clover. *See* King's clover; Red clover
Cnicus benedictus. See Holy thistle
Coca leaves, 134
Codonopsis pilosula. See Dang shen
Coffin, Albert Isaiah, 11
Cola nitida. See Kola nuts
Cold infusion, 145
Cold sores, 172–173
Colic, 230–231
Colitis, 190
Coltsfoot, 118, 236
Comfrey, 111, 154, 155, 217, 230
Comfrey ointment, 150
Commiphora molmol. See Myrrh
Commiphora mukul. See Guggul
Common cold, 130, 133, 134, 162–164
Compress, 147
Confusion, 225
Conjunctivitis, 171–172
Constipation, 186–187
Contraceptive, 135
Convallaria majalis. See Lily-of-the-Valley
Coptis chinensis. See Huang lian
Cordyceps sinensis. See Caterpillar fungus
Coriander, 4, 22, 226
Corms, 141
Cornflower, 254
Corn silk, 197, 213, 233, 254
Cornus officinalis. See Shan zhu yu
Couchgrass, 197, 198, 199, 213, 222
Cough, 165–166. *See also* Antitussive
Cowberry, 120
Cowslip, 92, 168, 204
Cradle cap, 230
Cramp, 159
Crataegus. See Hawthorn

Cream, 145–146, 148
Croup, 237
Curcuma longa. See Turmeric
Culpeper, Nicholas, 9
Cupressus sempervirens. See Cypress
Cynara scolymus. See Artichoke
Cyperus rotundus. See Xiang fu
Cypress, 224, 254
Cytisus scoparius. See Broom
Cystitis, 128, 197, 198, 213

D
Damask rose, 202, 217
Damiana, 203, 221, 227, 248, 250
Dandelion, 113, 181, 189, 190
Dandruff, 179
Dang gui, 164, 184, 209, 210, 214, 215, 224, 241, 242
Dang shen, 246
Dark ages, 9
Da zao, 242
Decoction, 142–143, 149
Demulcent, 23, 25, 31, 34, 72, 87, 91, 110, 111, 117, 118, 122
Dendrobium officinale. See Shi hu
Dendranthema x *grandiflorum. See* Ju hua
Depression, 202–203
Devil's claw, 60, 154, 155, 157
Diabetes, 136, 226, 227
Diaper rash, 229–237
Diaphoretic, 18, 22, 27, 29, 32, 34, 39, 40, 45, 47, 50, 51, 64, 65, 71, 76, 77, 78, 79, 95, 99, 103, 123, 127
Diarrhea, 130, 131, 137, 186, 187
Digestive problems, 185–193
Digestive stimulant, 18, 21, 24, 61, 62, 74, 77, 80, 96, 97–98, 99, 100, 108, 109, 112
Digestive tonic, 68, 78, 101, 117, 130
Digitalis purpurea. See Foxglove
Di huang, 244

Dill, 218–219, 230, 254
Dioscorea. See Yam
Dioscorides, Pedanius, 2, 132
Diuretic, 19, 20, 25, 26, 28, 29, 41, 47, 48, 50, 51, 52, 53, 55, 60, 61, 68, 72, 73, 74, 81, 90, 93, 94, 99, 100, 103, 104, 105, 108, 113, 114, 115, 116, 119, 121, 122, 125, 133
Doctrine of signatures, 9, 10
Dried herbs, 151
Drugs, 12
Drying, 140–141
Du huo, 7, 254
Duodenal ulcer, 188
Du zhong, 245–246
Dysmenorrhea, 210

E
Earache, 171
Echinacea, 10, 46, 163, 164, 170, 171, 172, 173, 176, 192, 193, 197, 206–207, 212, 213, 228, 235, 237
Eclecticism, 11
Eclipta prostata. See Bhringaraj
Eczema, 175–176
Edema, 133
Egypt, 2
Elder, 103, 167
Elderflowers, 163, 171, 172, 195, 235, 236
Elderly, 222–225
Elecampane, 4, 19, 65, 165, 166, 168, 169, 228, 236
Elements
in Ayurvedic medicine, 3
in Chinese medicine, 5–6, 8, 185
in Greek medicine, 3
Elettaria cardamomum. See Cardamom
Eleutherococcus senticosus. See Siberian ginseng
Elymus repens. See Couchgrass

Emblica officinalis. See Amalaki
Emetic, 73, 88, 103
Emetine, 12
Emmenagogue, 50, 102, 112
Emotional upset, 205
Emu berry, 131
Endocrine problems, 225–228
Energy tonics, 248–249
Ephedra sinica. See Ma huang
Epimedium grandiflorum. See Yin yang huo
Equisetum arvensis. See Horsetail
Erythroxylum catuaba. See Catuaba
Erythroxylum coca. See Coca leaves
Eschscholzia californica. See California poppy
Estrogenic, 116
Eucalyptus, 49, 157, 169, 237
Eucommia ulmoides. See Du zhong
Eupatorium. See Agrimony; Boneset; Hemp a Gravel root
Euphorbia. See Spurge
Euphrasia officinalis. See Eyebright
Europe, 9–10
Evening primrose, 176, 206, 209, 210, 254
Evening primrose capsule, 150
Evodia rutaecarpa. See Wu zhu yu
Exhaustion, 206
Expectorant, 22, 25, 27, 31, 34, 41, 42, 45, 50, 52, 58, 64, 65, 71, 73, 76, 79, 83, 87, 91, 92, 97–98, 103, 111, 114, 115, 118, 121, 122, 125, 127
Eyebright, 167, 171, 172, 194, 195, 235

F
Facial neuralgia, 161–162
Fagopyrum esculentum. See Buckwheat
False unicorn root, 210, 211, 214–215, 224, 254

Fang feng, 154

Febrifuge, 18, 29, 33, 34, 44, 47,
    49, 50, 56, 83, 95, 130. *See
    also* Antipyretic

Fennel, 4, 13, 22, 52, 186, 189,
    191, 193, 213, 215, 216, 250

Fenugreek, 117, 192, 196, 227

Feverfew, 112, 161

Figwort, 3, 104, 164, 176, 177, 178

Filipendula ulmaria. See
    Meadowsweet

First aid, 150–151

Flatulence, 191

Flax, 72

Fleming, Alexander, 132

Flowers, 140

Flu, 31, 163–164

Fluid extract, 149

Fly agaric, 10, 132, 247

Foeniculum officinalis. See Fennel

Fomes fomentarius. See Hoof fungus

Food, 13–15

Food intolerance, 195–196

Food poisoning, 129–130, 192

Forgetfulness, 225

Forsythia suspensa. See Lian qiao

Four-element model, 3

Foxglove, 13, 180

Fractures, 130

Fragaria vesca. See Strawberries

Fringe tree bark, 11, 254

Fruit, 141

Fucus vesiculosis. See Bladderwrack

Fu ling, 133, 209, 243

Fungal infection, 178

Fungi, 132–134

G

Galactagogue, 34, 52, 117, 119,
    123

Galangal, 24, 183, 207

Galega officinalis. See Goat's rue

Galen, 2, 3, 13–14

Galium aparine. See Cleavers

Gallbladder inflammation, 188–
    189

Gallstones, 189

Ganoderma lucidem. See Reishi
    mushroom

Gardenia jasminoides. See Zhi zi

Garlic, 22, 151, 163, 173, 175, 176,
    184, 192, 196, 226. *See also*
    Wild garlic

Gastric stimulant, 56

Gastritis, 187–188

Gastroenteritis, 192

Gelsemium sempervirens. See Yellow
    jasmine

Gentian, 56, 190

Geranium, 254

Geranium maculatum. See
    American cranesbill

Geranium robertianum. See Herb
    Robert

German chamomile, 75, 169, 190,
    192, 205, 215, 218, 231. *See
    also* Chamomile

German measles, 236

Ginger, 127, 151, 164, 166, 183,
    191, 199, 215, 234, 245

Ginkgo, 57, 206, 223, 227

Ginseng, 19, 85, 158, 160, 173,
    205, 206, 220, 221, 227, 242,
    243. *See also* Korean ginseng;
    Siberian ginseng

Glandular fever, 228

Glandular problems, 225–228

Glechoma hederacea. See Ground
    ivy

Glycyrrhiza. See Licorice

Gnaphthalium uliginosum. See
    Marsh cudweed

Goat's rue, 218, 227, 254

Gokshura, 4, 129, 240

Golden rod, 167, 170, 254

Goldenseal, 4, 10, 62, 164, 167,
    171, 182, 190, 193, 194, 195,
    196, 211

Gotu kola, 4, 191, 204, 206, 207,
    221, 241, 249

Gou qi zi, 181, 212, 244, 246

Gout, 134, 136, 156

Gravel root, 50, 156, 198

Gray hair, 179

Greater celandine, 10, 254

Green tea, 184

Grewia retusifolia. See Emu berry

Grindelia camporum. See Gumplant

Ground ivy, 163, 166, 168, 195,
    254

Guaiacum officinale, 134. *See also
    Lignum vitae*

Guarana, 135–136

Guduchi, 130

Guelder rose, 124, 157, 159, 181,
    186–187, 189

Guggul, 4, 129

Gui zhi, 183

Gumplant, 169, 254

Gynecological problems, 208–213

H

Hair, 174–179

Hair loss, 178–179

Halitosis, 193

Hamamelis virginianum. See Witch
    hazel

Haritaki, 4

Harpagophytum procumbens. See
    Devil's claw

Harvesting, 140–141

Hawthorn, 43, 181

Hay fever, 194, 195

Headache, 159–162

Head lice, 232–233

Heart, 180–185. *See also* Cardiac
    stimulant; Hypertensive;
    Hypotensive

Heartsease, 125, 176, 178, 196,
    230

Heart tonic, 86

Helleborus niger. See Christmas rose

Hemorrhoids, 193
Hemostatic, 20, 119
Hemp, 2
Hemp agrimony, 50
Henbane, 10
Herbalists, 257–258
Herb Robert, 254
Herpes, 32, 64, 129, 172–173
He shou wu, 179, 180, 184, 212, 221, 244
Hibiscus, 4, 206, 251
Hieracium pilosella. See Mouse-ear hawkweed
Hippocrates, 2
Hives, 196
Holy thistle, 191, 254
Honey, 151
Honeysuckle, 73, 164
Hoof fungus, 132
Hops, 61, 204
Horse chestnut, 182, 254
Horsetail, 48, 157, 168, 198, 222, 224
Hot infusion, 145
Huai jiao, 193, 254
Huai niu xi, 154, 254
Huang lian, 7, 254
Huang qi, 158, 163, 164, 173, 206, 207, 224, 243
Huang qin, 164
Humulus lupulus. See Hops
Huo ma ren, 222, 254
Hydrangea, 199, 220, 222, 254
Hydrastis canadensis. See Goldenseal
Hyperactivity, 233
Hypericum perforatum. See St. John's wort
Hypertensive, 41, 62, 102
Hypoglycemic, 22, 29, 49, 95, 102, 117, 119, 120, 132, 226, 228
Hypotensive, 22, 28, 38, 71, 73, 79, 84, 86, 93, 95, 104, 121, 128, 132
Hyssop, 3, 64, 157, 166, 169, 202,

235, 237
Hyssopus officinalis. See Hyssop
Hysterectomy, 200, 208, 213

I
Iberis amaria. See Bitter candytuft
Immune stimulant, 42, 85, 88, 133, 164
Impotence, 220–221
Incontinence, urinary, 224
Indian snakeroot. *See* Snakeroot
Indian tobacco, 159, 254
Indigestion, 189
Infections, 162–164. *See also* Antibiotic; Antimicrobial; Antiviral
Infertility
female, 214–215
male, 221
Influenza, 31, 163–164
Infused oils, 144, 148, 151
Infusion, 142, 145
Inhalants, steam, 148
Insecticide, 132
Insomnia, 133, 203
Inula. See Elecampane
Involution, 219
Ipecacuanha, 12
Ipomoea digitata. See Vidari
Irish moss, 255
Iris versicolor, 177
Iron-deficient anemia, 184
Irritable bowel syndrome, 186, 190
Islam, 2–3
Isphagula, 187
Ivy. *See* Ground ivy

J
Jaborandi, 12
Jamaican dogwood, 161, 201, 202, 210, 255
Jasmine, 66, 216. *See also* Yellow jasmine
Jasminum. See Jasmine

Jateorhiza calumba. See Calumba
Jesuit's bark, 134
Jie geng, 255
Jin yin hua, 235
Juglans. See Walnut
Ju hua, 44, 172, 181, 244
Juices, 149
Juniper, 68, 154, 157, 159, 198, 199
Juniperus communis. See Juniper

K
Kanda, 239
Kapha, 4
Katuka, 129, 191
Kava kava, 90
Khella, 26, 199
Kidney stones, 199
Kidney tonic, 45
King's clover, 182, 255
Kola nuts, 248, 250
Korean ginseng, 206, 221. *See also* Ginseng
Kudzu, 95
Kunzea ericoides. See New Zealand tea tree

L
Labor, 216–217
Lactation, 102, 107
Lactuca virosa. See Wild lettuce
Lady's mantle, 10, 21, 173, 192, 209, 211, 212, 215
Lamium album. See White deadnettle
Lavandula. See Lavender
Lavender, 69, 161, 162, 173, 201, 204, 212, 237
Lavender oil, 150
Laxative, 27, 29, 31, 50, 53, 62, 72, 73, 74, 79, 81, 91, 96, 100, 103, 104, 108, 113, 114, 123, 125
Leaves, 140–141
Lemon, 161, 189, 255

Lemon balm, 4, 22, 77, 160, 163, 186, 189, 190, 191, 192, 196, 201, 203, 204, 205, 207, 215, 216, 231, 235, 236, 250
Lemonwood, 131
Lentinus edodes. See Shiitake
Leonurus. See Motherwort
Lepista nuda. See Wood blewits
Leptandra virginica. See Black root
Leptosporum scoparium. See New Zealand tea tree
Lesser celandine, 10
Lesser periwinkle, 224, 255
Levisticum officinale. See Lovage
Lian qiao, 164, 255
Libido, 220–221
Lice, 232–233
Licorice, 4, 19, 58, 164, 166, 168, 186, 188, 189, 193, 196, 206, 209, 214, 236
Lignum vitae, 134, 156, 157, 255
Ligusticum. See AlpineLovage
Ligustrum luciden. See Nu zhen zhi
Lily-of-the-Valley, 182, 255
Linaria vulgaris. See Toadflax
Linden, 181, 201, 204, 223, 231, 255
Ling zhi, 163
Linseed, 187
Linum. See Flax
Liver protective, 114
Liver stimulant, 74, 93
Liver tonic, 113, 123
Lobelia inflata. See Indian tobacco
Lonicera. See Honeysuckle
Lonicera japonica. See Jin yin hua
Lotions, 149
Lotus, 82
Lovage, 71, 193, 255
Lumbago, 157
Lungwort, 10
Lycium chinense. See Gou qi zi
Lycopus virginicus. See Bugleweed
Lymphatic cleanser, 55

Lymphatic stimulant, 88
Lymphatic tonic, 46

M
Macerations, 149
Madagascar periwinkle, 12
Ma huang, 12, 47, 169
Mai men dong, 247, 255
Male reproductive problems, 219–222
Malus. See Apples
Mandrake, 10, 247
Marcus Aurelius, 2
Marigold. *See* Pot marigold
Marigold cream, 150
Marrubium vulgare. See White horehound
Marsh cudweed, 167, 174, 195, 255
Marshmallow, 25, 166, 187–188, 189, 192, 222
Massage oils, 148
Mastitis, 218
Matricaria chamomilla. See German chamomile
Meadowsweet, 51, 156, 158, 188, 192, 196
Meals, 13–15
Measles, 234–235, 236
Measurement, 142
Meda, 240
Medicinal herbs, 18–127
Melaleuca. See Paperbarks
Melaleuca alternifolia. See Tea tree
Melancholic, 3
Melilotus officinale. See King's clover
Melissa officinalis. See Lemon balm
Menopause, 136, 180, 211–212
Menorrhagia, 210–211
Menstrual pain, 210
Menstrual regulation, 134
Mentha. See Mint
Menyanthes trifoliata. See Bogbean
Metabolic stimulant, 54

Migraine, 159–162, 161
Milk insufficiency, 218–219
Milk thistle, 107, 189, 190, 207
Mind tonics, 250–252
Mint, 78
Mistletoe, 223, 255
Mitchella repens. See Squawvine
Modern medicine, 12–13
Monkshood, 12
Morchella esculenta. See Morels
Morels, 134
Morning sickness, 215
Morphine, 12
Morus. See Mulberry
Motherwort, 70, 182, 183, 211–212, 216, 228
Mouse-ear hawkweed, 255
Mouth ulcers, 172
Mu dan pi, 180
Mugwort, 30, 192, 205, 209, 217, 219
Mulberry, 79, 163, 166
Mullein, 122, 167, 171, 236
Mumps, 234
Muscle relaxant, 124
Mushrooms, 132–134
Myalgia, 156–157
Myrica cerifera. See Bayberry
Myristica fragrans. See Nutmeg
Myrobalan, 114
Myrrh, 4, 42, 172, 178, 193

N
Nardostachys grandiflora. See Spikenard
Nasturtium, 9
Native Americans, 10–11
Nausea, 191
Neem, 33, 232–233
Nelumbo nucifera. See Lotus
Nepeta cataria. See Catmint
Neroli, 202
Nervine, 19, 30, 66, 81, 82, 92, 99, 105, 109, 123, 126

Nervous disorders, 200–207
Nervous tonic, 61, 63, 69, 77, 99, 135
Nettle. *See* Stinging nettle
New Zealand tea tree, 132, 188. *See also* Tea tree
Niaouli, 224
Nightshade, 10, 12, 247
Nipple soreness, 217–218
Nits, 232–233
North America, 10–11
Notopterygium forbesii. See Qiang huo
Nutmeg, 4, 9, 80, 245
Nutritive, 32, 54, 119
Nu zhen zhi, 179, 212, 213, 222, 255

O
Oak, 255
Oats, 32, 160, 185, 203, 248, 250
Ocimum basilicum. See Basil
Oenothera biennis. See Evening primrose
Oils
infused, 144, 148, 151
massage, 148
Ointment, 146, 148
Onions, 151, 196, 226
Ooolong tea, 184
Ophiopogon japonicus. See Mai men dong
Orange, bitter, 41
Osteoporosis, 224–225
Oyster mushrooms, 134

P
Paeonia. See Peony
Palpitations, 183–184
Panax. See Ginseng
Panic attacks, 202
Paperbarks, 131
Paracelsus, 9
Paratudo, 136

Parietaria diffusa. See Pellitory-of-the-wall
Parotitis, 234–235
Parsley piert, 199, 255
Parturition, 66
Partus preparator, 100
Pasque flower, 160, 170, 171, 201, 202, 210, 212, 222, 251–252
Passiflora incarnata. See Passion flower
Passion flower, 86, 181, 190, 201, 203, 204, 233, 252
Patent medicine, 11
Pau d'arco, 136
Paullinia cupana. See Guarana
Pelargonium odorantissimum. See Geranium
Pellitory-of-the-wall, 198, 199, 255
Pelvic inflammatory disease, 136
Peony, 17, 19, 84, 176
Pepper, 4, 89, 166, 168, 191, 213
Peppermint, 163, 189, 190, 215, 234, 235
Peptic ulcer, 188
Perineal tears, 217
Periwinkle. *See* Lesser periwinkle; Madagascar periwinkle
Persea americana. See Avocado
Persia, 3
Peruvian bark, 12
Peruvian cat's claw, 135
Pessaries, 149
Peumus boldo. See Boldo
Peyote, 247
Pfaffia paniculato. See Paratudo
Phlegmatic, 3
Phyllostachys nigra. See Bamboo
Physiomedicalist philosophy, 11–12
Physiomedical movement, 11
Phytolacca americana. See Pokeroot
Picorrhiza kurroa. See Katuka
Picrasma excelsa. See Quassia

Piles, 193
Pilewort, 193, 217, 255
Pills, 12
Pilocarpine, 12
Pinellia ternata. See Ban xia
Piper. See Pepper
Piper methysticum. See Kava kava
Pippali, 4
Piscidia erythrina. See Jamaican dogwood
Pitta, 4
Pittosporum. See Lemonwood
Plantago major. See Plantain
Plantago lanceolata. See Ribwort plantain
Plantago psyllium. See Psyllium
Plantain, 91, 218, 230
Platycodon grandiflorum. See Jie geng
Pleurisy root, 10
Pleurotus ostreatus. See Oyster mushrooms
Plum, 94
Poke root, 88, 174
Polygonatum odoratum. See Solomon's seal
Polygonum bistorta. See Bistort
Polygonum multiform. See He shou wu
Polyporus officinalis. See Agaric
Poppy, 12, 204, 232, 253
Potentilla erecta. See Tormentil
Pot marigold, 36, 172, 178, 188, 189, 195, 211, 212, 217, 230, 234, 235, 236
Poultice, 147
Powders, 146–147
Prana, 4
Pregnancy, 213–219
Premenstrual syndrome, 208–209, 209–210
Prickly ash, 156, 157, 158, 183, 255
Primrose, 92

Primula. See Cowslip; Primrose
Primula veris. See Cowslip
Prostate problems, 219–220,
    221–222
Prunella vulgaris. See Self-heal
Prunus. See Plum
Prunus serotina. See Wild cherry
    bark
Psoralea corylifolia. See Bu gu zhi
Psoriasis, 177–178
Psyllium, 187
Pueraria lobata. See Kudzu
Pulmonaria officinalis. See Lungwort
Pulsatilla vulgaris. See Pasque
    flower
Purgative, 23, 67, 88, 103
Purple coneflower, 46, 163

Q
Qi, 6, 7
Qiang huo, 7
Qi tonics, 242–243
Quassia, 255
Quercus robur. See Oak
Quillaja saponaria. See Soap bark
Quinine, 12, 134

R
Ramsoms, 232, 255
Ranunculus ficaria. See Lesser
    celandine; Pilewort
Rasayana karma, 240–242
Raspberry, 100, 216, 219, 250, 251
Rauwolfia serpentina. See Snakeroot
Red clover, 116, 176, 178, 179,
    196, 215
Red peony, 19
Reduced alcohol tincture, 148
Rehmannia glutinosa. See Di huang
Reishi mushroom, 132–133
Relaxant, 26, 69, 70, 112, 123, 204
Repetitive strain injury (RSI), 158
Reproductive problems. *See*
    Infertility; Male reproductive

problems; Pregnancy
Rescue remedy, 150
Reserpine, 13
Resin, 141
Respiratory problems, 165–169
Rhamnus purshiana. See Cascara
    sagrada
Rheumatism, 155–156, 156–157.
    See also Antirheumatic
Rheum palmatum. See Rhubarb
Rhinitis, 195
Rhubarb, 3, 96, 186
Rhus aromatic. See Sweet sumach
Ribwort plantain, 165, 171, 187
Ritual herbalism, 10–11
Roman chamomile, 204. *See also*
    Chamomile
Rome, 2
Roots, 141
Rosa. See Rose
Rosa x damascena. See Damask rose
Rose, 4, 97–98, 202, 203, 251
Rosemary, 99, 154, 159, 172, 179,
    201, 206, 207, 225, 249
Rosmarinus officinalis. See
    Rosemary
Rou gui, 40
Rubefacient, 39, 89, 99, 115, 127
Rubella, 236
Rubus idaeus. See Raspberry
Rue, 4
Rumex crispus. See Yellow dock

S
Safflower, 255
Saffron, 4, 241
Sage, 102, 172, 173, 179, 206, 211,
    218, 225, 234, 236
Salerno school, 9
Salivation, 102
Salix alba. See Willow
Salvia officinalis. See Sage
Sambucus nigra. See Elder
Sandalwood, 4, 128, 202

Sanguine, 3
Santalum album. See Sandalwood
Saps, 141
Satureja montana. See Winter
    savory
Saw palmetto, 220, 221–222, 248,
    249, 250
Schisandra fruit, 7
Schizandra chinensis. See Wu wei zi
Sciatica, 158–159
Scrophularia. See Figwort
Scutellaria. See Skullcap
Seasonal affective disorder (SAD),
    136, 207
Sedative, 19, 23, 28, 31, 41, 60, 61,
    63, 66, 71, 75, 77, 84, 86, 90,
    92, 97–98, 102, 104, 109,
    122, 123, 124, 126, 133
Seeds, 141
Self-determination, lack of,
    200–201
Self-heal, 4, 93, 172, 233
Senna, 3, 106, 186
Serenoa serrulata. See Saw palmetto
Serturner, Friedrich Wilhelm, 12
Sesame, 238
Shan zhu yu, 180, 244, 255
Shatavari, 4
Shen Nong, 5, 44, 243, 244, 245,
    247
Shepherd's purse, 38, 199, 211
Shi hu, 247
Shiitake, 133, 158
Shingles, 32
Shock, 207
Shu di huang, 180, 184, 212, 214
Siberian ginseng, 158, 160, 173,
    205, 220, 248. *See also*
    Ginseng
Sida cordifolia. See Bala
Silybum marianum. See Milk thistle
Sinusitis, 167–168
Skin, 174–179
Skin ulceration, 132

Skullcap, 4, 105, 160–161, 201, 202, 204, 205, 210, 221, 232, 235, 248, 252

Sleep, 90, 203, 231–232

Slippery elm bark, 25, 188, 256

Snakeroot, 12, 13

Soap bark, 179, 256

Solanum lycopersicum. See Tomato

Solidago virgaurea. See Golden rod

Solomon's seal, 240

Soma, 4

Sophora japonica. See Huai jiao

Sore throat, 130, 173

South American herbs, 134–137

Southernwood, 179, 256

Spikenard, 81

Sprains, 155

Spurge, 131–132, 169

Squawvine, 216, 217, 256

Stachys officinalis. See Wood betony

Stachys palustris, 256

Star of Bethlehem, 154

Steam inhalants, 148

Stellaria. See Chickweed

St. George's mushroom, 132

Stinging nettle, 119, 158, 176, 177, 179, 184, 196, 222, 225, 227

St. John's wort, 10, 19, 63, 155, 157, 158, 159, 160, 161–162, 203, 207, 210, 217, 224, 227, 250

Strains, 155

Strawberries, 53

Stress, 205

Strophanthin, 12

Strophanthus kombé. See Strophanthin

Styptic, 23, 38, 48

Styrax benzoin. See Benzoin

Sumach, 233

Suppositories, 149

Sweating, 44, 102

Sweet sumach, 233, 256

Symphytum officinale. See Comfrey

Syrup, 144, 150

Syzygium aromaticum. See Clove

T

Tabebuia impetiginosa. See Pau d'arco

Tanacetum parthenium. See Feverfew

Tangerine, 41

Taraxacum officinale. See Dandelion

Taste, in Chinese medicine, 7

Tea, 37, 184, 251

Tea tree, 76, 173, 176, 197, 212, 230, 232

Tea tree oil, 150

Teething, 231

Tennis elbow, 157–158

Tenosynovitis, 157–158

Tension, 201–202

Tension headache, 160

Terminalia. See Myrobalan

Terminalia belerica. See Bibhitaki

Teucrium chamaedrys. See Wall germander

Teucrium scorodonia. See Wood sage

Theobroma cacao. See Chocolate

Thomson, Samuel, 10, 11

Thorn apple, 10

Threadworms, 232

Thrush, 197, 212

Thuja occidentalis. See Arbor vitae

Thyme, 3, 115, 155, 157, 196, 206, 225, 230, 233, 236, 249

Thyme oil, 150

Thymus. See Thyme

Thyroid problems, 227–228

Thyroid tonic, 54

Tibet, 5

Tila, 238

Tilia x europaea, 181

Tincture, 143–144, 148

Tinospora cordifolia. See Guduchi

Tiredness, 206

Tissue healer, 20, 48, 118

Toadflax, 10

Tomato, 108

Tonic wine, 149

Tonsillitis, 174

Tormentil, 187, 256

Tranquilizer, 121

Travel sickness, 234

Tribulis terrestris. See Gokshura

Trifolium pratense. See Red clover

Trigeminal neuralgia, 161–162

Trigonella foenum-graecum. See Fenugreek

Tropaeolum majus. See Nasturtium

True unicorn root, 11, 256

Tuckahoe, 133

Turmeric, 4, 129–130, 191

Turner, William, 9

Turnera diffusa. See Damiana

Tussilago farfara. See Coltsfoot

U

Ulcer, 188

Ulmus fulva. See Slippery elm bark

Unani, 2

Uncaria. See Peruvian cat's claw

Unicorn root. *See* False unicorn root; True unicorn root

Urinary antiseptic, 68, 90

Urinary disorders, 197–199

Urinary dysfunction, 133

Urinary gravel, 198–199

Urinary incontinence, 224

Urinary tract infection, 198

Urtica dioica. See Stinging nettle

Urticaria, 196

Uterine relaxant, 38, 124

Uterine stimulant, 30, 68, 70, 71, 102, 117, 123

Uterine tonic, 66

V

Vaccinium myrtillus. See Bilberry

Vaccinium vitis-idaea. See Cowberry

Vaginal itching, 212

Vaginal thrush, 212
Vajikarana, 239–240
Valerian, 4, 121, 157, 158, 159, 161, 181, 204, 205
Valeriana officinalis. See Valerian
Varicella, 235
Varicose veins, 182
Vasodilator, 18, 19, 26, 43, 44, 50, 57, 64, 77, 78, 86, 102, 112, 127
Verbascum thapsus. See Mullein
Verbena officinalis. See Vervain
Vermifuge, 41
Verrucas, 177
Vervain, 4, 123, 158, 160, 161, 162, 163, 190, 201, 202, 203, 204, 205, 212–213, 221, 227, 250
Viburnum opulus. See Guelder rose
Viburnum prunifolium. See Black haw
Vidari, 239
Vinca minor. See Lesser periwinkle
Vincristine, 12
Viola. See Heartsease; Violet
Violet, 3, 125
Viscum album. See Mistletoe
Vitex agnus-castus. See Chaste-tree
Vitiligo, 129
Vomiting, 33, 191

W
Wall germander, 156, 256
Walnut, 67
Warts, 177
Washes, 149
Western medicine, 10–11
Western tonics, 247–252
White bryony, 256
White deadnettle, 209, 211, 222, 256
White horehound, 165, 166, 168–169, 228, 236, 237, 256
White peony, 7. *See* Bai shao yao
Whooping cough, 19, 236

Wild cherry bark, 165, 166
Wild garlic, 232, 255
Wild indigo, 174, 256
Wild lettuce, 165, 166, 203–204, 236, 256
Willow, 12, 101, 154, 156, 157, 158
Wine, tonic, 149
Winter cherry. *See* Ashwagandha
Winter savory, 251
Witch hazel, 59, 150, 217, 235
Withania somnifera. See Ashwagandha
Withering, William, 13
Wolfiporia cocos. See Tuckahoe
Women. *See* Childbirth; Gynecological problems; Menopause; Menstrual regulation
Wood betony, 4, 109, 160, 181, 196, 201, 205, 206, 207, 209, 213, 216, 228, 252
Wood blewits, 132
Wood sage, 256
Worms, 22, 33
Wormwood, 30, 228
Wound herb, 21, 25, 36, 53, 93, 110, 111, 115, 122, 136
Woundwort, 256
Wu wei zi, 213, 244, 246, 247, 2345
Wu zhu yu, 245, 256

X
Xia ku cao, 233. *See also* Self-heal
Xiang fu, 256

Y
Yage. *See* Ayahuasca
Yam, 45, 159, 189, 190, 211, 219
Yang, 6, 8, 14
Yang tonics, 245–246
Yarrow, 18, 25, 156, 158, 163, 181, 210, 235

Yellow dock, 156, 176, 178, 186, 256
Yellow Emperor, 5
Yellow jasmine, 161, 256
Yin, 6, 8, 14
Yin tonics, 246–247
Yin yang huo, 246
Yucca, 9

Z
Zanthoxyllium americanum. See Prickly ash
Zea mays. See Corn silk
Ze xie, 197, 256
Zhi ke, 41, 193
Zhi shi, 41
Zhi zi, 256
Zhu li, 166
Zingiber officinalis, 127
Zizyphus jujube. See Da zao